FERTILITY AND FAMILY PLANNING
A WORLD VIEW

THE UNIVERSITY OF MICHIGAN
A SESQUICENTENNIAL PUBLICATION

FERTILITY
AND
FAMILY PLANNING

A WORLD VIEW

S.J. Behrman, M.D.   Leslie Corsa, Jr., M.D.
and Ronald Freedman
Editors

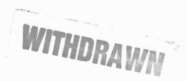
Ann Arbor
THE UNIVERSITY OF MICHIGAN PRESS

PREFACE

In 1967 The University of Michigan observed the one hundred and fiftieth anniversary of its founding. A year-long Sesquicentennial observance included five major university-wide conferences. The fifth and final program dealt with "Fertility and Family Planning"— one of the world's most important problems and one to which the University had made strong commitment with initiation of the University of Michigan Population Program in 1965. The conference began with the papers which constitute this volume. Nineteen of the world's most knowledgeable leaders in the field of population problems and family planning prepared the papers by mid-year at our invitation. The papers were made available to participants in advance so that they could be read in preparation for discussion at the conference on November 15-17. They were discussed in five sessions, each opened by a world authority with a summation of issues raised in the papers:

Philip Hauser: Fertility Trends in the Modern World
Edgar M. Hoover: Causes and Consequences of Fertility Trends
A. S. Parkes: Biologic Aspects of Fertility Control
Sir Colville Deverell: Public Programs for Family Planning
C. Chandrasekaran: Fertility Planning in the Developing World
During the Next Decade.

Panels of the following discussants then interacted with the authors on the podium and responded to questions from the audience: Paul Demeny, Otis Dudley Duncan, Moye W. Freymann, Alan Guttmacher, Oscar Harkavy, Paul A. Harper, Alexander Kessler, Milos Macura, R. T. Ravenholt, Roger Revelle, J. N. Spuhler, Paul Todd, Samuel Wishik, Emil Witschi, I. C. Yuan.

Mr. John D. Rockefeller III, chairman of the Population Council, addressed participants at a banquet honoring the authors and discussants. Significant contributions were also made by Harlan Hatcher, President of the University, Allan F. Smith, vice-president for Academic Affairs; William Haber, dean of the College of Literature, Science and the Arts; Charles W. Joiner, chairman of the

Sesquicentennial Committee; Frank W. Notestein, president of the Population Council; and Myron E. Wegman, dean of the School of Public Health.

A key person behind the scenes was Diane Mulvaney, cheerful secretary and expediter for the planning committee.

To all these persons we give our warmest thanks.

S. J. B.
L. C.
R. F.

CONTENTS

I. FERTILITY TRENDS IN THE MODERN WORLD

THE DECLINE OF FERTILITY IN EUROPE FROM THE FRENCH REVOLUTION TO WORLD WAR II

Ansley J. Coale

*Office of Population Research, Princeton University**

In EUROPE IN THE PAST two centuries virtually every region has experienced a substantial reduction in mortality (increase in the average duration of life) and a substantial reduction in fertility (decrease in the average number of children born per woman living through the childbearing years). Widely known generalizations about the typical population changes that occur during industrialization or modernization—the so-called demographic transition—are based to a large extent on European experience. Surprisingly enough, however, there has not been a systematic collation and comparison of the statistical records of various European populations to provide a thorough documentation of these changes and a possible basis for their explanation. We have begun a project along these lines at Princeton. The decline of fertility in each of the provinces of Europe will be recorded from the time in each province when marital fertility was essentially constant until it reached a minimum or until the present, if it is still declining. We are not attempting a similarly systematic study of mortality, and intend to use statistics on mortality only as an aid to the

* The author gratefully acknowledges the assistance of his collaborators on the research project of which this paper is essentially a progress report: Paul Demeny, Office of Population Research, Princeton, and Population Studies Center, Michigan; Erna Härm, John Knodel, and Etienne van de Walle, Office of Population Research; Massimo Livi-Bacci, Office of Population Research, and University of Florence. In addition we have enjoyed the generous cooperation of George Siampos, National Statistical Service of Greece, and Vasilios Valaoras, University of Athens, and of the Central Statistical Office under Egon Szabady, in Budapest. Many of the ideas, and most of the laborious research and calculations were made by these others. The figures were drawn by Mrs. Joan Westoff. The author is, of course, solely responsible for errors and other shortcomings.

3

indirect estimation of births where the registration of the latter is inadequate or as a possible explanatory variable for changes in fertility.

With very few exceptions, all of the provinces in Europe have by now experienced a decrease in marital fertility of large magnitude, usually 50 percent or more. The decrease in each province has occurred at diverse times and under widely different circumstances, and because data on population in Europe are unusually complete and accurate, we feel that Europe provides a unique statistical laboratory in which to investigate the conditions under which a population undertakes the voluntary restriction of fertility.

In attempting to summarize the fall of fertility in Europe, I shall inevitably cast the summary within the framework of analysis used in this research project, draw on the materials that have been assembled to date, and be limited essentially to the preliminary findings discovered so far. Unfortunately, this implies that much that I shall report will be tentative and incomplete since the work upon which it is based is probably no more than half done.

Fertility Measures Employed

Four interrelated indexes of fertility have been devised as the principal measures we plan to use to document levels and trends of fertility in Europe. The indexes are: (1) An index of overall fertility (I_f) that indicates the extent to which the women in a given population approach the flow of births they would achieve if all were subject to the highest rates of age-specific fertility on reliable record for a population of substantial size: the fertility of married Hutterite women. The Hutterites are a religious sect now settled in North America whose members have long scrupulously followed a number of special rules including one that forbids the use of any form of contraception. The married population of French Canada from the eighteenth century until the early twentieth approached the high age-specific fertility rates of this group, but most other recorded schedules are lower. Precisely, I_f is defined as follows: $I_f = \dfrac{B}{\Sigma w_i F_i}$, where B is the total births to the population in question in a given year (or the average annual number over a short period of years), w_i is the number of women in each 5-year age interval from 15 to 50, and F_i is the marital fertility of Hutterite women in each age interval. The average number of children born to a group of women passing through life, married at age 15 and subject to the Hutterite childbearing rates, would be 12.6. (2) An index of marital fertility (I_g) that indicates how closely married women approach the births they would produce if subject to the Hutterite age-specific fertility rates. Precisely, $I_g = \dfrac{B_L}{\Sigma m_i F_i}$, where B_L is the average annual number of legitimate births, and m_i is the number of married women in the 5-year age interval. (3) An index of the fertility of the nonmarried women (I_h) that indicates how closely the fertility of the unmarried approaches that of the married Hutterites. Specifically, $I_h = \dfrac{B_I}{\Sigma u_i F_i}$, where B_I is the average annual number of illegitimate births and u_i is the number of nonmarried women in the ith age interval. (4) An index of the proportion married among women in the childbearing ages (I_m) that indicates the extent to which marriage is contributing to the achievement of the highest potential of fertility of the population in question. It shows the number of births that would occur if married women experienced the Hutterite fertility schedule relative to the number that would occur if all women married and nonmarried experienced these fertility rates. Specifically, $I_m = \dfrac{\Sigma m_i F_i}{\Sigma W_i F_i}$.

There is an important interrelation among these indexes, namely: $I_f = I_m \cdot I_g + (1 - I_m)I_h$. When, as is common in Europe, I_h is no more than 3 or 4 percent, this relationship reduces essentially to: $I_f = I_m I_g$. Thus, in populations where illegitimate fertility contributes a negligible proportion of total births, these indexes provide a measure of overall fertility that can be factored into an index of proportion married and an index of marital fertility.

The three measures of fertility $(I_f, I_g, \text{and } I_h)$ embody a form of indirect standardization for age within the childbearing interval, since the age distribution of women is the same in the numerator and denominator. The numerator—the number of births actually occurring to the women in question—equals the sum of terms consisting of the number of women in each age interval times the actual fertility rate for that interval, and the denominator is the sum of terms consisting of the number of women in each age interval times the Hutterite fertility in that interval. Moreover, the age standardization thus achieved requires a minimum of demographic data: the actual average annual number of all births, of legitimate births, and of illegitimate births, and the distribution of women from 15 to 50 by age and marital status.

The index of the proportion married requires for its construction only data on the number of women in each 5-year age interval classified by marital status. It is an index of proportion married wherein more weight is given to marital status in the most fertile ages—i.e., the index is strongly affected by the proportion married at 20-24, but little affected by the proportion at 45-49. It can be rewritten in the fol-

lowing form: $I_m = \dfrac{\Sigma w_i F_i \cdot \dfrac{m_i}{w_i}}{\Sigma w_i \cdot F_i}$ —as the weighted average of the pro-

portions married in each age interval, where the weights $(w_i F_i)$ are the number of births that would occur in each age interval if the Hutterite marital fertility schedule prevailed. The number of births by interval depends on the age distribution of the women between 15 and 49, as well as on the fertility schedule of the Hutterites. This fact means that a high fertility population, which tends to have a steeply falling age distribution, assigns more weight to the proportion married at 15-19 and 20-24 than a low fertility population—ages at which the proportions married are usually low. Therefore even if both populations had the same proportions married in each age interval, the higher fertility population would tend to have a lower value of I_m. When it was likely that this feature of I_m might cause misleading conclusions, we have employed an alternative index I'_m

$(= \dfrac{\Sigma F_i \cdot \dfrac{m_i}{w_i}}{\Sigma F_i})$ that is independent of the age distribution. However, I_m and I'_m rarely differ consequentially. We have retained I_m as the usual measure of proportions married because of the convenience of the identity: $I_f = I_g \cdot I_m + (1 - I_m) I_h$.

The Initial Hypothesis about the Nature of the Fertility Decline in Europe

One of the reasons for devising and employing the fertility indexes just described was the realization in the early stages of planning our study of the decline of fertility in Europe that apparently prior to any widespread resort to voluntary birth control within marriage there had developed a nuptiality pattern in much of Europe that had reduced fertility well below that in any other area of the world. In other words, much of Europe in the eighteenth and early nineteenth centuries was characterized by low values of I_m. John Hajnal had called attention to this characteristic pattern of nuptiality in a number of articles.[1] In European populations west of a line that might be drawn from Trieste to Leningrad the proportion of women married at ages 15 to 50 was no more than 45 or 50 percent whereas east of this line in Europe, as well as in most populations of Africa and Asia, the proportion married among such women was 60 to 70 percent or higher. In other words, I_f (as well as other measures of overall fertility) was much reduced in a large proportion of European populations through what might be called Malthusian methods—"Malthusian" because abstinence from marriage (which Malthus referred to as moral restraint) was the method of fertility limitation he advocated.

It was a further part of our provisional hypotheses that every European population at some time in the not too remote past had "natural" fertility among its married couples. Natural fertility was a term invented by Louis Henry as a more realistic contrast to "controlled fertility" than such previous concepts as "the biological maximum fertility." "Natural" fertility implies the absence of a carefully defined kind of deliberately controlled fertility: "Control can be said to exist when the behaviour of the couple is bound to the number of children already born and is modified when this number reaches the maximum which the couple does not want to exceed; it is not the case for a taboo concerning lactation, which is independent of the number of children already born."[2] The natural fertility of married couples in different populations would be expected to differ because of differences in the extent and duration of breastfeeding, different customs governing abstinence, differences in the average frequency of intercourse, differences in health (especially in characteristics affecting pregnancy wastage), possible genetic differences in sterility and fecundity, etc. There might also be variations over time in I_g in a population in which there is no fertility control in Henry's sense because of changes in some of the above listed factors, for example, in the average duration of nursing. We also expected that there might have been substantial fluctuations in I_f in a population in which there was no voluntary control of fertility within marriage because of variations in I_m, and possibly in the frequency of illegitimate births.

Although the effect of low values of I_m and of low values of I_g on I_f are equivalent, variations in I_m among populations at a given period, and fluctuations in I_m over time within the same population do not reflect the same differences in social conditions or fluctuations in motivation as underlie the differential resort to voluntary birth control at different times or places. When birth control first appears among the married, fertility is usually reduced initially among women of high parity, and among women over 35 or 40. This tendency clearly shows that voluntary birth control is usually employed at first to avoid children in excess of the number the couple wishes. A deliberate restrictive motive is implied by the age pattern of the change in fertility. On the other hand, it is highly dubious that if a couple gets married when the bride is 26 instead of 25, the purpose is to reduce the number of children they will have by one. It seems more plausible that couples postpone marriage because they do not command the resources conventionally needed for marital union in the western European "stem family" tradition. The couple may feel that it should have property or at least separate living quarters before being able to marry and may in this way postpone marriage to an extent that fertility is substantially reduced without, however, being consciously motivated by this implication of the postponement. In hard times— crop failure, military defeat, social disorder, or the like—the marriage rate may fall and the average age of marriage increase, not because couples feel that they can afford fewer children in the long run, but because they feel they cannot afford the short-run cost of an immediate marriage, including, of course, immediate pregnancy. In contrast, in a population in which there is voluntary fertility control people who feel they can afford only a certain number of children reduce their fertility (ideally to zero) when this number is reached, and the tie between motivation and fertility control is immediate.

According to our provisional hypothesis, at dates which vary from one European population to another there began to develop within the past two centuries in each of the more than 700 provinces of Europe a degree of voluntary control of marital fertility that caused a significant reduction in I_g. Because of the work of earlier demographers, we suspected that in much of Europe the initial means of birth control employed was withdrawal or coitus interruptus. What is required for the development of effective birth control utilizing these means is, first, knowledge of the method, which must surely be known to some members of every society and seems rather easily susceptible to independent invention, although to some degree its use by many couples may be expedited by the diffusion of knowledge from those who have used it successfully to those ignorant of it; second, an attitude toward intercourse and reproduction that permits (i.e., sanctions) this modification of behavior; and third, a strong desire, shared by the male, for the avoidance of further pregnancy and births so that the considerable degree of self-discipline required to make this method effective will exist.

When the circumstances causing this mode of behavior arise, there has tended to be—so the provisional hypothesis ran—a spread of the control of fertility through the population. Because control affects the fertility of the women in the later ages of childbearing and with the largest number of children first and the women at lower parity and ages below 30 at a later stage, the most sensitive indicator of the control of marital fertility would be the decline in the age-specific rates above 30. However, recorded age-specific rates are rare, and we are forced to depend on the fact that the decline should be evident in any population with accurate birth statistics because of a decline in I_g. A decline in *marital* fertility is the characteristic form of decline expected during the demographic transition, i.e., accompanying modernization.

The separation of the effects of nuptiality and contraception in the indexes of proportions married and of marital fertility helps to clarify comparisons both between areas, and within the same area at different times. Differences in I_m may be the result of major underlying differences in social structure, such as systems of inheritance, that may have influenced family relationships without any direct association with the number of children people want, or any change in their attitude toward the range of permissible behavior. We know that the control of marital fertility has developed both in populations characterized by late marriage and a substantial proportion of spinsterhood on the one hand and in populations in which marriage is virtually universal and at an early average age on the other. The development of low values of I_m in western Europe apparently preceded the reduction in marital fertility by a century or two, and has not occurred yet in some countries of eastern Europe. Consequently, England had a birth rate in 1870 that was lower than any recorded in Hungary until after 1910. However, marital fertility in the two populations began to decline at about the same time and at about the same pace, and the higher birth rate in Hungary was caused by the consistently higher proportions marrying.

Qualifications of the Initial Hypothesis
Our work to date has shown (as might be expected) that our initial framework of thought was oversimplified. This framework suggests that there should have been in every province during a pre-decline period of "natural fertility" a plateau of essentially constant I_g; then, with the onset of fertility control within marriage, I_g should begin a sustained and continuous decline cumulating to a fall of some 50 percent. Indeed, such a pattern is a very common one, and even some exceptions, for example where I_g appears to rise before control is instituted, are really the result of faulty data; i.e., there is reason to believe that the apparent increase is really the result of increasing completeness of the recording of births. But there are disturbing genuine indications that natural fertility is not as clear-cut a concept —the absence of control was never as universal—as our preliminary framework of analysis suggests. First of all, the range in the value of I_g in different parts of Europe prior to the onset of a systematic decline is very large—from about .65 to 1.00. We have not succeeded in explaining differences of this order by differential behavior with regard to breastfeeding, nor does it appear readily attributable to

differences in health, since some of the highest fertility populations are to be found in impoverished provinces of Russia where infant mortality was extremely high and one would guess average income and conditions of life to be very low. An explanation that cannot be dismissed of the strong correlation that Knodel and van de Walle found between infant mortality and marital fertility in geographical areas of Germany where few women nursed their children is that sexual behavior was deliberately modified in a way that reduces the probability of conception following a live birth.[3]

Indeed, there are a number of suggestions, direct or indirect, that the deliberate control of fertility in some form is latent in populations that have not begun a sustained and extended decline, opening up the possibility that there is a fraction, not changing in size, that for a long time practiced some form of deliberate fertility limitation. From an analysis of genealogies of the leading families of Geneva and of the French nobility, demographers at the Institut National d'Etudes Démographiques in Paris have shown conclusively that marital fertility was controlled to a substantial extent during the seventeenth century by these groups;[4] and analysis of data from the parish register in Colyton (East Devon) by members of the Cambridge Group for the History of Population and Social Structure shows that beyond any reasonable doubt there was a tangible degree of voluntary control of fertility in that community in the last half of the seventeenth century, a control that was subsequently relaxed.[5] Finally, a member of our project, Professor Massimo Livi-Bacci of Florence, has found persuasive if not wholly conclusive evidence of a 10-12 percent decline in the fertility of Spain between the late eighteenth century and about 1860. This decline (indicated by recorded age distributions in the censuses of 1787 and 1797 that are demographically consistent only with higher fertility than prevailed before the censuses of 1860 and 1887) appears to have been at a very gradual pace and was not the initial part of the sharp and sustained decline that we are in the process of documenting for almost every province in Europe. In short, we are less sure than we were at first that the plateau in I_g that we consider typical of the pre-decline period is a perfectly level plateau or that "natural fertility" in the sense of a negligible resort to contraception or abortion to limit family size was in fact as ubiquitous in Europe as our preliminary hypothesis held.

Nevertheless, the general outline of typical fertility experience in European populations seems solid enough: namely, that against different backgrounds of nuptiality experience and trends, almost all European populations departed from essentially constant or only gradually varying marital fertility (at levels that vary from perhaps 65-100 percent of Hutterite marital fertility), departed in a sustained decline accomplished by an increasing use of deliberate birth control. A nice illustration of such a history is indicated in Figure 1, showing on the same graph the crude birth rate of the population of Tuscany from 1819 until 1960 and the average of the crude marriage rate during the 10 years preceding each date. Note that the crude birth rate fluctuated over a range of approximately 25 percent of its maximum value between 1819 and about 1880. However, there were also extreme fluctuations in the marriage rate. We do not have data on the marital status of the population of Tuscany by age and cannot calculate I_m, but the proportion of the population consisting of women in the first 10 years of marriage is adequately represented by the average of the marriage rate during the preceding ten years. Since the mean age of marriage in Tuscany is about 25 years for women, the vast majority of births take place to women in the first 10 years of marriage. If marital fertility were constant, we would expect the birth rate to fluctuate very nearly in proportion to the average marriage rate during the peceding 10 years. Note how closely the two curves conform until about 1875 or 1880, after which the fluctuations of the marriage rate continue about a horizontal average while the birth rate falls ever lower. It seems clear that if we had the data for calculating our indexes, I_f and I_m would have varied together (with I_g approximately constant) up until about the ¾ mark of the nineteenth century after which I_g followed a steady and fairly rapid decline.

Results
I shall organize my summary of what we have learned so far in our study about the decline of fertility in Europe around three maps that show the indexes of overall fertility, marital fertility, and proportions married in 1900 for the provinces of all of the countries in Europe except a few in the Balkans. At a later stage we expect to complete these maps with data for all areas except the European part of the Ottoman Empire. These maps represent a small fraction of those that we expect to draw before the project terminates. For 1900 we expect to prepare additional maps showing the index of illegitimate fertility and possibly separate maps for rural and urban populations of the provinces. We shall have a full series of maps for 1870, 1930, and 1960 as well as for 1900. Finally, one or more maps are contemplated on which the code assigned to each province will indicate the approximate date at which I_g reached 10 percent below its "plateau" level in a sustained decline. The maps for 1900 have a special interest because

1900 is not far from the median date at which European national populations had experienced a 10 percent decline in marital fertility —in other words, in 1900 about half of the populations had experienced such a fall and the other half had not.

We shall first comment on the map of the index of proportion married. John Hajnal's selection of a line from Leningrad to Trieste as the dividing point between populations with and without what he called a "European pattern of marriage" seems nicely confirmed, if an I_m of .55 is accepted as the division between European and non-European marriage patterns, and if one overlooks some areas in western Europe that are above this proportion. The high proportions married in France appear to be related to the special fertility history of France, in particular the early date at which the decline in marital fertility began in France and the low levels reached before the end of the nineteenth century. We shall return to this point later. A somewhat fanciful explanation of the divergence of parts of Spain from the "European pattern" of nuptiality is the Moorish component of the Spanish cultural tradition.

There is a very striking pattern of variation of I_m in Russia.[6] The 4 provinces on the Baltic (St. Petersburg, Latvia, Lithuania, and Estonia) are the only Russian provinces with an I_m below .55, and on the map they appear a natural extension of the patterns along the southern Baltic in Germany and Denmark. Adjacent to the Baltic provinces is a ring with I_m in the lowest "non-European" category, .60 to .649. Then more or less systematically as the distance from the Baltic provinces increases, the value of I_m rises until in the southeastern provinces I_m has values above .75—a level attained when virtually every woman marries and the mean age of marriage is not above 20 years. For example, the index of proportions married in India at about this time was .80, a value approached by the 5 provinces of Russia with the highest proportions married. Figure 2 presents this geographical relationship in a different form. It shows the value of I_m for each province in European Russia in 1897 plotted against the number of provinces that must be traversed in going from the province in question to the Baltic. Thus, the 4 Baltic provinces have a distance index of 0, the 5 provinces bordering on the Baltic provinces have an index of 1, the 2 provinces bordering on these, an index of 2, and so on. The relationship is startling, the correlation coefficient being .91. It is difficult to avoid an interpretation of the map of proportions married in Russia and of Figure 2 as a crosssectional picture, at a moment of time, of a diffusion across Russia of western nuptiality patterns. Unfortunately, it will be difficult if not impossible to document the development during the years

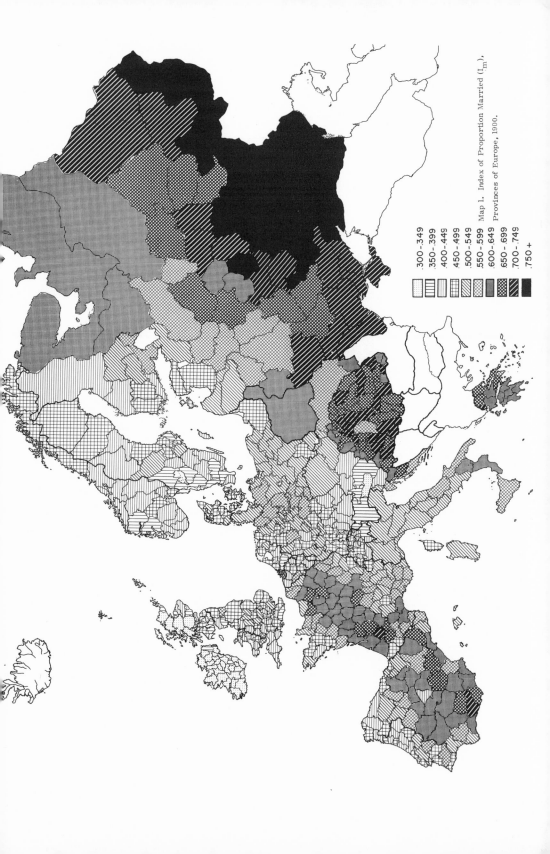

Map 1. Index of Proportion Married (I_m), Provinces of Europe, 1900.

.300 - .349
.350 - .399
.400 - .449
.450 - .499
.500 - .549
.550 - .599
.600 - .649
.650 - .699
.700 - .749
.750 +

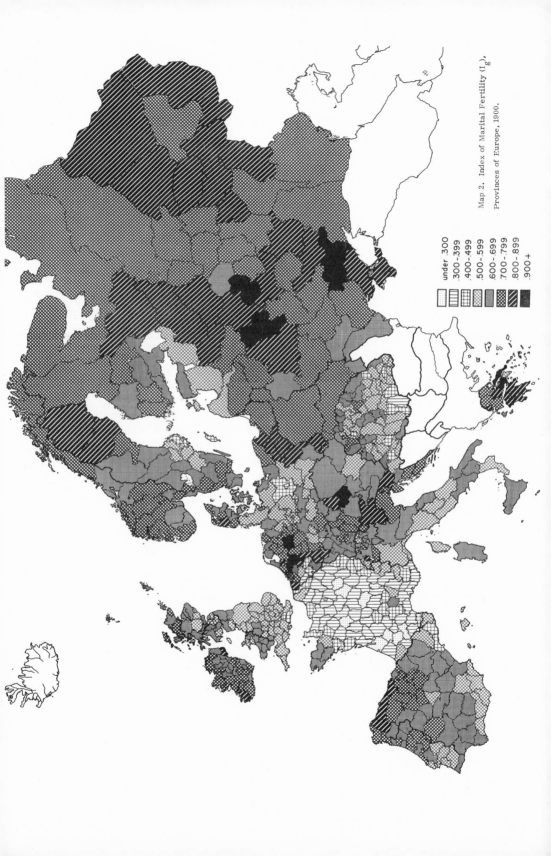

Map 2. Index of Marital Fertility (I_g), Provinces of Europe, 1900.

under .300
.300 - .399
.400 - .499
.500 - .599
.600 - .699
.700 - .799
.800 - .899
.900 +

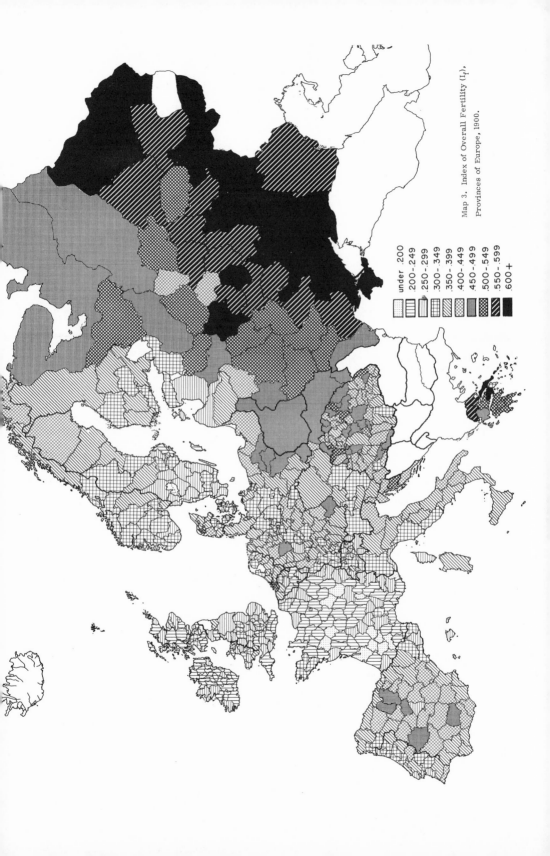

Map 3. Index of Overall Fertility (I_f), Provinces of Europe, 1900.

under .200
.200- .249
.250- .299
.300- .349
.350- .399
.400- .449
.450- .499
.500- .549
.550- .599
.600 +

prior to the 1897 census because this was the first census of Russia that provided the requisite data of a cross-tabulation of age and marital status. By 1959 the I_m values were much more nearly uniform and at a substantially lower level, but interpretation is complicated by the turbulent history of Russia in the interval, including a reduction of I_m in 1959 because of the loss of life among males during World War II.

At the other end of the scale, the very low proportions married in Ireland that developed in the last half of the nineteenth century have been the object of much comment. Explanations have cited the effect of the famine, of special inheritance laws and customs, of male emigration, and of religion. It is interesting to note, then, that the proportions married in northwestern Scotland and in a county of Wales on the Irish Sea are at the same general level.

A map of the index of marital fertility in 1900 shows the effects of differences in I_g previous to any sustained decline combined with the decline itself in provinces where it had occurred. In reading this map it is useful to consider an I_g of .6 as the dividing point between the gradations that delineate the various degrees of low fertility and those that delineate high fertility. Indeed, it is reasonable to assert that any instance of marital fertility less than 60 percent of the Hutterites must almost certainly connote some form of deliberate birth control. The converse is not true: areas whose pre-decline I_g was approximately the same as the Hutterites could have experienced a very substantial decrease and still be above the division point of .6 in 1900.

We were surprised to find that marital fertility was within 10 percent of the Hutterite schedule in several provinces—3 in Russia, 2 in Germany, and 2 in the Netherlands. (In 1870 there were 2 in Germany with I_g's above .9, 2 in the Netherlands and 2 in Belgium). The geographical pattern in this map has a number of features that should be noted. First, there is a clear general tendency for the fertility in a province to be at a level not too dissimilar from its neighbors. In other words, there is a high degree of inter-connectedness. The areas with I_g above .6 in Scandinavia are connected through Finland to the Russian provinces, which with the exception of 3 of the 4 Baltic provinces are all above .6, through Poland and Prussia to Austria, northeastern Italy, Switzerland, southern and western Germany, to Holland and parts of Belgium. The isolated province with a lower I_g in Austria contains Vienna; a map of marital fertility of the rural population would show this to be well above .6 The extraordinarily low fertility of France is no surprise, and the fact that the lowest marital fertility in Spain is in Catalonia as well as the strip of low fertility extending from the French border down into Italy might be the result in part of some degree of French cultural influence. Some of the examples of low fertility in 1900 are surprising. The extent to which marital fertility had fallen in some of the French départements is impressive: several had I_g's in 1900 lower than the level reached by the German Reich in 1933. Low marital fertility in southern Spain and at the boot of Italy is unexpected. Perhaps the greatest surprise on this map is an I_g below .4 in the province of Krasso-Szörény, a wholly rural province in southern Hungary. In fact, the index of overall fertility (I_f) for this province was the lowest in Hungary with the exception of the province containing Budapest, in spite of the fact that in Krasso-Szörény I_m was approximately the same as for Hungary as a whole and that unmarried women had a fertility 21 percent as high as the married Hutterites—the highest index of illegitimate fertility in Hungary; in spite of the fact, to put it in other terms, of a high proportion married and of extramarital fertility ⅔ as high as among married women. Note that low marital fertility in Hungary in 1900 covered about the same proportion of the area as in England and Wales. A source of milder surprise is the fact that fertility in St. Petersburg and two other Baltic provinces was lower than in any province of Finland or in eastern Prussia. One final comment on geographic pattern. One could make a more or less irresponsible case for a Mediterranean pattern of low fertility (parts of Italy, France, of course, Catalonia, and southern Spain), a Baltic pattern of low fertility (in Russia and Sweden), and an Atlantic pattern of moderately high fertility (Norway, northern Scotland, Ireland, Brittany, and the Atlantic provinces in Iberia).

The map of the index of overall fertility shows primarily the combined effect of nuptiality and marital fertility. The areas of eastern Europe, especially in Russia, that combined high values of both indexes have an overall fertility well above that anywhere in the west. Because the areas in France that had the lowest marital fertility were also characterized by high values of I_m and because the provinces of western Europe that had the highest marital fertility had characteristically low proportions married, there is a general tendency for more uniformity in I_f in the west than in either of the constituents.

Fertility Trends
Because the collection of data is far from complete and the calculation of indexes, including as it does adjustments for incompleteness of birth registration, is in an even earlier stage, I cannot proceed as I would like to a detailed description of when the western pattern of

marriage that produced the low values of I_m was formed in each province, and when in each province the decline in marital fertility began. In fact, the former point is beyond the scope of our project, because data on marital status did not exist for most of the populations when the fall in I_m began.

As a somewhat disappointing substitute for a detailed description of fertility trends, I shall present the sequence of I_m's and I_g's calculated for a few interesting national populations in Europe from some time in the nineteenth century up until 1960. These countries are France, Sweden, England and Wales, Ireland, Finland, and Bulgaria. The calculated values of I_m are shown in Figure 3 and for I_g in Figure 4. The I_m sequences of England and Sweden illustrate the pattern common to many western European populations (especially Scotland and Norway). The pattern is that of essential constancy from whatever point the calculations begin in the nineteenth century until about 1930, at which point there begins a marked increase in proportions married continuing until 1960. Because of our restriction to the period between the French Revolution and World War II, I shall not comment on the well-known marriage boom in the post-World War II era in many of these countries. What is striking is the increase in I_m recorded in several countries in the 1930's (as in Sweden and France). Bulgaria is characterized by a very high index of proportion married that dropped in censuses taken after World War I and World War II only to recover in a subsequent census, giving a clear indication that the "normal" proportion married has remained solidly immune from the western European customs of late marriage and abstinence from marriage. In the first Finnish census that cross-classified age and marital status (in 1880), the index of proportion married was about .5, at the high end of western European levels, at least above other northern countries. By 1910, the index had fallen and by 1930 to a level slightly below that of Sweden. During the 1930's and on into the post-war period, Finland shared the marriage boom characteristic of other countries with low indexes of I_m during this era. Somewhat less satisfactory evidence shows that in the eighteenth century the proportion married in Finland may have been on a more nearly non-European pattern. The demographic data for Finland up until 1880 includes an age distribution and a distribution of the population by marital status though not cross-classified by age. The ratio of married women to the total women over age 20 declined from over 65 percent in 1751 to about 58 percent in 1880, although the changes in the age composition of the married population that one would expect on the basis of the recorded decline in fertility and mortality would have increased the proportion of the married who were beyond age 50. We may conjecture, then, that between the mid-eighteenth and mid-nineteenth centuries and continuing into the twentieth, Finland was adopting a west European pattern of nuptiality, which at the end of the nineteenth century was still spreading across Russia. Ireland's decline in I_m appears to have begun from a level not very different from that of England and Wales, but fell to the lowest values recorded for a national population. Ireland has shared only to a limited extent in the marriage boom during and after World War II.

The index of proportion married for France is of special interest since it shows a general upward trend from 1850 that faltered in the latter part of the nineteenth century, and fell after World War I, but that by 1936 was nearly 15 points higher than in the middle of the preceding century. Aside from the effect of the war, the rise was fairly steady from 1890 on.

An earlier look at these data had led me to believe that the increase in the proportions married in France was a more or less direct effect of the control of marital fertility that France achieved so much earlier than other populations. I_g fell below .4 before the turn of the century. The more recent rise in marital fertility in other western countries occurred not long after *their* marital fertility fell below .4. However, every simple hypothesis about European fertility seems to encounter obstacles or at least qualifications. I_m has also risen since the middle of the last century in Belgium and Holland and to a lesser extent in Denmark, areas in which a significant fall in I_g did not occur until much later than in France.

There is an additional support for the presumption of a causal relationship between the achievement of a highly effective control of marital fertility and a rise in proportions married. By 1870 in France, a number of provinces had reduced marital fertility below .4 and one at least (Lot-et-Garonne) below .3. The proportions married in these low fertility départements were mostly above .65 and in Lot-et-Garonne above .7. Figure 5 shows a scatter diagram of I_g against I^*_m (the age-distribution-free index of proportion married).

Summary of Comparative Trends
Within a matrix of overall fertility differences caused to a major extent by differential resort to marriage, a differential resort with origins too remote for exact statistical documentation and certainly prior to our period of reference, there has developed in essentially all of Europe a control of fertility within marriage effective enough to reduce marital fertility by at least 50 percent. The few exceptions are in Ireland, some provinces of Spain and Portugal, Albania, and one or two areas in Yugoslavia. If we stop our observations at the begin-

ning of World War II, the list of areas that had not reduced marital fertility by 50 percent would be greatly lengthened, including parts of Italy, more of Spain and Portugal, much of Russia, and additional areas in the Balkans. The decline began in France where it is clear several départements had started to reduce their fertility before the end of the eighteenth century. At the moment, we cannot show with certainty that the decline began in any area (except Geneva) outside of France before the middle of the nineteenth century. By 1900 an unmistakable downturn had occurred in Scandinavia, Great Britain, Germany, Italy, Spain, Austria, Switzerland, Holland, Belgium, and Hungary, and before World War I in Bulgaria, Romania, Poland, and Russia. There is a stronger parallel than we had suspected between the trends in Eastern and Western Europe—less of a lag in the east in the decline in marital fertility. The parallelism may have escaped notice in part because the consistently higher proportions married east of Hajnal's line meant that measures of overall fertility at any given moment of time showed Eastern Europe at higher levels, until in the post-World War II period the decline in fertility reached such an extreme point in some eastern countries that, especially with the concurrent rise in I_m in the west, their indexes of overall fertility became the lowest in Europe.

Explanation of the Decline in Fertility

In 1965, I listed the following factors as representative of explanations given by demographers for the decline of marital fertility:

"(1) The decline in mortality. With more children surviving, fewer births are needed to achieve a given family size.

(2) The rising cost and diminished economic advantages of children in urbanized industrial societies. In rural families children assist in production at an early age and are a source of support for parents in their old age; in an urban environment children contribute less and cost more, especially after the establishment of universal primary education and the prohibition of child labor, both characteristic of advanced industrialization.

(3) Higher status of women. The extension of education to women, women's suffrage, and the employment of women in occupations formerly reserved for males are objective indications of wider opportunity and higher status for women. Since the burdens of pregnancy, parturition and child care are all women's burdens, these changes in opportunity and status promote the spread of birth control.

(4) Religious changes and differences. The early reduction of marital fertility in France compared to Spain and Italy on the one hand, and England and Scandinavia on the other, has been explained

by the fact that Italy and Spain remained under the direct influence of the Vatican, and the Protestant countries had willingly accepted their religion, but France had dissented from Catholicism without breaking away. The unique continuation after 1900 of high marital fertility in Ireland has been attributed to the character of Irish religion.

(5) The development of a secular, rational attitude. Such an attitude favors the voluntary control of fertility, and has been considered as a natural part of industrialization and modernization, and also as a feature of revolutionary and pre-revolutionary France."
I then continued:

"Examples can be found illustrating the presumed influence of each of these factors, but counter-examples or exceptions are nearly as prevalent. Every nation in the world today in which no more than 45% of the labor force is engaged in extractive industry, in which at least 90% of the children of primary school age attend school, and which is at least 50% urban has experienced a major decline in fertility. But France reduced its fertility before attaining any of these characteristics, and England had most of them before its marital fertility fell at all.

Fertility fell in Spain, Bulgaria, and other Southern and Eastern European countries when mortality was still very high; in many countries rural fertility declined as early and as much as urban fertility; in some countries industrialization was far advanced before marital fertility fell, in others a major decline preceded substantial industrialization. Catholics in the United States and the Netherlands have higher fertility than Protestants, but some Catholic populations, e.g. in North Italy—have fertility as low as any other in the world.

In European national experience, the only factor apparently always changing at the same time that fertility declined was literacy, but the onset of fertility decline has no consistent relationship with the proportion literate at the time.

Fertility reduction seems to be a nearly universal feature of the development of modern secular societies, but its introduction and spread cannot yet be explained by any simple, universally valid model or generalized description."[7]

Two years later, two members of our research project examined indexes of the proportion married, of total fertility, of infant mortality, of urbanization, of industrialization, and of literacy in a number of European countries at the time marital fertility began to fall, and concluded:

". . . The range of each index is broad, so that there appears to be little in the statistical record for Europe which confirms the existence of an association between the beginning of the fertility decline and any specific level, or threshold, of economic and social development."[8]

It should be noted that we are still in the midst of collecting data and documenting the history of fertility itself for a much finer geographic study than one based on national units. Perhaps we shall through a stroke of insight or good fortune discover a grand generalization that will provide a compact and widely valid explanation of the decline of marital fertility in Europe. But at the moment it appears that the process was more complex, subtle, and diverse than anticipated; only an optimist would still expect a simple account of why fertility fell.

Notes

1. The articles culminate in J. Hajnal, "European Marriage Patterns in Perspective," in D. V. Glass and D. E. C. Eversley, eds., *Population in History* (London: Arnold Press, 1964).

2. L. Henry, "Some Data on Natural Fertility," *Eugenics Quarterly*, VIII (1961) 81-91.

3. J. Knodel and E. van de Walle, "Breastfeeding, Fertility, and Infant Mortality: An Analysis of Some Early German Data," *Population Studies* (forthcoming).

4. L. Henry, *Anciennes Familles Genevoises* (Paris: Presses Universitaires, 1956); C. Levy and L. Henry, "Ducs et Pairs sous l'Ancien Régime," *Population*, xv (1960) 807-30.

5. E. A. Wrigley, "Family Limitation in Pre-industrial England," *The Economic History Review*, second series, Vol. xix (1966) 82-109.

6. Data taken from the census of 1897.

7. A. J. Coale, "Factors Associated with the Development of Low Fertility: An Historic Summary," in United Nations, *World Population Conference, 1965*. ii, 205-9.

8. E. van de Walle and J. Knodel, "Demographic Transition and Fertility Decline: The European Case." Paper presented at the 1967 conference of the International Union for the Scientific Study of Population, Sydney, Australia.

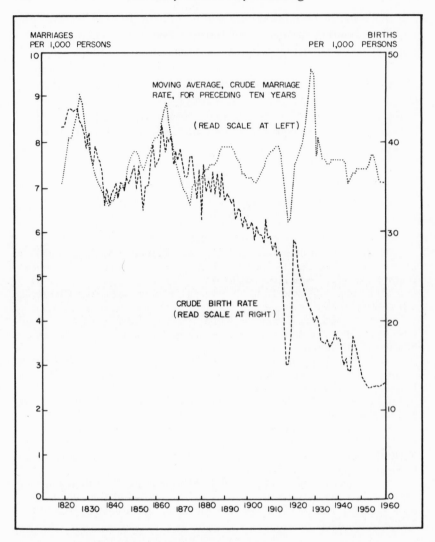

Figure 1. Tuscany. Births per 1,000 persons, average number of marriages per 1,000 persons, preceding ten years; 1819-1959.

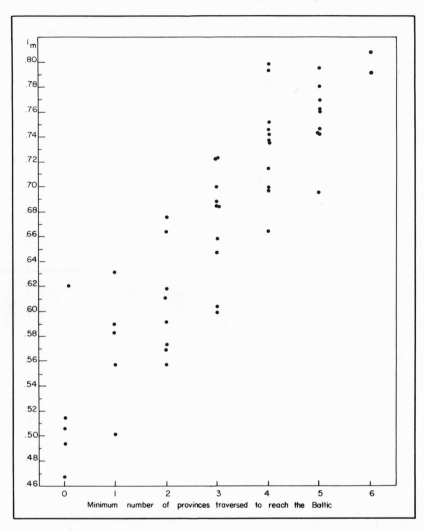

Figure 2. Index of proportion married and "distance" from the Baltic, provinces of Russia, 1897.

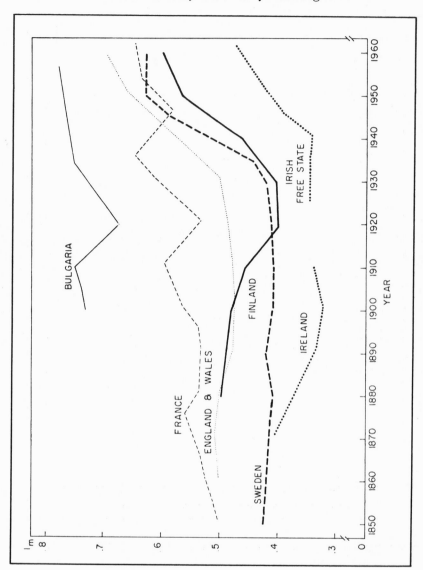

Figure 3. Index of proportion married (I_m), selected countries of Europe, 1850-1960.

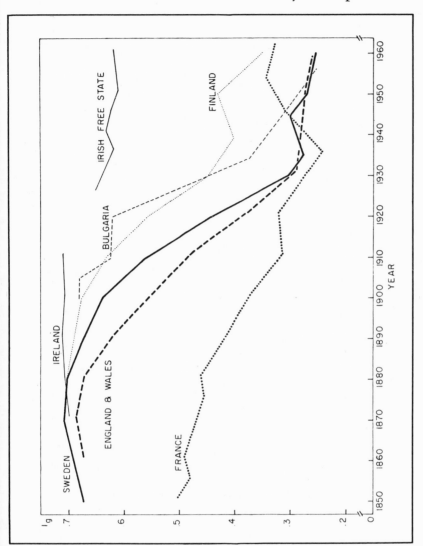

Figure 4. Index of marital fertility (I_g), selected countries of Europe, 1850-1960.

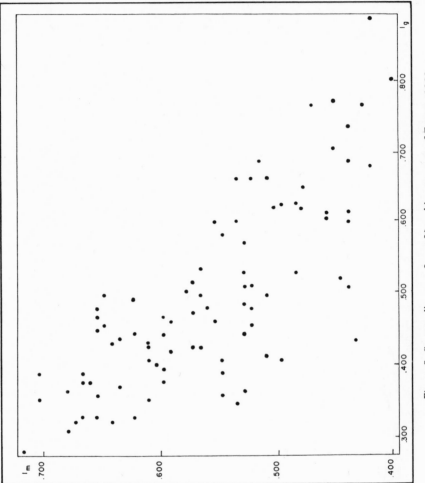

Figure 5. Scatter diagram: I$_g$ vs. I*$_m$, départements of France, 1866.

FERTILITY TRENDS IN EUROPE SINCE THE SECOND WORLD WAR

D. V. Glass

The London School of Economics and Political Science,
University of London

BEFORE DISCUSSING THE MOVEMENTS in fertility in Europe since World War II, it is necessary to consider, both as a background and a yardstick for measurement, the general situation around the mid-1930's. This period has been chosen for several reasons. First, it was at about this time that the crude birth rates and other period indices of fertility in most western and northwestern countries of Europe reached their lowest points. The decline initiated in the 1870's and 1880's had proceeded without interruption except for the years immediately after World War I, and had gathered momentum in the 1920's. Only in France, in which the birth rate had been falling throughout the nineteenth century, did there appear to be some approach to stabilization. Secondly, pro-natalist policies began to expand in France, Belgium, and Italy, and were initiated in Germany with the Nazi take-over. The very expansion of such policies reinforced the feeling of impending depopulation in other Western countries, a feeling made more intense by the increasingly frequent use of period net reproduction rates as indicators of national "vitality." ("True" rates of natural increase were much less frequently cited: they required more elaborate computations and appeared to be less striking.) Such rates were regarded as sophisticated and meaningful measures of replacement tendencies, and they were given a semi-official status by inclusion in the League of Nations Statistical Yearbooks. The apparent implications of these rates were made even more sharply visible by the publication of population projections constructed on a component basis, and using essentially the same approach as that embodied in net reproduction rates—that is, with fertility measured in terms of age-specific fertility rates, and with no regard paid to nuptiality. Thirdly, the early thirties saw the great economic depression, with its correlate of mass unemployment, appearing to provide an economic explanation for at least part of the apparent demographic depression.

Finally, though World War II brought with it in some countries civilian mortality on a scale not formerly seen, save as a result of devastating pandemics, and was followed by a major reshuffling of populations within Central and Eastern Europe, the trend of fertility as such showed less discontinuity than might have been expected. What became fully visible in the fifties and sixties was often already implicit in the trends of the later thirties and continued during World War II in several Western European countries. These trends might have been detected before World War II if better demographic data had been available and if marriage cohort or birth generation techniques of analysis had been applied. At any rate, postwar analysis showed that fertility had begun to stabilize in many Western countries during the thirties, while in most of Eastern and Southern Europe the downward movement had continued. The net result—and this has been reinforced by the fact that in some Western countries marital fertility has actually increased in the last twenty years—has been to even out the levels of fertility in Europe as a whole. Before, and shortly after World War II, most of Eastern and Southern Europe had a high marital fertility and crude birth rates near or over 25 per 1000. By the 1960's, high fertility—defined by Livi-Bacci as corresponding to a crude birth rate of 25 per 1000 and a legitimate fertility rate of 178 live births per 1000 married women aged 15 to 49 years—was shown only by Albania, parts of Yugoslavia, parts of Italy and Portugal, and a few areas in Switzerland and Austria.[1] In some other areas—in parts of Poland, for example—the crude birth rates were high, but primarily because of a high nuptiality. In Eire, always unique, marital fertility continued to be high, but was coupled with a very low nuptiality, thus producing a crude birth rate of under 25 per 1000. For much of Western and Central Europe, on the other hand, with generally low crude birth rates in the 1930's—mostly below 18 per 1000—the rates have risen, largely because of changes in nuptiality, but also in some countries associated with a rise in marital fertility, too. These generalizations need to be amplified. Unfortunately, even for Europe the official demographic data are by no means adequate. Too few countries have comprehensive data on fertility and even where such data exist, analysis is not always satisfactory or up-to-date. Thus only a low order of amplification is possible for most countries. It will be necessary to resort to illustrative cases to round out the picture, and the bias thereby incurred must be taken into account.[2]

It is appropriate to begin by considering the changes in nuptiality which have occurred since the thirties and these are summarized in Table 1. In the 1930's little regard was paid to marriage as an independent variable. There had been studies of the relationship between marriage rates and the trade cycle. But it was generally assumed—at least implicitly—that because the long period decline in the birth rates was not in any major sense the consequence of changes in marriage habits, marriage as such could be discounted in looking at the present or the near future. In fact, as Table 1 shows, most European countries have experienced some change in marriage levels and patterns since the 1930's. The change has been least in the Southern countries, though three of these—Spain, Portugal, and Yugoslavia—have maintained relatively high crude birth rates. In Eastern Europe, the ultimate proportions ever married, in the age group 45-49 years, have remained more or less unchanged, but the proportions ever married at the younger ages have increased, and in three of the countries quite substantially. In most Western and Central countries, however (though hardly at all in France), both types of change have occurred in varying degrees. Even Eire has shared in this general movement, though it still shows the highest proportions of elderly bachelors and spinsters in the whole of the continent. But in some countries the change has been quite radical, in marked contrast to the pattern which had been customary for two centuries or more. This is especially so in the Fenno-Scandian area and in Britain, and the change in the proportions ultimately marrying is even greater than is indicated in the table, since the full effect of changes at the younger

Table 1. European countries—Men and Women: percentage single in selected age groups and ratio of men aged 25-49 years to women aged 20-44 years

Country	Year	Males Age (Years) 20-24	25-29	45-49	Females Age (Years) 20-24	45-49	Ratio M.25-49: F.20-44
England &							
Wales	1931	86	47	11	74	17	835
	1961	69	29	10	42	11	1020
Eire	1936	96	82	35	86	26	961
	1961	93	67	31	78	22	1010
Sweden	1935	94	66	17	78	23	917
	1960	82	41	15	57	11	1045
Denmark	1930	90	51	10	71	16	847
	1960	77	32	10	46	9	986
Finland	1930	90	60	28	76	26	875
	1960	75	37	10	54	14	927

Fertility and Family Planning

Table 1. (Cont.)

Country	Year	Males Age (Years) 20-24	25-29	45-49	Females Age (Years) 20-24	45-49	Ratio M.25-49: F.20-44
Norway	1930	94	65	15	81	23	837
	1960	79	41	13	50	13	1053
W. Germany	1933*	90	54	6	74	12	841
	1946	88	52	6	73	13	709
	1961	79	36	5	55	9	844
Netherlands	1930	90	49	11	75	15	866
	1960	83	37	8	59	11	952
France	1930	57		10 (40-49)	37 (20-29)	12 (40-49)	
	1962	60		11 (40-49)	37 (20-29)	9 (40-49)	
	1962	84	38	11	56	9	989
Belgium	1930	80	38	11	60	13	936
	1961	71	27	9	44	9	998
Switzerland	1930	93	60	15	82	19	833
	1960	86	46	12	65	15	981
Italy	1931	88	49	10	67	13	792
	1961	89	55	9	61	14	974
Spain	1940	93	63	9	79	14	816
	1960	93	53	7	73	15	904
Portugal	1930	83	44	12	69	17	756
	1960	81	39	12	62	16	865
Yugoslavia	1931	60	27	5	35	5	801
	1953	64	23	4	41	6	781
Greece	1928	83	52	7	56	4	821
	1961	89	57	(7)	65	(6)	
Poland	1931	83	41	4	61	7	760
	1960	72	29	4	41	(9)	858
Czecho-	1930	88	43	6	62	10	810
slovakia	1961	74	26	5	33	6	974
Hungary	1930	81	39	5	52	6	822
	1960	71	23	5	31	7	938
Bulgaria	1934	56	20	3	35	1	868
	1956	61	19	2	27	2	957
E. Germany	1946	82	40	4	68	10	604
	1950	71	(24)	(4+)	60	(9+)	763
Romania	1956	71	22	(3−)	34	(4−)	866

*Whole of Germany, 1933 frontiers.

Source: Various issues of the United Nations *Demographic Yearbook,* and national census reports.

Table 2. European countries: Crude birth rates (live births per 1000 population)

	1930-34	1935-39	1950-54	1955-59	1960-64
England & Wales	15.3	14.9	15.5	16.0	17.9
Eire	19.5	19.4	21.4	21.1	21.9
Sweden	14.4	14.5	15.5	14.5	14.5
Denmark	17.9	17.9	17.9	16.8	17.0
Finland	20.0	20.2	22.8	19.9	18.1
Norway	15.7	15.0	18.7	18.1	17.3
W. Germany	16.3[1]	19.4[1]	16.1	16.8	18.3
Netherlands	21.7	20.3	22.1	21.2	20.9
France	17.3	15.1	19.5	18.4	18.0
Belgium	17.6	15.5	16.7	17.0	17.0
Switzerland	16.7	15.4	17.3	17.5	18.5
Austria	15.1	14.7	15.0	16.8	18.5
Italy	24.5	23.2	18.4	18.1	18.9
Spain	27.5	22.0	20.3	21.4	21.6
Portugal	29.3	27.1	24.0	24.2	24.1
Yugoslavia	33.0	27.9	28.8	24.8	22.0
Greece	(30.0)	(26.5)	(19.5)	(19.3)	(18.1)
Poland	(28.9)	(25.4)[2]	30.1	27.1	20.0
Czechoslovakia	19.7	17.1	22.0	18.5	16.3
Hungary	23.2	20.1	21.1	17.8	13.6
Bulgaria	30.3	24.1	21.7	18.7	16.9
E. Germany	—	18.4[3]	16.6	16.1	17.5
Romania	32.9	30.2	24.9	22.9	16.7

[1] Pre-1938 territory
[2] 1935-38
[3] 1938-39

Source: United Nations, *Demographic Yearbook 1965,* New York, 1966, Table 12. Rates in parentheses are referred to as being less reliable than others cited in the table.

ages is not yet visible in the age group 45-49 years. The case of England and Wales may be taken as an example, and the proportions ever married in each age group in 1963 are shown in Table 3. In the span of time between 1931 and 1963—and still more if the implications of continued marriage rates at the 1963 level are taken into account—there has been a fundamental change in marriage propensity and patterns, with marriage as such no longer acting, as it did for some centuries, as a brake on natural increase.[3]

In general, looking at the data for Europe, the increase in marriage propensity has been greater for women than for men, and this is partly associated with changes in the ratio of women to men in the

Table 3. England and Wales, 1963: Percentage ever married by age group, men and women separately.

Age group (years)	Actual position in 1963		Ultimate position if 1963 marriage rates continue		Actual position in 1931	
	Men	Women	Men	Women	Men	Women
20-24	32	59	30	59	14	26
25-29	72	86	75	88	53	59
30-34	84	92	88	94	78	75
35-39	89	92	91	95	86	79
40-44	90	92	93	96	89	82
45-49	91	91	94	96	89	83

(*Source: Registrar General's Statistical Review of England and Wales . . . . . 1963,* Part III, Commentary, London, 1966, p. 53, Tables C23 and C24)

marriageable ages. In many West European countries, these changes began to show themselves in the 1930's, with the elimination from the marriage market of the age groups affected by World War I, and with the decline in overseas migration during the economic depression. For any given country the relationship is undoubtedly a complex one, since it is affected by the varying numbers of births occurring each year, by immigration as well as emigration, and also by changes in the customary differences between the ages of brides and grooms, these changes themselves being at least in part influenced by the relative supply of unmarried men and women at various ages. In England and Wales, for example, by 1965 the mean difference in age at marriage of bachelors who married spinsters had increased by about half a year since 1926-30, and this means confronting the survivors of birth cohorts 2.5 years apart, instead of the former two years. The modification of the sex ratio is certainly not the full explanation of the changes. There have been similar modifications in countries in which marriage patterns have shown little alteration. In any case, the marriage propensities of men have also increased, and the fall in the age at marriage is too large to be explained solely in such terms.[4] So far, however, no firm explanation in terms of economic and social factors has been established, though it is true that very little has been done to investigate the spread of the new marriage pattern—in contrast to the increased attention given to the spread of birth control. At the same time, the possible cumulative effect of a change initiated in part by demographic factors should not be overlooked.

Given this recent history of marriage, some portion at least of the movement in birth rates and period fertility rates since World War II can be easily understood.[5] With more marriage, even if ultimate family size were to remain unchanged, crude birth rates will tend to rise, other things being equal. And with falling age at marriage, additional cohorts of men and women will marry in a given year and thus, other things being equal, be responsible for further increases in annual births. Further, earlier marriage increases the length of exposure to the chances of conception, again other circumstances being equal. Of course, other circumstances have not remained constant. In particular, there has been a marked increase in the access to, and use made of, various means of family limitation in many countries. It is also necessary to bear in mind the possibility that earlier age at marriage may carry with it not only a longer period of exposure to conception—which might be counterbalanced by greater and more effective use of family limitation—but also a different willingness to have children. On the other hand, in some countries, still only halfway along the road to low birth rates (as compared with Britain and Sweden, for example) before the war, the very change in the availability and in the legitimation of birth prevention may partly explain the movements in marriage. With the data available at present, these hypotheses cannot in general be confirmed. Indeed, even the movements in marital fertility as such are by no means clear for all European countries, for with the new role of marriage it is all the more important to be able to examine cohort rates and to compare them with period rates in order to see how far what is happening reflects a change in timing or in ultimate family size, or in both. But it is especially cohort rates over a relatively long period (say, since 1930) which are lacking for much of Europe. Thus from Table 4 it is possible to conclude only that the period rates in Western and Central Europe were generally higher in the 1960's than in 1935-39, with the converse generally being the case in Southern and Eastern Europe. Table 5, on the other hand, shows that in some countries in Western Europe the rise in general fertility rates has also involved an increase in period marital fertility since World War II. It is thus not simply the change in the proportion of women ever married which accounts for the new trend, but other circumstances such as the proportion of marriages of relatively short duration—since these have the highest childbearing rates—and also the age at marriage—since women marrying at the earlier ages tend to bear larger numbers of children. Again, these are demographic elements which should be examined with the help of detailed cohort analyses—and in particular by marriage cohort statistics which are shown separately by age at marriage. Few countries normally produce such statistics, either on the basis of vital registration or by means of fertility censuses.

Some general statistics based on marriage cohort analyses are

Fertility and Family Planning

Table 4. European countries. Live births per 1000 women aged 15-49 years for selected periods

| | *Approximate periods* | | | |
	1935-39	*1950-54*	*1955-59*	*1960-64*
England & Wales	54	62	67	77
Eire	84[8]	94[8]	96	103
Sweden	54	64	61	62
Denmark	66	73	71	72
Finland	74	88	80	74
Norway	55	76	78	76
W. Germany[1]	68[2]	60*	64*	75
Netherlands	77	90	90	89
France[3]	60	80	82	82
Belgium	60	68	72	76
Switzerland	55	68	70	76
Austria	. . .	58	67	80
Italy	90	70	. . .	73
Spain[4]	90	72	. . .	84
Portugal	105	90	91	94
Yugoslavia	132[5]	106	94	88
Greece	. . .	. . .	. . .	(69)
Poland	(90)[6]	109	106	84
Czechoslovakia	(60)[7]	87	78	70
Hungary	(75)	. . .	70	55
Bulgaria	(95)	76	72	66
E. Germany	. . .	61[10]	64	76
Romania	(161)[9]	. . .	(90)[9]	(60)

[1]Single year rates for 1936, 1951, 1956, and 1961.
[2]Pre-war territory of Germany, 1937.
[3]It is not clear whether live-born children who died before registration are included.
[4]Single year rates for 1940, 1950, and 1960.
[5]1931.
[6]1938.
[7]1937.
[8]Single year rates for 1936 and 1951.
[9]Single year rates 1931 and 1956.
[10]1950.
*rates are for 2nd year of each period.
. . . not available at the time of writing.

Source: Partly from United Nations, *Recent Trends in Fertility in Industrialized Countries,* New York, 1957, and partly calculated from national data.

summarized in Table 6. Because the basis varies between one country and another, the data are not fully comparable as between countries. But intertemporal comparisons for a given country are more reliable, and they show a rather different situation, as between Eng-

Table 5. European countries: Legitimate live births per 1000 married women under 50 years of age

	About 1930	About 1950	About 1960	About 1965
England & Wales	102	90	102	105
Eire	. . .	. . .	195	214
Sweden	107	94	80	93
Denmark	119	106	98	103
Finland	166	155	122	120
Norway	125	121	110	. . .
W. Germany	. . .	96	111	113
Netherlands	166	154	139	132
France	100	116	(119)	119
Belgium	108	104	106	. . .
Switzerland	125	120	117	. . .
Austria	. . .	84	(116)	. . .
Italy	171	120	119	. . .
Spain	. . .	. . .	142	. . .
Portugal	197	154	149	. . .
Yugoslavia	190	162	122	. . .
Greece	. . .	. . .	(100)	. . .
Poland	189	. . .	130	. . .
Czechoslovakia	128	. . .	92	101
Hungary	169	110	79	(71)
Bulgaria	(160)	. . .	(90)	. . .

. . . not available at the time of writing.

land and Wales, France and Norway, on the one hand, and the two eastern European countries on the other, with West Germany occupying an intermediate position. The first three countries all show fairly systematic increases in the total fertility of postwar marriages. The increase in France is somewhat larger than the table suggests—and especially at the longer durations of marriage—because the cohort rates for France are *net* rates, based upon the number of marriages originally contracted and not upon the surviving, intact first marriages. In West Germany, the levels of fertility for the postwar marriages seem to be back at about the same position as those of 1930. For Hungary and Czechoslovakia, comparable data for prewar and postwar marriages are not as yet available. But the postwar marriages show some decline in total fertility at each of the marriage durations specified. A falling marital fertility is also indicated by the net rates for Italy.

The ultimate total fertility of fairly recent cohorts is, of course, conjectural. When projections of ultimate family size are based on data for marriages of less than 10 years' duration, the speculative element is particularly large, for—as the statistics for Norway and for Britain indicate—there has been some tendency for a compensating variation between fertility in the first 5 years of married life and in the next 5-year segment. But with the now relatively low ultimate

Table 6. Cumulated duration-specific fertility rates by marriage duration (Equivalent to average number of live births per married woman) by date of marriage and by specified duration of marriage

Country	Year of marriage	5	5½	8	8½	10	10½	15	15½	19	19½	20
Austria	1951	1.04		1.31								
(net rates)	1955	1.19		1.48								
	1958	1.29		1.58								
	1960	1.35										
	1961	1.36										
Belgium	1939	0.94		1.30		1.45		1.69		1.79		1.80
(net rates)	1943	1.23		1.60		1.77		2.03		2.13		2.15
	1945	1.05		1.35		1.50		1.74		1.82		
	1950	1.15		1.51		1.69						
	1955	1.24		1.64								
	1959	1.30										
Czecho-	1950	1.33		1.68		1.80						
slovakia	1952	1.34		1.66								
	1953	1.33										
	1955	1.26										
Denmark	1945	1.47		1.77		1.89		2.05		2.10		
(net rates)	1950	1.29		1.56		1.67		1.82				
	1955	1.43		1.72		1.84						
	1957	1.45		1.75								
	1960	1.48										
England &	1931	1.10		1.45		1.61		1.91		2.04		2.05
Wales	1945	1.24		1.62		1.79		2.06		2.15		2.16
	1950	1.25		1.67		1.84		2.12				
	1955	1.29		1.78		1.99						
	1960	1.45										
Finland	1941	1.27		1.64		1.79		2.03		2.10		2.11
(net rates)	1945	1.24		1.51		1.64		1.82		1.88		
	1949	1.70		2.07		2.23		2.46				
	1950	1.64		1.98		2.13						
	1955	1.64		1.96								
	1959	1.64										

Country	Year of marriage	5	5½	8	8½	10	10½	15	15½	19	19½	20
France (net rates)	1943	1.32		1.73		1.91		2.20		2.30		2.32
	1945	1.31		1.69		1.86		2.11		2.19		2.20
	1950	1.35		1.77		1.96		2.26				
	1955	1.39		1.83		2.03						
	1957	1.39		1.84								
	1960	1.44										
W. Germany (gross rates)	1930		1.29		1.67		1.88		. . .		2.18	
	1933		1.39		. . .		. . .		2.13		2.20	
	1940		. . .		1.42		1.58		1.77		1.83	
	1950		1.25		1.54		1.67					
	1955		1.33		1.67		1.82					
	1960		1.38									
Hungary (gross rates)	1947	1.27		1.70		1.89						
	1950	1.29		1.67		1.79						
	1953	1.26		1.55								
	1955	1.16										
Italy (net rates)	1930	1.66		2.19		2.48		2.97				3.22
	1938	1.51		1.97		2.23		2.58				2.72
	1942	1.48		1.92		2.12		2.44				
	1945	1.55		1.93		2.12		2.43				
	1950	1.43		1.81		2.00						
	1956	1.47										
Netherlands (net rates)	1937	1.49		2.03		2.40		2.83		2.97		2.98
	1940	1.59		2.25		2.51		2.89		3.02		3.03
	1945	1.71		2.21		2.45		2.78		2.89		2.90
	1950	1.51		1.97		2.18		2.48				
	1955	1.53		2.00		2.21						
	1960	1.57										
Norway (gross rates)	1931	1.36		1.75		1.94		2.31		2.48		
	1940	1.32		1.83		2.04		2.36		2.49		
	1945	1.58		2.00		2.19		2.50				
	1950	1.49		1.93		2.13						
	1955	1.53										
Sweden (a) gross rates	1931	1.22		1.53		1.68		1.97		2.07		2.08
	1936	1.12		1.50		1.70		1.95				
	1940	1.25		1.62		1.77						
	1945	1.25		1.56								
(b) gross rates	1940	1.28		1.62		1.76		1.94		2.00		2.00
	1945	1.27		1.53		1.64		1.81		1.85		1.86
	1950	1.25		1.53		1.65		1.81				
	1955	1.30		1.58		1.71						
	1960	1.36										

Country	Year of marriage	Duration of marriage (years)										
		5	5½	8	8½	10	10½	15	15½	19	19½	20
Switzerland	1945	1.54		1.90		2.05		2.24		2.29		
(net rates)	1947	1.52		1.89		2.04		2.24				
	1950	1.50		1.87		2.02						
	1954	1.56		1.94		2.10						
	1955	1.57		1.96								
	1956	1.60		2.00								
	1959	1.70										
Yugoslavia	1950	1.58		1.93		2.09				2.33		
(net rates)	1953	1.67		2.00		2.16						
	1955	1.61		1.94								
	1958	1.46		1.75								
	1960	1.50										

Sources: (1) Austria. Computed from net duration-specific rates given in *Die natürliche Bevölkerungsbewegung* (Austrian Statistical Office) for 1957-66 inclusive (Vienna, 1958-67). Duration by subtraction of calendar years. All ages at marriage, all marriages. No allowance for pre-marital births.

(2) Belgium. From J. Morsa, "Tendances récentes de la fécondité belge." *Population et Famille,* No. 1, 1964, pp. 43-44, and unpublished data kindly supplied by Professor Morsa. All marriages, all ages at marriage, calendar year duration. Before 1961 children born alive but dying before registration were excluded from the statistics of live births.

(3) Czechoslovakia and Hungary. From E. Szabady, K. Tekse, and R. Pressat, "La population des pays socialistes européens." *Population.* Sept.-Oct. 1966, p. 960.

(4) Denmark. Computed from data in *Befolknings Bevaegelser* for the years 1940 to 1965 inclusive. The rates are partly estimates. For 1949-53, interpolation was necessary to obtain single-year duration within the duration group 5-9 years. Similarly, for the years 1959-65, interpolation was necessary within the duration group 15-19 years. All marriages, wife's age at marriage under 45 years.

(5) England and Wales. *Registrar General's Statistical Review . . . . 1965,* Part II, Tables, Population (London, 1966), p. 170. Women married once only, all marriages ages under 45. Marriage duration, exact years.

(6) Finland. Computed from data in *Vital Statistics (Väestonmuutokset)* for the years 1941 to 1964 inclusive. All marriages, wife's age at marriage under 45 years.

(7) France. *Etudes et Conjoncture.* No. 2, 1967, p. 63. All marriages, all ages at marriage. Duration—completed years of married life.

(8) W. Germany. *Bevölkerung und Kultur: Reihe 2. Natürliche Bevolkerungsbewegung 1961.* Appendix, and unpublished data kindly supplied by Dr. Karl Schwarz.

(9) Italy. From D. Moriconi, "La fecondità matrimoniale italiana nel decennio 1951-1961." *Statistica,* 24, 3, 1964, Table VI, p. 40. All marriages, all ages at marriage. Calendar year duration.

family size in most European countries, and also with the contraction of the childbearing period, 80 percent or more of ultimate fertility may be achieved within ten years of married life. (The situation in this respect for England and Wales is shown in Table 7). For marriages of 10 years' duration or longer, the speculative element in a projection of ultimate family size is relatively small.

(10) Netherlands. Computed from unpublished data of the Netherlands Central Statistical Office, kindly supplied by Dr. T. Van den Brink. All marriages, all ages at marriage. Calendar year duration.

(11) Norway. From (J.E. Backer), *Ekteskap Fodsler og Vandringer i Norge 1856-1960.* Oslo 1965, p. 143. Existing marriages, with wife under 45 years of age. Duration—completed years of married life.

(12) Sweden. (a) Gross rates, with allowance for pre-marital births, from J.R.L. Schneider. *"Fertility Changes During and After the Second World War,"* (Ph. D. thesis, University of London, 1963). Table 8, p. 182. All marriages, age of wife at marriage under 50 years. Duration —exact years. Pre-marital births included.

(b) Gross rates (no allowance for pre-marital births) computed directly from published duration-specific fertility rates (all ages at marriage under 50 years) kindly supplied by Dr. E. von Hofsten of the Swedish Central Statistical Office. The time-base is slightly different from that used by Dr. Schneider, but the results are almost identical. Since pre-marital fertility, like marital fertility, is now fairly low, the allowance for pre-marital births would probably not raise the cumulative rates for recent cohorts by more than about 0.1 births per married woman. Duration 20 years in the table actually represents "20 years and over," but the difference is not more than about 0.002 births per married woman. Finally, up to and including 1954, the duration-specific rates refer to legitimate maternities, while for later years they refer to legitimate live births. But the double analysis provided for the 1955 data shows that the differences involved are far too small to have any visible effect on the cohort rates.

(13) Switzerland. Net rates computed from annual data published in *Mouvement de la Population en Suisse,* for the years 1944 to 1964 inclusive. All marriages, wife's age at marriage under 45 years. Calendar year duration.

(14) Yugoslavia. Computed from data in *Demografska Statistika.* 1950 to to 1965 inclusive and unpublished data for 1966 (kindly supplied by the Federal Statistical Office). Some interpolation within duration groups was necessary and adds to the errors of the estimates. All marriages, wife's age at marriage under 45 years.

Notes: 1. Most of the tables give net cohort rates—that is, the births in a given calendar year are classified by the calendar years of marriage from which they derive and are then related to the original number of marriages in the cohort. (Gross rates are based upon calculations of the appropriate exposed-to-risk population each year). Reduction of the original number

In Table 8, projections for England and Wales, Norway and Hungary are given—the calculations having been made by official statisticians of the countries concerned.

For Norway, the estimate is—as Dr. Backer points out—very close to the level actually shown by the marriage cohorts of 1931-41. The estimates for England and Wales yield totals not very different from those for Norway, save in the case of the upper limit of the projection for the 1963 cohort. This latter estimate is, however, extremely speculative, since there was almost no actual experience of the cohort, and the level of 2.75 live births per marriage of completed fertility is higher than has been shown by any cohort in Britain since the marriages of 1914. Even so, the figure is still well below 3 live births per married woman; there is certainly no suggestion of a return to large families. For Hungary, the projected figures confirm the very low level of postwar marital fertility.

Since the projections in Table 8 relate to only three countries, I

---

of marriages by widowhood or divorce means that the longer the duration, the greater the understatement of the net duration-specific fertility rates, and of the cumulated rates. Unpublished Netherlands statistics show, in that country, that of the original cohort of first marriages in 1950, 93.6 percent were still in existence in 1960; and of the cohort of 1940, 82.6 percent were still in existence in 1960. Thus net and gross cohort rates can only be compared in broad terms. However, since there has been no radical change in dissolution rates during the past 20 or 30 years, comparisons between net cohorts within a given country are less subject to error. Certainly any major changes in fertility levels or patterns would be visible.

2. For some countries, ultimate fertility is also understated to some extent because of high illegitimacy. The duration-specific rates are based on legitimate births and pre-marital fertility is usually excluded (even if pre-marital births are legitimated). This factor would be especially important in respect to Austria and Sweden. For the latter country, Schneider (*op.cit.*, p.103) has estimated the number of pre-marital maternities per marriage to be 0.22 for the 1911 cohort; 0.14 for the 1938 cohort; and 0.12 for the 1945 cohort. (These estimates are included in the (a) rates for Sweden.)

3. The comparability of the data by duration for some countries (e.g. Sweden, Switzerland, and France) may be affected by postwar immigration—that is, if the rates include births to immigrants but if the population exposed to risk does not include the marriages of immigrants. It is clear that immigration now needs to be taken much more explicitly into account in several countries. It is therefore highly desirable that efforts should be made—primarily by the appropriate statistical offices in the various European countries—to prepare sufficiently reliable inter-censal estimates of the married female population exposed to risk of childbirth, in order that gross cohort rates on a comparable basis may be computed.

Table 7. England and Wales: average number of live births per marriage by specified duration (years) and proportion of total fertility (at 20 years' duration) achieved by specified duration (uninterrupted first marriages, wife's age at marriage under 45 years)

Year of marriage	Average number of live births by specified duration (years)				Percentage of total fertility at 20 years' duration achieved by specified duration (years)		
	5	10	15	20	5	10	15
1920-24	1.28	1.85	2.15	2.28	56	81	94
1930	1.13	1.64	1.92	2.06	55	80	93
1940	0.95	1.63	1.87	1.97	48	83	95
1945	1.24	1.79	2.06	2.16	57	83	95
1950	1.25	1.84	2.12	(2.22)*	56	83	95
1955	1.29	1.99	(2.27)*	(2.37)*	54	84	96

*Projected figures, assuming fertility in incomplete segment equivalent to that of most recent marriage cohort for which the actual data are available.

Source: Derived from *Registrar General's Statistical Review of England and Wales . . . 1965,* Part III, Tables, Population, London, 1967, Table QQ(b), pp. 170-75.

have tried to extend the coverage in Table 9. The projected figures have been arrived at by splicing on to the actual data for fertility at 10 years' duration, an estimate of the likely additional fertility for duration 10-20 years. This estimate in turn is based on the actual experience of the most recent cohorts which have completed 15 and

Table 8

Country	Year of marriage	Projected total number of births per marriage of completed fertility
Norway	1942-51	2.5
England & Wales	1953	2.33 - 2.36
	1955	2.36 - 2.43
	1963	2.35 - 2.75
Hungary	1947	2.18
	1950	2.01
	1951	1.95

Source: Norway: Backer, *op.cit.,* p. 216

England & Wales: *Registrar General's Statistical Review . . . . 1963,* Part III, Commentary, p. 75.

Hungary: Szabady, Tekse, & Pressat, *loc.cit.,* p. 960.

(The estimates relate to all ages at marriage within the limits used in the particular country for fertility analysis.)

20 years of exposure. (That is, the estimate is in two stages; the elements for 10-15 and 15-20 years relating to different cohorts.) Again, these figures are conjectural. As was indicated in Table 8, the element of conjecture beyond a duration of 10 years is relatively small, and that beyond a duration of 15 years amounts at most to only about 5 percent of ultimate marital fertility. But the projections do not take into account (for the necessary data are not yet available) the renewed fall in the crude birth rate in England and Wales and France, which may reflect a lower fertility at the later durations of marriage than has been assumed.

Two other points should be made in connection with current tendencies in Europe—at least with regard to those countries in which marital fertility is relatively low. First, even where fertility has risen somewhat as compared with the position of the marriages of the 1930's, there is no evidence of a return to large families. On the contrary, the proportions of married women having 4 or more live births have generally continued to fall. By contrast, there is now less childlessness and also a shift to

Table 9. Marriage cohort fertility rates: Projected total number of live births per married woman at 20 years' duration of marriage

Country	Year of marriage	Total number of live births per married woman	
		10 years' duration (actual)	20 years' duration (projected)
Belgium (net rates)	1950	1.69	2.04
England & Wales	1950	1.84	2.22
	1955	1.99	2.37
France (net rates)	1950	1.96	2.35
	1955	2.03	2.42
W. Germany	1950	1.67	1.94
	1955	1.82	2.09
Hungary	1950	1.79	2.01
Italy (net rates)	1950	2.00	2.45
Netherlands	1950	2.18	2.60
(net rates)	1955	2.21	2.63
Norway	1950	2.13	2.58
Sweden	1950	1.65	1.86*
	1955	1.71	1.92*
Switzerland	1950	2.02	2.27
(net rates)	1955	2.05+	2.37

*An allowance for pre-marital births would probably raise these figures by about 0.1 births per married woman.
+9 years' duration.
Source: Derived from data used in compiling Table 6.

2 and 3 births instead of 1. These changes are illustrated in Table 10, which summarizes the data for Norway and for Britain. For the former country, a convenient series of fertility censuses makes it possible to show for several points of time the distributions of total numbers of live births to marriages of 20 years' duration, while for Britain a similar series has been obtained by linking together the data of the 1946 Family Census with those of 1961 censuses of England and Wales and Scotland. On the other hand, statistics for Britain and England and Wales for marriages of 10 years' duration, also given in Table 10, suggest that among the more recent marriages there may have also been some slight shift to 4-birth marriages, though above that number the trend is still downwards. Secondly, childbearing continues to be compressed into a shorter period. The proportion of total fertility achieved by 10 years' duration of marriage has been increasing and the interval between marriage and first birth has contracted somewhat, though this may be partly a function of the shift from 1 to 2- and 3-child marriages—since birth intervals in general contract fairly systematically with increasing ultimate family size. The contribution to total fertility of each 5-year segment of married life is shown in Table 11 for England and Wales, the data being presented separately for three groups of age at first marriage. Even for the younger ages at marriage—20-24 years—fertility beyond the tenth year of married life is lower for the postwar marriages than it was for the marriages of 1930, and this also applies to marriages at 25-29 and at 30-34 years of age.

So far as fertility differentials within countries are concerned, fully comparable material is even scarcer than that for national units. But such recent data as are available suggest a continuation of the

Table 10. Marriages with various total numbers of live births.

(1) *Norway: Marriages of 20 years' duration.*

| | Year of marriage | | | | |
Percent of marriages with:	1900	1910	1926	1930	1940
0 births	7.1	9.4	11.6	12.0	10.4
1	6.4	8.7	18.6	20.5	16.8
2 or 3	19.6	27.7	42.3	43.6	50.6
4 or more	66.9	54.2	27.5	23.9	22.2
Total	100.0	100.0	100.0	100.0	100.0

Source: G. S. Lettenstrøm, *Ekteskap og Barnetall Xen Analyse av Fruktbarhetsutviklingen i Norge,* Statistisk Sentralbyrå, Artikler 14, Oslo, 1965, p.8.

Table 10.   (Cont.)

(2) *Great Britain: Marriages of 20 years' duration (uninterrupted marriages, age of women at first marriage under 45 years)*

Percent of marriages with:	Year of marriage			
	1900-09	1910	1925	1941
0 births	10.5	12.2	16.9	14.5
1	14.1	16.6	24.7	25.4
2 or 3	33.9	37.2	39.4	46.8
4 or more	41.5	34.0	19.0	13.3
Total	100.0	100.0	100.0	100.0

Source: D. V. Glass and E. Grebenik, *The Trend and Pattern of Fertility in Great Britain,* Part II, Tables, London 1954, Tables 1-37; England and Wales, *Census 1961,* Fertility tables, London, 1966, Table 7, p. 29; and Scotland, *Census 1961,* Fertility, Edinburgh 1966, Table 7, p. 29.

(3) *Great Britain and England and Wales: Marriages of 10 years' duration (uninterrupted marriages, ages of women at first marriage under 45 years),*

Percent of marriages with:	Year of marriage.				
	Great Britain			England & Wales	
	1920	1930	1935	1951	1955
0 births	15.5	18.8	19.2	16.2	12.9
1	24.5	30.3	31.0	24.1	24.7
2 or 3	44.3	41.4	41.7	50.4	51.2
4 or more	15.7	9.5	8.1	9.3	11.3
Total	100.0	100.0	100.0	100.0	100.1

Source: Great Britain, Glass & Grebenik, *op.cit.* (not adjusted for understatement of childlessness; England and Wales, 1951 - 1961 Census, *op.cit.* Table 7; England and Wales, 1955 - *Registrar General's Statistical Review* . . . . . *1965,* Part II, Tables, Population, p. 176, women married once only.

developments indicated by Gwendolyn Johnson in 1960.[6] Where fertility has stabilized—either at a very low level or at one somewhat higher than in the 1930's—regional variations appear to have been reduced. Sizable differences persist, however, where there are still pockets of high fertility in countries in which the trend has been generally downwards. Differences in fertility by socioeconomic status now tend to be somewhat narrower than were found formerly. It should be remembered, however, that these narrower differences can be seen in two rather distinct types of society. First, they continue to apply to Catholic populations, at least where, as in Eire and Northern Ireland, religious beliefs are relatively deeply imbedded, and

Table 11. England and Wales: Average number of live births per marriage in successive segments of married life (uninterrupted first marriages)

Year of marriage	20-24 Duration of marriage (years)				25-29 Duration of marriage (years)				30-34 Duration of marriage (years)			
	0-5*	5-10	10-15	15-20	0-5*	5-10	10-15	15-20	0-5*	5-10	10-15	15-20
1920-24	1.39	0.67	0.37	0.17	1.15	0.50	0.19	0.04	1.03	0.33	0	0
1930	1.23	0.58	0.34	0.17	0.97	0.47	0.19	0.06	0.85	0.25	0.06	0.01
1940	0.98	0.75	0.27	0.12	0.88	0.62	0.16	0.03	0.80	0.36	0.04	0
1945	1.28	0.57	0.31	0.13	1.19	0.50	0.17	0.03	1.03	0.30	0.04	0
1950	1.25	0.64	0.31		1.17	0.49	0.17		1.07	0.25	0.03	
1955	1.26	0.74			1.22	0.61			1.05	0.35		
1960	1.40				1.38				1.20			

Source: Derived from *Registrar General's Statistical Review of England and Wales . . . 1965*, Part II Tables, Population, London 1967, Table QQ (b) pp. 170-75.

*Including pre-marital births to the women

where contraception has had less impact than in most areas of western Europe. The data from the 1961 censuses for the two countries mentioned show this relatively narrow range of marital fertility for Catholics at each of the marriage durations specified. (Unfortunately, it is not possible to say whether the more restricted range for the shorter durations is merely a function of incomplete fertility or whether it suggests any further closure.) On the other hand, such societies tend to show a fairly wide gap between the fertility of Catholics and of other religious denominations. In Eire, for example, at 20-24 years' duration of marriage, the lowest level of Catholic fertility is higher than the highest level for other denominations, and this also applies to the shorter durations and is generally the case, too, in Northern Ireland.[7]

Secondly, in countries which have experienced a fall and then a rise—or at least a stabilization—in the fertility of marriage, there appears to have been a quite considerable shift in the previous pattern of socioeconomic differences. This, again, can only be illustrated by citing a few examples, one of the clearest cases being that of England and Wales. Taking a marriage duration of 15-19 years in 1961 as representing almost completed fertility but nevertheless reflecting the experience of relatively recent marriage cohorts (1941-46 ca), the 1961 census results show small differences between rural and urban areas (extreme ratio 1.04 : 1.0); between regions (extreme ratio 1.26 : 1.0) and socioeconomic groups. For the latter, the extreme range is 1.43 : 1.0, scarcely larger than the ratio of manual to non-manual categories for the marriages of the inter-war years. The splicing of the data of the 1911 censuses and of the 1946 Family Census had suggested that this latter ratio (of manual to non-manual categories) had increased from about 1.2 : 1.0 for the marriages of the 1870's to about 1.4 : 1.0 for the marriages of 1910-19. The 1961 Census shows for England and Wales, however, a ratio of under 1.2 : 1.0, a range slightly smaller than that applying to the late nineteenth century marriages. The analysis of fertility by terminal age of full-time education of husband and wife in England and Wales is also of considerable interest, exhibiting a U-shaped curve, the highest fertility being found in marriages in which both partners left school before the age of 15 years (2.09 live births), and in the very different circumstances in which the husband completed his education at the age of 20 or above and the wife at the age of 17 years or above (2.15-2.17 live births). The lowest fertility, on the other hand, was that of marriages in which the husband completed schooling at 15-16 years and the wife at 20 or over (1.55 live births).

For Norway, there are comparative data on socioeconomic differences for three censuses for women whose age at first marriage was 20-29 years and whose marriages had lasted for 17 years by the date of the census. Here, again, there has been a compression of fertility levels, the ratios of extremes having fallen from 1.60 : 1.0 at the 1930 census to 1.40 : 1.0 at the 1960 census. The 1962 "Microcensus" shows a similar reshuffling of relationships in West Germany, as far as broad socioeconomic groups are concerned. In addition, within each of these groups there was a positive correlation between total fertility and net monthly income. Only within the group of "workers" (i.e. manual workers in industry and commerce) did the correlation break down at the top end of the income scale, but that topmost band must cover a very small fraction of the working class.

One final aspect of socioeconomic differentials is worth noting, namely that relating to economically active married women (that is, gainfully employed). In some recent censuses separate data have been given for such women, treated as a group (though unfortunately they are not reported separately for each socioeconomic category). The statistics for Norway, Switzerland, and England and Wales

Table 12. Eire. 1961: Marital fertility by religion, socioeconomic status and duration of marriage. Number of live births per current marriage; all ages at marriage of women concerned.

	Duration of marriage (years)					
	10-14		15-19		20-24	
	Religion					
Socioeconomic status	*R.Cath.*	*Others*	*R.Cath.*	*Others*	*R.Cath.*	*Others*
Farmers, relatives, and managers	3.63	2.73	4.14	3.09	4.26	3.13
Other agricultural and fishermen	3.67	2.46	4.25	2.93	4.47	3.21
Higher professional	3.55	2.10	3.71	2.22	3.63	2.15
Lower professional	3.24	1.74	3.63	2.19	3.63	2.10
Employers and managers	3.49	2.05	3.68	2.20	3.60	2.22
Salaried employees	3.40	1.97	3.65	2.03	3.61	2.22
Intermediate non-manual	3.22	1.88	3.71	1.89	3.66	1.94
Other non-manual	3.49	2.12	4.10	2.55	4.30	2.91
Skilled manual	3.61	2.10	4.20	2.42	4.45	2.59
Semiskilled manual	3.76	2.44	4.39	2.71	4.70	2.86
Unskilled manual	3.83	2.93	4.65	3.32	4.96	3.57
Ratio of highest to lowest (lowest = 1.0)	1.19	1.68	1.28	1.76	1.38	1.84

Source: Eire, *Census of Population 1961*, Vol. 8, Fertility of Marriage, Table 15A.

Table 13. Northern Ireland, 1961: Marital fertility by religion, socioeconomic status (selected groups), and duration of marriage—Number of live births per marriage, women married once only, before age 45 at marriage and age 45 or over on census day

	Duration of marriage (years)			
	15-19		20-24	
	Religion			
Socioeconomic status	R.Cath.	Others	R.Cath.	Others
Employers and managers (large establishments)	2.87	1.57	3.62	1.99
Employers and managers (small establishments)	3.32	1.76	4.36	2.14
Professional—independent	3.42	1.85	3.80	1.98
Professional—employees	2.00	1.71	3.67	1.92
Intermediate non-manual	3.31	1.55	3.54	2.06
Junior non-manual	2.85	1.39	3.76	1.91
Foremen and supervisors	3.60	1.59	4.61	2.22
Skilled manual	3.35	1.66	4.45	2.31
Semiskilled manual	3.25	1.60	4.09	2.41
Unskilled manual	3.17	1.72	4.54	2.59
Farmers and managers	3.43	2.42	4.37	2.94
Agricultural workers	3.32	2.08	4.40	2.81
Ratio of highest to lowest (lowest = 1.0)	1.80	1.74	1.28	1.54

Source: Previously cited, Table 7.

show that the economically active women constitute a very important element in differential fertility. Indeed, in England and Wales such women exhibit a lower fertility as a group than any of the seventeen socioeconomic categories into which the husband's employment is classified. This kind of situation suggests that much more attention should be—and should have been—given to the analysis of married women's employment in fertility censuses, and also that it would be eminently worthwhile undertaking a study of the impact of such employment on overall trends in fertility since the 1930's. For the growth of this employment introduces—at least in theory—two possibilities: first, by providing additional income, it may facilitate earlier marriage and the earlier onset of childbearing; but second, it may help to set a more powerful upper limit on family size, since the circumstances in most of our societies are not such as to encourage gainfully employed married women to have large families. At any rate, when, as is the case in Britain, a third or more of married women are gainfully employed, it is quite unrealistic not to take this factor

Table 14. England and Wales: Marital fertility, by socioeconomic status and duration of marriage in 1961. Women married once only and enumerated with their husbands, and with age at marriage under 45 years. Number of live births per marriage

Socioeconomic status	Duration of marriage (years)		
	10-14	15-19	20-24
Employers and managers—large establishments	1.81	1.85	1.79
Employers and managers—small establishments	1.78	1.83	1.80
Professions—self-employed	2.17	2.18	2.04
Professions—employees	1.86	1.90	1.84
Intermediate non-manual workers	1.76	1.80	1.76
Junior non-manual workers	1.68	1.76	1.72
Personal service workers	1.90	2.00	1.86
Foremen and supervisors—manual	1.90	1.99	1.92
Skilled manual workers	2.00	2.11	2.06
Semiskilled manual workers	2.02	2.15	2.11
Unskilled manual workers	2.30	2.34	2.30
Own account workers—not professionals	1.88	1.92	1.81
Farmers—employers and managers	2.22	2.25	2.30
Farmers—own account	1.99	2.05	2.01
Agricultural workers	2.10	2.24	2.29

Source: Census 1961. England and Wales, Fertility Tables, table 14.

Table 15. Norway: Marital fertility by socioeconomic status and duration of marriage. Number of live births per marriage, age at marriage of women 20-29 years (selected socioeconomic groups)

	Census date					
	1930	1950	1960	1930	1950	1960
Socioeconomic status	Duration of marriage (years)					
	10 years			17 years		
Farmers	3.35	2.68	2.63	4.72	3.33	3.22
Agricultural workers	3.24	2.54	2.27	4.98	3.18	2.62
Workers in manufacture	(2.59)	(2.07)	2.14	(3.93)	(2.36)	2.39
Managers and administrative civil servants in manufacturing	2.27	2.16	2.18	3.20	2.33	2.53
Clerical and sales workers etc.	2.27	1.99	2.00	3.15	2.05	2.32
Employers and administrative civil servants in govt., community, and business services	1.97	2.31	2.14	2.73	2.40	2.42
Professionals in govt., community, and business services	2.70	2.29	2.24	3.52	2.65	2.57
Economically active women	2.10	1.17	1.17	3.13	1.53	1.78

Source: G. S. Lettenstrøm, *op.cit.,* Table 13, p. 21.

Table 16. Germany, Federal Republic: Marital fertility by socioeconomic status,
duration of marriage, and net monthly income in 1962 (current marriages,
all ages of women at marriage)

(a) Number of live-born children per marriage by socioeconomic status and
duration of marriage

	Duration of marriage (years)	
Socioeconomic status	*10-16*	*17-22*
Independents: all	2.04	2.07
In agriculture & forestry	2.60	2.73
Others	1.72	1.85
Officials	1.74	1.97
Salaried employers	1.51	1.76
Workers: all	1.78	1.98
In agriculture & forestry	2.29	2.27
Others	1.77	1.97
All categories	1.75	1.91

(b) Number of live-born children per marriage by socioeconomic status, net
monthly income (in DM), and duration of marriage, excluding husbands
engaged in agriculture or forestry

		Duration of marriage (years)	
Socioeconomic status	*Monthly income (DM)*	*10-16*	*17-22*
Independents	Under 600	1.63	1.77
	6-800	1.66	1.76
	8-1200	1.74	1.80
	1200 & over	1.79	1.99
Officials	Under 600	1.28	1.58
	6-800	1.71	1.81
	8-1200	1.89	2.07
	1200 & over	2.60	2.53
Salaried employees	Under 600	1.38	1.56
	6-800	1.49	1.71
	8-1200	1.59	1.85
	1200 & over	1.54	1.93
Workers	Under 600	1.64	1.88
	6-800	1.99	2.20
	8-1200	2.35	2.36
	1200 & over	2.26	1.59

Source: Statistisches Bundesamt, Wiesbaden, *Bevölkerung und Kultur, Reihe 2:
Natürliche Bevölkerungsbewegung,* October 1962, Table 6, pp. 34-43. Averages
standardized on the duration of marriage and age at marriage of women in the
total population.

Table 17. Netherlands, 1960: Marital fertility by occupational group, religious denomination, and duration of marriage. Total live-born children per existing first marriage (wife's age at marriage—all ages)

Occupational group	Duration of marriage (yrs.)	All	Religious denomination of wife			
			Roman Catholic	Dutch Reformed	Calvinist	None
1. Farmers	10-14	3.60	4.56	2.64	3.61	2.37
	15-20	4.24	5.62	3.15	4.34	2.74
	21-25	4.50	6.21	3.28	4.52	2.46
2. Other employers and own account workers with employees	10-14	2.90	3.46	2.42	3.33	2.08
	15-20	3.50	4.27	2.91	4.12	2.41
	21-25	3.68	4.64	3.02	4.31	2.36
3. Other heads of businesses and own account workers without employees	10-14	2.63	3.07	2.30	3.00	2.02
	15-20	2.96	3.45	2.57	3.48	2.44
	21-25	3.00	3.79	2.51	3.45	2.49
4. Professions	10-14	2.90	3.61	2.61	3.23	2.20
	15-20	3.19	4.10	2.90	3.71	2.45
	21-25	3.04	4.17	2.67	3.70	2.25
5. Senior managing employees	10-14	2.83	3.57	2.51	3.27	2.54
	15-20	3.18	4.18	2.84	3.83	2.44
	21-25	3.12	4.26	2.75	3.82	2.34
6. Other salaried employees with annual income of D fl. 5500 and over	10-14	2.62	3.20	2.28	3.06	2.00
	15-20	3.04	3.83	2.66	3.71	2.26
	21-25	2.99	4.00	2.56	3.75	2.15

Table 17.—Cont.

Occupational group	Duration of marriage (yrs.)	Religious denomination of wife				
		All	Roman Catholic	Dutch Reformed	Calvinist	None
7. Other salaried employees with annual income under D fl. 5500	10-14	2.65	3.14	2.33	2.98	2.02
	15-20	3.13	3.81	2.76	3.70	2.31
	21-25	3.16	4.04	2.74	3.61	2.27
8. Farm workers	10-14	3.27	4.06	2.80	3.57	2.70
	15-20	4.06	5.17	3.44	4.41	3.25
	21-25	4.25	5.51	3.61	4.70	3.77
9. Other workers with annual income D fl. 5500 and over	10-14	2.69	3.11	2.40	3.12	2.10
	15-20	3.45	4.07	3.01	4.71	2.60
	21-25	3.28	4.18	2.87	3.92	2.38
10. Other workers with annual income D fl. 3750-5500	10-14	2.86	3.30	2.56	3.20	2.27
	15-20	3.49	4.23	3.08	3.95	2.61
	21-25	3.64	4.53	3.22	4.16	2.65
11. Other workers with annual income under D fl. 3750	10-14	2.87	3.17	2.54	3.08	2.38
	15-20	3.53	4.04	3.14	3.75	2.87
	21-25	3.79	4.51	3.34	4.04	2.94

Source: Computed from unpublished tabulations of the 1960 Census, kindly supplied by Dr. T. Van den Brink and used here with the agreement of the Netherlands Central Statistical Office.

Notes: Religious denomination is that of the wife, but in the three main denominations shown, there is a high degree of religious endogamy. The Dutch Reformed Church is the largest Protestant denomination. The Calvinist group consists of five denominations. Taking only the endogamous

Table 17.—Cont.

marriages, and not distinguishing socioeconomic status, the fertility rates (number of live births per existing first marriage, all ages at marriage of wife) by duration of marriage are as follows:

Denomination:	Duration of marriage (years)				
	5-9	10-14	15-20	21-25	
Roman Catholic	2.48	3.43	4.28	4.62	
Dutch Reformed	1.98	2.50	2.98	3.05	
Calvinist	2.47	3.26	3.98	4.13	
None	1.74	2.16	2.47	2.48	

The 1960 census shows the following distributions of the population by religious denomination (data from Dr. T. Van den Brink):

Religious Denom.	Total population Percent	Existing marriages (wife's denom.) Percent
Roman Catholic	40.4	36.4
Dutch Reformed	28.3	31.1
Calvinist	9.3	9.0
Other	3.6	4.3
No denom.	18.4	19.2
	100.0	100.0

Table 18. Marital Fertility—All married women and "economically active" married women

(a) Number of live births per married woman (marriage ages under 45 yrs)

Country & Census	Category	Duration of marriage (years)		
		10-14	15-19	20-24
England & Wales,	All women	1.96	2.03	1.97
1961	"Active"	1.42	1.68	1.75
	Percent of women "active"	33	39	38
Scotland, 1961	All women	2.26	2.32	2.34
	"Active"	1.58	1.88	2.06
	Percent of women "active"	25	31	28
Switzerland, 1960	All women	2.24	2.48	2.53
	"Active"	1.32	1.66	1.80

(b) Percentage of childless marriages

Country & Census	Category	Duration of marriage (years)		
		10-14	15-19	20-24
England & Wales,	All women	15	14	15
1961	"Active"	26	17	16
Scotland, 1961	All women	13	13	14
	"Active"	24	15	15

Sources and definitions:

(1) England and Wales and Scotland: Sources cited previously. Data for all women relate to uninterrupted first marriages; i.e. intact until the woman reaches 45 years of age. Data for "active" women relate to women married once only—a smaller universe than covered by the previous definition. Proportions "active" are minimum, since they are arrived at by relating the second universe to the first. But the "true" proportions are unlikely to be seriously larger. The tabulations published are not strictly comparable, but the upper limit may be estimated by relating the "active," once-married women to all women married once only and enumerated with their husbands. The proportions would then be 34, 41, and 41 per cent for England and Wales for duration 10-14, 15-19 and 20-24 years respectively.

(2) Switzerland: 1960 *Recensement Fédéral de la Population,* Vol. 27, Part 1, Berne 1964 pp. 148-55. The analysis relates to women currently married and to legitimate and legitimated live births to the current marriage. Women marrying at 45 years of age or more have been excluded and so have their births (this involves the assumption that no such woman had more than one child—information on childlessness is given—but the error involved is minute).

explicitly into account in investigating marital fertility. For the Socialist countries of Eastern Europe, it may be even more important to pay specific attention to this factor in examining the trend of fertility since the 1930's.

Table 19. Hungary, 1960 Census: Marital fertility by socioeconomic status and employment status of women (number of live births per married women)

Age of women at census

Socioeconomic status	30-39 years			40-49 years		
	All	*Gainfully employed*	*Not gainfully employed*	All	*Gainfully employed*	*Not gainfully employed*
Manual agriculture	2.50	2.20	2.76	3.08	2.69	3.42
Manual non-agriculture	2.18	1.83	2.38	2.42	1.90	2.72
All manual	2.31	2.01	2.52	2.73	2.31	3.03
Non-manual	1.71	1.45	2.08	1.86	1.55	2.17
All	2.19	1.86	2.46	2.59	2.18	2.91

Source: 1960 Census of Hungary, Fertility Report (see reference in notes to Table 21). Definition: women married at Census date, all ages at marriage.

To sum up, the incomplete—often highly incomplete—evidence upon which it has been possible to draw suggests several lines of convergence in Europe in respect to fertility. First, marriage patterns have changed, and in general most sharply in those countries in which fairly late marriage was customary before World War II and in which the proportions of women ever married in the age group 45-49 years tended to be not much above 85 percent. More marriage and earlier marriage explain in part the stabilization or rise of general fertility in such countries, but there have also been some increases in duration-specific marital fertility—especially at the shorter durations—and in ultimate family size. By contrast, in countries in which, before World War II, levels of fertility were relatively high, marital fertility has often fallen sharply. In some of these countries overall fertility—and crude birth rates—would have declined to a still greater extent but for the fact that there, too, marriage patterns have shifted to earlier marriage (though not in any major degree to more marriage). Changes in the age at marriage, the earlier onset of childbearing, and the contraction of the effective childbearing period combine to make the use of conventional period replacement rates very hazardous either for inter-country or for inter-temporal comparisons. Rough estimates suggest that for many countries replacement rates based upon the most recent marriage cohorts and allowing for the illegitimacy component are likely to be at or slightly above 1.0. This must clearly be so with marriage probabilities (by age 50) of 90 percent or higher, and with mortality wastage before the age of 45 years now

Fertility and Family Planning

Table 20. Czechoslovakia: 1961 census. Marital fertility by socioeconomic status and employment status of women (Number of live births to present marriage) for marriages of 10-14 years' duration

Socioeconomic status	All women	Active women	Percent of women active
Workers	2.28	2.00	48
Employees	1.83	1.60	58
Members of united agricultural co-ops	2.39	2.41	88
Members of popular production co-ops	1.93	1.81	74
Individual farmers	2.79	2.95	67
Learned professions and independent.	1.42*	1.21*	30

*The numbers of women in this category are very small—namely 214 "active" and 712 "All."

Source: Computed from data in 1961 Census of Czechoslovakia, *Demografické Charakteristiky Obyvatelstva.* Prague 1965, Table 10, pp. 262-309. Dr. M. Žďárský, Head of the International Division of Statistics, the Czechoslovak Statistical Office, kindly provided both the census volume and a translation of the main table headings.

Definition: All ages at marriage, marriages existing at Census date, fertility of current marriage.

Table 21. The fertility of marriage: Census data on number of live births per married woman, by duration of marriage

Country	Census year	Number of live births per married woman Duration of marriage (years)		
		10-14	15-19	20-24
Belgium	1947	1.82	2.46	
	1961	1.93	2.15	2.35
Czechoslovakia	1961	2.16	2.39	2.46
Eire	1946	3.49	4.09	4.44
	1961	3.56	4.08	4.21
Finland	1950	2.74	3.20	3.48
France	1946	2.11	2.31	2.31
W. Germany	1950	1.78	2.14	2.23
	1962	1.72	1.89	1.94
Hungary	1949	2.29	2.73	3.66 (20 & over)
	1960	2.14	2.46	3.23 (20 & over)
Netherlands	1947	2.75	3.22	3.46
	1960	2.86	3.40 (15-20)	3.52 (21-25)

Norway	1950	2.17	2.40	2.59
	1960	2.10	2.38	2.47
Portugal	1960	2.49 (10)	3.05 (15)	...
Spain	(1966)	2.63 (8-15)	2.84 (16-20)	3.48 (over 20)
Switzerland	1950	2.21	2.37	2.47
	1960	2.24	2.48	2.53
United Kingdom:				
Britain	1946	1.82	2.09	2.34
	1961	1.99	2.06	2.00
England & Wales	1961	1.96	2.03	1.97
Scotland	1961	2.26	2.32	2.34
N. Ireland	1961	2.85	3.10	3.26
Yugoslavia	1953	3.1	3.8	4.3 (20-29)

Sources and Definitions:

A. Census data for 1946-50 are from United Nations, *Recent Trends in Fertility in Industrialized Countries,* New York 1958, p. 60, Table 15.

Belgium: Including families headed by widow or widower.

France: First marriages only (including marriages in which wife widowed or divorced at age 45 or over). All live births to the woman, including pre-marital. Duration 11-15, 16-20, and 21-24 years.

West Germany: Including stillbirths.

Great Britain: First marriages unbroken until wife aged 45 or over. All live births to wife, including pre-marital. Wife's age at marriage under 45.

Netherlands: First marriage only.

Norway: Wife's age at marriage under 45.

Switzerland: Legitimate and legitimated live-born children.

B. Census data for 1960-62.

Belgium: 1961 Census. *Recensement de la Population,* vol. 7, p. 26. Live births to married couples. Age range at marriage not specified (all ages).

Czechoslovakia: 1961 Census, Part I, *Demografické Charakteristiky Obyvatelstva,* Prague 1965, Table 4a, p. 125. Computed from frequency distributions by duration of marriage. Definition: present marriages, total number of live-born children, all ages at marriage.

Eire: 1961 Census. *Census of Population 1961,* Vol. 8, *Fertility oj Marriage,* Dublin 1965, Table 9. Existing marriages and total live births to those marriages. Computation excludes women aged 45 years or over at marriage.

at a very low figure.[8] Replacement rates for birth generations for those countries in which fertility fell continuously from the late nineteenth century will, however, in many cases only now be approaching one, since such generations have been exposed to higher mortality and lower marriage probabilities, as well as to the relatively low age-specific legitimate fertility rates of the early 1930's.[9] A few

---

West Germany: 1962 Microcensus. Computed from single year data in *Bevölkerung und Kultur*, Reihe 2 (Kinderzahlen der Ehen, October 1962), 1966, p. 23. All live births to existing marriages (including legitimated), all ages at marriage of wife.

Hungary: 1960 Census. *Termékenységi Adatok*, Budapest 1966, p. 16. I am indebted to Dr. E. Szabady, who sent me the report, and to John Hajnal, who translated the relevant sections of the text. For purposes of comparison, it may be of interest to note that the 1930 census reported the following numbers of live births per married woman—10-14 years, 2.82; 15-19, 3.52; 20 & over, 4.99. All women married at census date, all ages at marriage, total live births to the marriage.

Netherlands: 1960 census. Computed from unpublished tabulations kindly supplied by Dr. T. Van den Brink, Netherlands Central Statistical Office. Live births to existing marriages, wife's age at marriage under 45 years.

Norway: 1960 census. *Folketelling 1960*, Vol. VII, Oslo 1964, Table 1. Computed from single year data. Total live births to existing marriages, wife's age at marriage 16-45 years.

Portugal: 1960 Census. Vol. 1., Part III, Table 3—photo-copy kindly supplied by U.N. Statistical Office. Figures are estimates. Data tabulated by age at marriage and age at census, 5-year groups, age at census being distinguished only up to 50 years & over. For 10 and 15 year durations, it was thus necessary to estimate proportions of women married at ages 35 years and over, and fertility of those women. However, the error involved is small, since marriages in which age of wife is under 35 years constitute 95 percent of all marriages. Total live births to existing marriages, wife's age at marriage under 45 years.

Spain: Although the 1960 Census of Spain asked a question on total live births to married women, the results so far are not available. The data in the table derive from a stratified random sample investigation, undertaken in 1966 on behalf of the Fundacion Foessa, and covering some 2500 households. The table covers married women only, all ages at marriage, total live births to the marriage. See Fundacion Foessa, *Informe sociológico sobre la situación social de España*, Madrid 1966, pp. 30-34 and 44-47; and M. Gómez Reino y Carnota, "La familia rural y urbana en España," *Anales de Moral Social y Económica*, Vol. XIV, 1967. Information regarding the coverage of the sample survey, as well as copies of the various reports and

countries stand out fairly sharply from this general picture. One is, of course, Albania, with the highest level of fertility in Europe—an average of over 6 live births per woman (all marital conditions) aged 45-49 years at the 1960 Census. But the Netherlands, Eire, and to a lesser extent Northern Ireland are also countries of above average fertility, with the Catholic population being especially fertile—though in the Netherlands, van Heek has argued, it is high Catholic fertility which has also provoked emulation by the more rigorous Protestant groups.[10] However Eire and Northern Ireland both have late marriage and low marriage propensity and these counteract high marital fertility. In the Netherlands, on the other hand, relatively high marital fertility is combined with a relatively high marriage propensity and with ages at marriage which are considerably below those obtaining in the 1930's.

Within countries, reproductive behavior has become somewhat more uniform. Though special studies of marriage as such are rare, the overall figures indicate that marriage changes must have affected the bulk of the population. A specific study undertaken for Britain confirms that the fall in age at marriage has occurred in all socioeconomic groups.[11] Marital fertility has become compressed into a narrower band of family sizes; childlessness has tended to fall, but so, too, has the frequency of families with 4 or more live births. Some, at least, of the former distinct regional and socioeconomic differences have been reduced. The data on religion show a continuing, consid-

---

papers based upon it, were kindly supplied by Dr. Amando de Miguel, manager of DATA S. A., who directed the inquiry.

Switzerland: 1960 Census. *1960 Recensement fédéral de la population,* Vol. XXVII, Part 1, Berne 1964, pp. 148-55. Women currently married, legitimate and legitimated live births to current marriage. Women aged 45 or over at marriage excluded (see note to Table 9).

United Kingdom:
Britain: 1961 Censuses of England and Wales and Scotland. England and Wales, *Fertility Tables* (London 1966) p. 25; Scotland, Vol. X, *Fertility* (Edinburgh 1966) p. 25. Uninterrupted first marriages (until wife aged 45 or over), wife's age at marriage under 45 years, total live births to marriage.

Northern
Ireland: 1961 Census. *Census of Population 1961,* Fertility Report (Belfast 1965) Table 5, p. 20. Same definitions as for Britain.

Yugoslavia: First marriages only, wife's age at marriage 15-49 years. Data kindly supplied by Dr. Z. Aničič, Federal Inst. for Statistics, Belgrade.

erably higher marital fertility of Catholic couples, but these data relate mainly to countries in rather special situations. A recent sample investigation in Britain suggests that the difference there may amount to about 0.5 children per married woman in favor of Catholic couples —a much smaller difference than is evident in Eire or Northern Ireland.[12] The survey undertaken by the Population Investigation Committee in 1959-60 showed that substantial proportions of Catholic couples in Britain were practicing birth control and were, in fact, using methods prohibited by their Church.[13] And this must undoubtedly apply generally to Catholics in France and to the Orthodox families in Greece.[14] Paralleling these changes in fertility have been changes in access to, and in the use of, contraception and abortion— contraception especially in Western Europe, illegal abortion in Greece and, to a considerable extent, in France; and legalized abortion, especially in Eastern Europe, where it has helped to bring down the crude birth rates to the lowest levels in the Continent. To consider these developments and also the question of trends in family size norms would require a separate paper.[15] It should, however, be emphasized that though family limitation is now widely practiced in most European countries, it does not at all follow that the full effects of fertility control as such have already been displayed. There is not only the question of prevalence—of the extent to which couples ultimately use some form of control—but also that of the stage in family building at which control is initiated, and that of the effectiveness of the methods used. On the latter point, it should be remembered that, apart from abortion, the methods of family limitation generally used in Europe are not of the most up-to-date or efficient kinds. Socially, their effectiveness has been of a high order. But at the individual level, accidental pregnancies are by no means uncommon. The spread of more advanced means of contraception may thus have a substantial effect on the timing of births, even if it has a much smaller effect on ultimate family size. And given the fact that in most European societies the ultimate family size of fairly recent marriage cohorts is relatively modest, changes in timing may give rise to a proportionately larger variation in period fertility rates and in short-term population growth. So, too, will even small absolute changes in family size norms. At the level of demographic analysis, it may become more difficult to disentangle the components involved in short-term movements in the birth rate, as may be seen from discussions of the recent fall in the birth rate in the U.S.A., Canada, Australia, England and Wales, and France. Certainly it will be necessary to have much fuller official data on marriage and fertility than are now usually available and to provide for a much speedier analysis of those data.[16]

Notes

1. M. Livi Bacci, "Communication sur les régions de l'Europe ou la fécondité demeure élevée," European Population Conference, 1966, *Official Documents*, Vol. I. (henceforth referred to as *European*).

2. For previous general surveys of recent trends of fertility in Europe, see: United Nations, *Recent Trends of Fertility in Industrialized Countries* (New York 1958); H. Gille, "An International Survey of Recent Fertility Trends," and G. Z. Johnson, "Differential Fertility in European Countries," both in National Bureau of Economic Research, *Demographic and Economic Change in Developed Countries* (Princeton, N.J., 1960); J. N. Biraben, Y. Péron, and A. Nizard, "La situation démographique en Europe occidentale," *Population*, No. 3 (1964); J. N. Biraben, "Prevailing Fertility Situation and Its Causes in Western Europe," G. Acsádi, "Demographic Variables as a Source of Differences in the Fertility of Low Fertility Countries," and N. B. Ryder, "Fertility in Developed Countries During the Twentieth Century"; all in United Nations, *World Population Conference, 1965* (New York 1967) Vol. II (henceforth referred to as *Belgrade*).

3. For the historical background of marriage patterns in Europe, see J. Hajnal, "European Marriage Patterns in Perspective," in D. V. Glass and D. E. C. Eversley (eds.), *Population in History* (London 1965). Recent developments as such are discussed in T. H. Hollingsworth, "Communication on the Marriage Rate in Pre-Malthusian Europe etc.," in *European*, Vol. I.

4. See J. A. Rowntree, "Communication on the Falling Age at Marriage and Decrease of Celibacy," in *European*, Vol. I.

5. There is very little discussion in this paper of the extent to which changes in period rates in the years 1930-50 were explained by the postponement or "making-up" of births. This problem is considered in great detail in earlier studies, and especially in the contributions of John Hajnal to the work of the British Royal Commission on Population (see, in particular, Hajnal's contributions in Papers of the Royal Commission on Population, *Reports and Selected Papers of the Statistics Committee*, Vol. II (London 1960); see also J. Hajnal, "The Analysis of Birth Statistics in the Light of the Recent International Recovery of the Birth-Rate," *Population Studies*, I, 2, 1947).

6. *Op. cit.*, pp. 70-72.

7. Information on religious differentials in the Netherlands and W. Germany is given by C. D. Witt, "Communication on Differential Fertility," *European*, Vol. I. A survey based largely on the vital statistics of Switzerland, especially as analyzed in *Mouvement de la Population en Suisse 1949—1956-57*, text (Berne, 1959), is given by J. W. Nixon, "Some Demographic Characteristics of Protestants and Catholics in Switzerland," *Revue de l'Institut Internationale de Statistique*, xxix, 2 (1961). For 1959-62, Monsieur A. Gross, of the Swiss Federal Statistical Office, kindly supplied tables of age-specific legitimate birth rates by religion.

8. For Europe as a whole (excluding Albania and Northern Ireland), Keyfitz has constructed life tables for 1961. These yield a female expectation of life at birth of 72.22 years and a probability of survival from birth to age 15 of 0.955 and to age 45 of 0.923. For women who reach age 15,

the probability of survival to age 45 is 0.966 (see N. Keyfitz, "Une table de vie européenne et sa version stochastique," (forthcoming).

9. See the table of generation fertility rates in Appendix I. Of course, the mortality factor in generation rates will depend upon the definition of the generation. A generation from birth to birth (that is, following women from their birth to the end of their childbearing period) will have been subject to the relatively high infant mortality of the period in which they were born. A generation spanning women from age 15 to their children at that age will have been exempt from the high infant mortality of the earlier period. Similar questions of definition may arise in using conventional period replacement rates or marriage cohort rates. In this paper, the generation used is a birth-to-birth one (and excludes the migration factor).

10. F. van Heek, "Roman-Catholicism and Fertility in the Netherlands," *Population Studies* (Nov. 1956).

11. E. Grebenik and G. Rowntree, "Factors Associated with Age at Marriage in Britain," *Proceedings of the Royal Society*, Series B, CLIX, 974 (10, December 1963). This paper was based upon a sample survey undertaken by the Population Investigation Committee in 1959-60.

12. The investigation was undertaken in 1966 for the Population Investigation Committee by Social Surveys (Gallup Poll) Ltd. The results are published in *Population Studies*, March 1968 (Ru Chi Chou and S. Brown, "A Comparison of the Size of Families of Roman Catholic and Non-Catholics in Great Britain").

13. Of the Catholic couples married in the 1940's and interviewed in 1959-60, almost half had used methods prohibited by their Church. See R. M. Pierce and G. Rowntree, "Birth Control in Britain," II, *Population Studies* (November 1961), 144-45.

14. On the role of coitus interruptus and abortion in Greece, see V. G. Valaoras *et al.*, "Control of Family Size in Greece," *Population Studies* (March 1965). In France, an investigation of birth control practice among 1200 maternity cases in the Grenoble public hospital in 1961-62 found that almost 70 percent had used birth control, coitus interruptus being by far the most important method—and among practicing Catholics, too. (S. Siebert and J. Sutter, "Attitudes devant la maternité: une enquête à Grenoble," *Population*, October-December 1963).

15. I have dealt with this to some extent in two earlier papers: "Family Limitation in Europe," in C. V. Kiser, ed., *Research in Family Planning* (Princeton, N.J., 1962); and "Family Planning Programmes and Action in Western Europe," *Population Studies* (March 1966). An interesting discussion of the relation between ideal and actual family size will be found in R. Pressat, "Opinions sur la fécondité et la fécondité effective," *European*, Vol. I. See also K.-H. Mehlan, "The Socialist Countries of Europe," in B. Berelson *et al.*, eds., *Family Planning and Population Programs* (Chicago 1966). In one East European country, Romania, access to abortion has again been restricted, no doubt because of concern with the continued fall in the birth rate. Mr. J. Berent, of the Economic Commission for Europe, has provided me with a summary of the monthly birth statistics published in the *Revista de Statistica*, No. 9, 1967, p. 101, which suggests that the withdrawal of free access to abortion has resulted in a marked increase in the number of births, the implication being that induced abortion

was formerly the primary method of birth prevention. But more detailed analysis of the data would be required to confirm this.

16. In this paper I have followed the usual practice of excluding the Soviet Union from the discussion of fertility trends in Europe. This is not unreasonable, for in any case to include the Soviet Union would require a major addition to the discussion. It is, however, worth drawing attention to some of the material on the Soviet Union: B. T. Urlanis ("Dynamics of the Birth Rate in the Union of Soviet Socialist Republics and Factors Contributing to It," *Belgrade,* Vol. II; A. M. Vostrikova "Female Fertility and Methods of Studying It in the Union of Soviet Socialist Republics," *Belgrade,* Vol. II; D. P. Mazur, "Reconstruction of Fertility Trends for the Female Population of the U.S.S.R.," *Population Studies* (July 1967); A. M. Vostrikova, "Examination of Fertility, Marriages and the Family in the U.S.S.R.", in E. Szabady, ed., *Studies on Fertility and Social Mobility,* Budapest, 1964; D. M. Heer, "Abortion, Contraception and Population Policy in the Soviet Union," *Demography,* Vol. II (1965); and a new collection of data on recent trends in fertility in the Soviet Union—referred to in a document prepared for the first meeting of the Working Group on Social Demography, established by the U.N. Office at Geneva to consider the comparative demography of Europe. (*Vital statistics concerning fertility*—UN/SOA/W6/2/WP.6.) The data were presented in a series of appendix tables in *Vestnik Statistiky* (Statistical News), 1967, No. 8, pp. 87-95.

Appendix I

Generation Total Fertility Rates

The purpose of this appendix is to bring together such generation total fertility rates for Europe as could be computed from the data available at the time of writing. A generation rate is defined here in the same way as in the text of the paper—that is, the span of a generation is from birth to birth, and the rates purport to show the number of live births occurring to 1000 women born in a specified period, experiencing no mortality, and subject to the age-specific fertility rates of the years through which they pass during the childbearing period. Other sets of generation rates have been published—notably those by Depoid for France, Vogt for Norway, Hjortkjaer and Kjeldgaard for Denmark, and von Hofsten for Sweden—and some of these rates have been made use of in the present tables.[1] But the general aim here is to present a series of rates on a standard basis. Thus, save in the case of the U.S.S.R., the tables have all been constructed first on the basis of 5-year age-specific fertility rates, and then by splicing the rates along the diagonals. For the U.S.S.R., the data have been taken directly from the tables of D. P. Mazur and are on the time scale which he used.

In order to present estimates for fairly recent generations of women, it was necessary to extrapolate in the case of generations in which the women have not yet reached the age of 50. The main extrapolation applies to the women born in 1916-25 or 1921-30—that is, women whose mean age at maternity would have fallen roughly in the periods 1944-53 or 1949-58. In a few cases, the extrapolation is also extended to the generation of 1926-35—women whose mean age at maternity would have occurred, approximately, during the period 1954-63. The method of extrapolation is a very simple one. The fertility rates were cumulated and it was assumed that the proportion of ultimate fertility reached by a given age was the same as that shown by the most recent completed generation. Although arbitrary,

62

the method cannot result in major errors in the estimates for the generations of 1916-25 or 1921-30, since the extrapolation is only beyond age 45 in the former and beyond age 40 in the latter generation. As is evident from the tables, over 99 percent of total fertility is achieved by age 45 in fairly recent generations for most countries, and over 95 percent by age 40. The exceptions are the Netherlands, Portugal, and the U.S.S.R., and even for these countries over 90 percent of total fertility is achieved by age 40. The estimates of total fertility for the 1926-35 generation are naturally more tentative, since extrapolation beyond age 35 is involved. Even so, the available data indicate that, for the countries concerned, at least 80 percent of total fertility is achieved by that age, and over 85 percent in 4 of the 7 cases.

It would have been useful to complete the tables by showing generation net replacement rates. Unfortunately, few generation life tables have so far been published and those that have are generally on a different time basis from that used here and do not cover relatively recent generations. However, a reasonable idea of the situation can be gained by considering the data for Sweden, for which a full series of tables has been prepared by Keyfitz.[2] The relevant statistics are summarized in Table 1. Mortality in Sweden has, of course, been among the lightest in Europe for some time. Delaporte's calculations, for example, show that the expectation of life at birth of females born around 1860 was 49.5 years for Sweden; 51.4 years for Norway; 46.5 years for England and Wales; 42.9 years for the Netherlands; and 42.7 years for France.[3] Even so, as in the case of England and Wales, mortality for the generation born around the beginning of the twentieth century was such that about 2.7 live births per woman would have been necessary to yield a net replacement rate of 1.0. And for the most recent generation covered by the table, the requirement would still be about 2.35 live births, a figure substantially larger than the actual number of births per woman for the 1920 generation. But mortality has continued to fall and fertility has risen. Légaré has shown, basing his analysis on the data for England and Wales, that generation mortality up to age 30 years is roughly equal to the mortality displayed for the same ages by a current life table for a point of time 5 years later than the date of birth of the generation.[4] Further, the ratio of the N.R.R. to the G.R.R. is roughly equal to the probability of a female surviving from birth to age 30 years. Working with these approximations, the net replacement rate for Sweden for the generations of 1921-30 and 1926-35 would be very roughly 0.90 and 0.97 respectively. Again, handling the data in an extremely rough manner, the net rates for the 1926-35 generation

Table 1. Sweden: Generation female life tables, fertility rates and net replacement rates

Approx- imate date of birth	Expectation of life at birth (yrs)	Total fertility by age 50	Generation gross reproduction rate	net reproduction rate	Minimum total fertility needed for net reproduction rate of 1.0
1850	48.61	4.171	2.030	1.326	3.145
60	49.54	3.978	1.935	1.290	3.086
70	49.67	3.722	1.809	1.206	3.086
80	52.25	3.336	1.621	1.128	2.959
85	53.99	3.055	1.484	1.064	2.874
90	55.80	2.689	1.307	0.963	2.793
95	57.70	2.338	1.135	0.859	2.755
1900	59.25	2.033	0.987	0.761	2.674
05	62.35	1.821	0.884	0.712	2.558
10	64.66	1.815	0.881	0.733	2.475
15	66.23	1.915	0.929	0.791	2.421
20	(67.87)*	(2.032)*	(0.986)*	(0.863)*	(2.353)

*Based partly on projections

Source: From the detailed computer output kindly provided by Professor N. Keyfitz (see references).

in the various countries for which the total fertility of that generation has been estimated in Table 2, would be about:

Denmark:	1.05
England & Wales:	1.03
Finland:	1.04
France:	1.13
Norway:	1.12
Switzerland:	about 1.0

For the Soviet Union, it is doubtful if the net replacement rate for the 1928-32 generation was above 0.85 or 0.9. Fertility was not high, while mortality must have been at least as high as that implied by the 1926-27 life table for the European areas of the U.S.S.R.—probably considerably higher, allowing for war mortality.

However, levels of mortality have been falling fairly rapidly during the past 30 years, and the range of variation between countries in Europe has become much narrower than it was. Keyfitz has prepared life tables for almost every country in Europe (excluding

Table 2. Generation fertility rates for selected countries in Europe

Country	Period of birth	Cumulative rates per 1000 women per year			Percent of total fertility by		Total fertility by age 50 (cumulative ×5)
		to age 40	to age 45	to age 50	age 40	age 45	
Belgium	1916-25	412.4	428.4	429.0*	96.1	99.9	2145*
Denmark	1901-10	411.6	433.0	434.0	94.8	99.8	2170
	1906-15	433.4	448.7	449.6	96.4	99.8	2248
	1911-20	452.0	464.1	464.7	97.3	99.9	2324
	1916-25	458.5	468.5	469.1*	97.7	99.9*	2346*
	1921-30	462.3	. . .	473.2**	97.7**	99.9**	2366**
	1926-35	. . .	. . .	. . .	. . .	. . .	(2453)[1]

[1]Extrapolated beyond age group 30-34, assuming cumulative fertility by age 35 represents 89.5 percent of total fertility by age 50, as in 1921-30 cohort.

Country	Period of birth	to age 40	to age 45	to age 50	age 40	age 45	Total
England & Wales	1901-10	344.0	361.0	361.9	95.1	99.8	1810
	1906-15	353.4	366.3	367.1	96.3	99.8	1836
	1911-20	378.1	390.6	391.4	96.6	99.8	1957
	1916-25	409.7	423.2	424.0*	96.6	99.8*	2120*
	1921-30	430.2	. . .	445.3**	96.6**	99.8**	2227**
	1926-35	. . .		. . .	. . .	. . .	(2441)[1]

[1]Extrapolated beyond age group 30-34, assuming that cumulative fertility by age 35 represents 85.7 percent of total fertility, as in 1921-30 cohort

Country	Period of birth	to age 40	to age 45	to age 50	age 40	age 45	Total
Finland	1846-55	834.2	948.9	967.5	86.2	98.1	4838
	1856-65	838.9	950.1	966.3	86.8	98.3	4832
	1866-75	826.6	929.8	943.1	87.6	98.6	4716
	1876-85	732.1	806.1	815.6	89.8	98.8	4078
	1886-95	579.4	625.7	630.8	91.9	99.2	3154
	1891-1900	517.0	561.7	567.1	91.2	99.0	2836
	1896-1905	468.2	510.0	515.0	90.9	99.0	2575
	1901-10	437.5	480.8	484.7	90.3	99.2	2424
	1906-15	459.0	494.1	496.6	92.4	99.4	2485
	1911-20	488.7	516.2	518.4	94.3	99.6	2592
	1916-25	502.3	524.8	527.0*	95.3	99.6*	2635*
	1921-30	502.6	. . .	527.4**	95.3**	99.6**	2637**
	1926-35	. . .	. . .	. . .	. . .	. . .	(2599)[1]

[1]Extrapolated beyond age group 30-34, assuming that cumulative fertility by age 35 represents 84.8 percent of total fertility by age 50, as in 1921-30 cohort.

General Note: * = Total rate based on extrapolation beyond 40-44 years age group
                 ** = Total rate based on extrapolation beyond 35-39 years age group

Table 2. Generation fertility rates for selected countries in Europe

Country	Period of birth	Cumulative rates per 1000 women per year			Percent of total fertility by		Total fertility by age 50 (cumulative ×5)
		to age 40	to age 45	to age 50	age 40	age 45	
France	1846-55	610	648	654	93.3	99.1	3270
	1856-65	571	604	607	94.1	99.5	3035
	1866-75	509	532	534	95.3	99.6	2670
	1876-85	451	473	475	94.9	99.6	2375
	1886-95	395	412	413	95.6	99.8	2065
	1891-1900	379	394	396	95.7	99.5	1980
	1896-1905	407	427	429	94.9	99.5	2145
	1901-10	416	442	444	93.7	99.5	2220
	1906-15	444	465	467	95.1	99.6	2335
	1911-20	475	494	495	96.0	99.8	2475
	1916-25	488	506	507*	96.3	99.8	2535*
	1921-30	505	...	524**	96.4**	99.8**	2620**
	1926-35	...	...	...	...	...	(2695)[1]

[1]Extrapolated beyond age group 30-34, assuming that cumulative fertility by age 35 represents 86.1 percent of total fertility by age 50, as in 1921-30 cohort.

Netherlands	1906-15	535.5[1]	577.6	580.6	...	...	2903
	1911-20	558.8	594.2	596.7	93.6	99.6	2984
	1916-25	553.8	583.5	586.0*	94.5	99.6*	2930
	1921-30	537.3	...	568.6**	94.5**	99.6**	2843

[1]15-19 age group estimated by assuming same percent higher for 1911-20 as 1911-20 higher than 1916-25

Norway	1901-10	372.3[1]	408.6[1]	411.5	...	...	2058
	1906-15	387.6[1]	416.1	418.5	...	...	2093
	1911-20	408.9	433.7	435.1	94.0	99.7	2176
	1916-25	422.1	441.1	442.5*	95.4	99.7*	2213*
	1921-30	438.7	...	459.9**	95.4**	99.7**	2300**
	1926-35	...	...	...	...	...	(2670)[2]

[1]Interpolated from J. Vogt's estimates—see references.
[2]Extrapolated beyond age group 30-34, assuming cumulative fertility by age 35 represents 80.1 percent of total fertility by age 50—as in 1921-30 cohort.

Portugal	1906-15	622.4[1]	670.9	675.9	...	...	3380
	1911-20	573.4	616.3	619.5	92.6	99.5	3098
	1916-25	556.5	603.6	606.8*	91.7	99.5*	3034*

[1]15-19 age group estimated by assuming same percent higher than next generation as 1911-20 generation higher than 1916-25.

General Note: * = Total rate based on extrapolation beyond 40-44 years age group

** = Total rate based on extrapolation beyond 35-39 years age group

Table 2. Generation fertility rates for selected countries in Europe

Country	Period of birth	Cumulative rates per 1000 women per year			Percent of total fertility by		Total fertility by age 50 (cumulative ×5)
		to age 40	to age 45	to age 50	age 40	age 45	
Sweden	1856-65	694.9	782.7	792.7	87.7	98.7	3964
	1861-70	672.9	751.8	759.9	88.6	98.9	3800
	1866-75	656.3	725.5	732.8	89.6	99.0	3664
	1871-80	637.5	696.2	702.2	90.8	99.1	3511
	1876-85	589.8	638.0	642.4	91.8	99.3	3212
	1881-90	534.6	571.1	574.1	93.1	99.5	2871
	1886-95	473.8	499.5	501.8	94.4	99.5	2509
	1891-1900	408.3	430.1	432.0	94.5	99.6	2160
	1896-1905	354.6	378.2	380.0	93.3	99.5	1900
	1901-10	344.3	366.3	367.6	93.7	99.6	1838
	1906-15	364.0	379.9	380.8	95.6	99.8	1904
	1911-20	386.3	399.2	399.9	96.6	99.8	2000
	1916-25	398.4	409.1	409.8*	97.2	99.8*	2049*
	1921-30	406.1	. . .	417.8**	97.2**	99.8**	2089**
	1926-35	. . .	. . .	. . .	. . .	. . .	(2216)[1]

[1]Extrapolated beyond age group 30-34, assuming that cumulative fertility by age 35 represents 87.8 percent of total fertility by age 50, as in 1921-30 cohort.

Switzerland	1911-20	413.3	431.2	432.4	95.6	99.7	2162
	1916-25	426.9	444.5	445.7*	95.8	99.7*	2229*
	1921-30	428.0	. . .	446.8**	95.8**	99.7**	2234**
	1926-35	. . .	. . .	. . .	. . .	. . .	(2309)[1]

[1]Extrapolated beyond age group 30-34, assuming that cumulative fertility by age 35 represents 83.6 percent of total fertility by age 50, as in 1921-30 cohort.

U.S.S.R.(A)	1911-15	2694.7	2986.3	3048.7	88.2	98.0	3049
	1916-20	2499.5	2748.9	2819.3	88.7	97.5	2819
	1921-25	2359.6	2583.2	2647.0*	91.3	97.6*[1]	2647*
	1926-30	2435.8		2710.0**	92.1**[2]	97.6**	2710**
	1928-32	2417.2		2690.0**	92.1**	97.6**	2690**

[1]Based on 1918-22 cohort. [2]Based on 1923-27 cohort.
Source: D. P. Mazur—see references.

U.S.S.R.(B)	1890-94	4430	4920	5120	86.5	96.1	5120
	1895-99	4550	5030	5140	88.5	97.9	5140
(a) All women	1900-04	4130	4380	4450	92.8	98.4	4450
	1905-09	3600	3810	3850	93.5	99.0	3850

General Note: * = Total rate based on extrapolation beyond 40-44 years age group

** = Total rate based on extrapolation beyond 35-39 years age group

Fertility and Family Planning

Table 2. Generation fertility rates for selected countries in Europe

Country	Period of birth	Cumulative rates per 1000 women per year			Percent of total fertility by		Total fertility by age 50 (cumulative ×5)
		to age 40	to age 45	to age 50	age 40	age 45	
	1910-14	3190	3350	3380*	94.3*	99.0*	3380*
	1915-19	2800	. . .	2970**	94.3**	99.0**	2970**
	1920-24	. . .	. . .	(2750)[1]	. . .	. . .	(2750)[1]
(b) Urban areas	1890-94	4410	4610	4640	95.0	99.4	4640
	1895-99	3890	4050	4080	95.3	99.3	4080
	1900-04	3200	3310	3320	96.4	99.7	3320
	1905-09	2660	2780	2790	95.3	99.6	2790
	1910-14	2560	2640	2650*	96.6*	99.6*	2650*
	1915-19	2250	. . .	2360**	96.6**	99.6**	2330**
	1920-24	. . .	. . .	(2060)[1]	. . .	. . .	(2060)[1]
(c) Rural areas	1890-94	4550	5130	5380	84.6	95.4	5380
	1895-99	4620	5190	5310	87.0	97.7	5310
	1900-04	4330	4620	4700	92.1	98.3	4700
	1905-09	4020	4260	4310	93.3	98.8	4310
	1910-14	3510	3710	3760*	93.4*	98.8*	3760*
	1915-19	3230	. . .	3460**	93.4**	98.8**	3460**
	1920-24	. . .	. . .	(3330)[1]	. . .	. . .	(3330)[1]

[1]Extrapolation beyond age group 30-34, assuming cumulative fertility by age 35 represents 81.8, 87.1, and 79.5 percent of total fertility for all women, urban areas and rural areas respectively, as in 1915-19 cohort.

Source: Vestnik Statistiky—see references. The rates have been expressed as per 1000 women in line with the other data in this Appendix.

General Note: * = Total rate based on extrapolation beyond 40-44 years age group

** = Total rate based on extrapolation beyond 35-39 years age group

Sources of data in Table 2: Generally, the various issues of the United Nations *Demographic Yearbook,* and especially the issues for 1954, 1959, and 1965. Also, League of Nations, *Statistical Yearbook* for 1939-40, 1940-41, 1941-42, 1942-44.

In addition:—

Denmark: *Befolkningens Bevaegelsen, 1959 and 1965 and Egteskaben Fødte og Døde i Aarens 1926-30.*

England and Wales: *Registrar General's Statistical Review, 1946-50,* Text,—Civil; *1964 & 1965* (Tables, population).

Finland *Annuaire Statistique de Finlande,* for 1952 and 1956.

France: P. Depoid, *op. cit.,* and *Annuaire Statistique de la France* for 1966.

Albania and Northern Ireland) for 1961 and reaches an expectation of life at birth for Europe as a whole (not including the U.S.S.R.) of around 72.2 years for females. And for the U.S.S.R., too, the expectation of life at birth for females in 1960-61 was 73 years. When these high expectations of life have become established as the generation pattern, net replacement rates of 1.0 will be achieved with only around 2.1 live births per woman.

Notes

1. P. Depoid, *Reproduction Nette en Europe depuis l'Origine des Statistiques de l'État Civil* (Paris, 1941); J. Vogt, "En undersokelse over generasjonenes frugtbarhet i Norge," *Statsøkonomisk Tidsskrift* (September 1956); T. Hjortkjaer and E. Kjeldgaard, "Frugtbarheden i Danmark," *Nationaløkonomisk Tidsskrift*, 1-2 (1956); E. v. Hofsten, "Fertility for Birth Cohorts of Swedish Women, 1870-71—," *Statistisk Tidsskrift*, 1966, No. 4. See also N. H. Carrier, "An examination of generation fertility in England and Wales," *Population Studies* (July 1955); and Denmark, Statistisk Tabelværk, 1962:1, *Ægteskaber, Fødte og Døde 1941-1955* (Copenhagen 1962).

2. I am greatly indebted to Professor N. Keyfitz, who let me have a copy of the full computer print-out of all these tables.

3. P. Delaporte, *Evolution de la Mortalité en Europe depuis l'Origine des Statistiques de l'Etat Civil* (Paris, 1941), p. 62.

4. J. Légaré, "Quelques considérations sur les tables de mortalité de génération," *Population* (September-October 1966), esp. pp. 935-38.

Norway: J. Backer, *op. cit.* and the relevant issues of *Folkmengdens Bevegelse* (for fertility rates for 45-49 years age group).

Sweden: *Folkmängdens Förändringar 1965.*

U.S.S.R. (A) D. P. Mazur, "Reconstruction of fertility trends for the female population of the U.S.S.R.," *Population Studies* (July 1967).

U.S.S.R. (B) Official data—rates published in *Vestnik Statistiky*, No. 8, 1967, p. 88, Table 2.

Appendix II

Additional Factors in Fertility Trends

In the text of the paper, the analysis has been concerned primarily with marital fertility and the discussion of differentials has been limited to regional, urban-rural, religious, and socioeconomic levels. In some countries, however, extra-marital fertility is an important component of total fertility, while in other countries immigrants have contributed significantly to total fertility (in some cases both to extra-marital and to marital fertility). It is not possible to consider these additional factors in detail here—not only because they would require quite substantial studies, but also because the information available varies very greatly from country to country. Few countries have undertaken serious inquiries into the social demography of extra-marital fertility; the subject often gives rise to more heat than light. And data on the fertility of immigrant groups are scanty. However, a note has been prepared bringing together illustrative material on this subject. Copies may be obtained by writing to the Population Studies Center, University of Michigan, 1225 S. University Avenue, Ann Arbor, Michigan 48105.

Appendix III

Urban-rural fertility differences in Europe. Fertility rates: children under 5 years of age per 1000 women 15 to 49 years of age (from census data)

Country	Year	Total	Urban	Rural	Ratio Rural : Urban
Albania	1955	725	692	738	1.07
Bulgaria	1956	346	312	366	1.17
Czechoslovakia	1961	359	315	403	1.28
Denmark	1960	338	310	436	1.41
Finland	1960	382	348	435	1.25
France	1962	329	307	375	1.22
Greece	1961	362	287	442	1.54[1]
Hungary	1960	332	263	382	1.45
Ireland	1961	503	474	535	1.13
Netherlands	1960	432	382	517	1.35[3]
Norway	1960	378	327	438	1.34[2]
Poland	1960	477	406	553	1.36
Portugal	1960	398	274	441	1.61
Romania	1956	392	303	437	1.44
Sweden	1960	286	279	310	1.11
Switzerland	1960	332	274	404	1.47
U.K.: England & Wales	1961	336	329	361	1.10
Scotland	1961	385	380	398	1.05
N. Ireland	1961	443	412	484	1.17
Yugoslavia	1961	415	323	456	1.41

[1]There is also a semi-urban category, with a rate of 374 per 1000.
[2]There is also a semi-urban category, with a rate of 466 per 1000.
[3]There is also a semi-urban category, with a rate of 423 per 1000.

Source: United Nations, *Demographic Yearbook 1965,* Table 8, pp. 238-39.

References and Acknowledgments

For those readers who wish to look more closely at developments in fertility in Europe since World War II, it may be useful to have some notes on studies additional to those cited in the text of the paper.

To begin with, where official publications contain commentaries and special analyses beyond the normal basic annual vital statistics, they are often of the greatest value. The commentaries published by the Registrar General of England and Wales are a very good example, and the discussions of changes in marital fertility in those volumes are among the best available. The text volumes which appear from time to time in conjunction with the vital statistics of Switzerland are also very helpful, and it is to be regretted that there is no text dealing with recent years. For West Germany there are often useful contributions in *Wirtschaft und Statistik* as well as in the series *Bevölkerung und Kultur:* and for Austria in *Statistische Nachrichten.* Equally valuable are the historical compilations, the outstanding example being the three volumes on Norway by Dr. Julie Backer, published by the Norwegian Statistical Office—the volume most relevant here being *Marriages, Births and Migrations in Norway, 1856-1960,* Oslo, 1965 (Samfunnsøkonomiske Studier No. 13). In Eastern Europe, the official demographic journals provide comparable textual commentaries in the form of articles on specific topics (especially *Demografie* for Czechoslovakia and *Demográfia* for Hungary, both containing some summaries in English). *Études et Conjoncture,* the publication of the Institut National de la Statistique et des Études Économiques, provides analyses of developments in France. For the Netherlands, a brief study of fertility trends in the period 1960-65 will be found in the official Bulletin of Population and Health Statistics, xv, 5 (May 1967).

As for individual contributions, apart from those referred to in the text, I have found the following very helpful. *Belgium:* J. Morsa, "Tendances récentes de la fécondité belge," *Population et Famille* (1963), No. 1; G. Wunsch, "Les méthodes d'analyse de la nuptialité: leur application au cas de la Belgique," *Recherches Économiques de Louvain* (1965), No. 2; G. Wunsch, *Les Mesures de la Natalité:*

Quelques Applications à la Belgique (Louvain 1967). *Denmark:* P. C. Matthiessen, *Fertilitetsforskelle i Danmark* (Copenhagen, 1965). *France:* The journal of I.N.E.D., *Population,* is an indispensable reference. The following articles represent only a very small sample of the relevant contents: "Rapport de l'Institut national d'études démographiques . . . sur la régulation des naissances en France" (July-August, 1966); A. Girard and E. Zucker, "Une enquête auprès du public sur la structure familiale et la prévention des naissances" (May-June, 1967); R. Pressat, "Les aléas de la natalité française" (July-August, 1967); G. Calot and S. Hémery, "L'évolution de la situation démographique française au cours des années récentes," (July-August, 1967).

Hungary: Dr. E. Szabady and his colleagues have contributed valuable studies not only of developments in Hungary but also in the Socialist countries of Eastern Europe in general. See, e.g., E. Szabady, *Basic Fertility Tables for some East-European Socialist Countries,* Budapest, 1967; and G. Acsádi and A. Klinger, "Result of Inquiries Concerning Family Planning and Birth Control," reprinted from *Statisztikai Szemle* (Hungarian Statistical Review), March, 1963, with a long summary in English.

Italy: A particularly useful survey is given by M. Livi-Bacci, "Modernization and Tradition in the Recent History of Italian Fertility," (forthcoming in *Demography.*) See also: L. di Comite, "Sull'evoluzione regionalle della fecondità in Italia," *Atti Della XXIII Riunione Scientifica* (Società Italiana di Statistica), Rome, 29/30 Oct. 1963; D. Moriconi, "La fecondità matrimoniale italiana nel decennio 1951-1961," *Statistica,* xxiv, No. 3, 1964; M. de Vergottini, "Natalità e fecondità," *Annali di Statistica,* Series viii, 17, Rome, 1965.

Norway: G. Jahn, *Barnetallet i Norske Ekteskap* (1950 Census of Norway, Vol. v), Oslo, 1957.

Sweden: J. R. L. Schneider, *Fertility Changes during and after the Second World War in England and Wales and Sweden,* Ph.D. thesis, University of London, 1963; E. v. Hofsten, "Fertility for Birth Cohorts of Swedish Women 1870-71," *Statistisk Tidskrift* No. 4, 1966; C.-E. Quensel, "Fruktsamheten 1951-1955 samt medelbarntalet 31/12 i skilda kohorter," *Statistisk Tidskrift,* July, 1958.

Switzerland: W. Bickel, "Zur neueren Entwicklung der ehelichen Fruchtbarkeit und Fruchtbarkeitsunterschiede in der Schweiz," *Schweizer. Ztschr. f. Volkswirtschaft und Statistik,* No. 4, 1958; and in the same journal, No. 2, 1961, A. Miller, "Die Fruchtbarkeit der schweizerischen Bevölkerung von 1932 bis 1956."

Many colleagues have been generous with information and with comments on the content and coverage of demographic statistics in their countries. I am especially indebted to Dr. Z. Aničič; Professor W. Bickel; Dr. T. Van den Brink; Monsieur G. Calot; Monsieur A. Gross; Dr. Helczmanovski; Dr. E. v. Hofsten; Professor N. Keyfitz; Professor M. Livi-Bacci; Professor J. Morsa; Dr. K. Schwarz; Dr. E. Szabady; and Dr. M. Žďárský. And I am equally indebted to Dr. S. Thapar for her help in preparing several of the tables, a task which absorbed a great deal of her time.

NATALITY IN THE DEVELOPING COUNTRIES: RECENT TRENDS AND PROSPECTS

Dudley Kirk

Food Research Institute, Stanford University

WELL OVER TWO-THIRDS of the human race live in the "developing" or less industrialized countries.[1] These contain the larger part of the world's people today, and this share is growing. United Nations projections suggest that some 85 percent of the world's population growth to the end of the century will be occurring in these areas. The biological future of the human race is largely dependent on what happens here.

The major population trends in the underdeveloped areas, and their first order causes, are well-known. Mortality is declining in all of the non-industrial countries for which data are available. Aside from temporary reversals (e.g., due to war, civil disorder, or catastrophe) it is doubtful if there is any country in the underdeveloped world where mortality is rising or even constant.

Furthermore, mortality is generally declining *more rapidly* than it did historically in the industrial countries. There is every prospect that, barring a major world catastrophe, mortality will continue to decline rapidly in the non-industrial countries.

In the non-industrial countries, as in the West, declines in mortality have preceded declines in natality, which have thus far occurred in relatively few of these countries. The result has been a widening gap of births over deaths, rapidly expanding population growth, and what has been popularized as the world's "population explosion."

In the industrial nations birth rates, as well as death rates, are much reduced. The number of children is largely determined by the wishes of the parents; effective birth control is practiced by a very large percentage of the total populations. Population growth is now modest, generally 1 percent or less per annum.

75

The "world population problem" is essentially whether or not the non-industrial countries will follow Europe and North America in reducing birth rates and rates of population growth.

Present Levels of Natality

Measurement of existing levels of natality, much less of trends, is hazardous and approximate for most of the less developed countries. Quite understandably, the accuracy of population data is highly correlated with general development. According to a United Nations compilation[2] 99 percent of the population in the developed areas are covered by satisfactory registration data on births. Only 10 percent of the population in the less developed areas are so covered.

In the absence of reliable vital statistics, birth rates and reproduction rates are commonly estimated indirectly from census reports of the age structure or from information obtained in sample surveys. This has been done for some 54 percent of the population living in less developed countries. These estimates do not permit year-by-year comparisons, especially for most recent periods. Furthermore, the vagaries of census reporting often make it unsafe to posit trends in natality from inter-censal comparisons. The methods are usually too crude to detect trends with any assurance. Finally, in some 28 countries, containing 36 percent of the population, the United Nations compilation found "no satisfactory data."

The Population Division of the United Nations nevertheless did undertake the monumental task of estimating birth rates and reproduction rates for most countries for 1960 or the most recent earlier date for which data were available. A summary for major regions is given in Table 1, including data for some countries of special interest.[3]

Several generalizations may be made from this table and from the data for some 116 countries presented in the source given.

1. *Natality is almost universally high* in the less developed countries, commonly twice as high as in the developed countries.

2. There is a sharp *dichotomy* between the natality of the developed and the less developed countries. No unequivocally "less developed" country of major consequence yet has a birth rate under 30.[4] No developed country has a birth rate of over 25, and few have a birth rate over 20.[5] Natality is itself perhaps the best single socioeconomic variable distinguishing developed and less developed countries. This holds with more refined measures such as the gross reproduction rate or total fertility rate. In the less developed countries the gross reproduction rates cluster around 3. No developed country has a rate above 2 and very few less developed countries fall below this figure.

Table 1. Estimated crude birth rates and gross reproduction rates for regions and selected countries of the world, about 1960

Region	Crude birth rate[1]	Gross reproduction rate[2]
World Total	35-36[3]	2.25-2.31[3]
Developing Regions	41-42[3]	2.6 -2.7[3]
Africa	48	3.0
North Africa	46	2.9
United Arab Republic	(45)	(2.8)
West Africa	54	3.4
Nigeria	(53-57)	(3.6-3.8)
South and East Africa	45	2.7
Kenya	(50)	(2.9-3.4)
South Africa (Bantus)	(46)	(3.0)
Asia (excluding USSR)	40-41[3]	2.5-2.6[3]
Southwest Asia	45	3.0
Turkey	(43)	(2.9)
South central Asia	44	2.9
India	(39)	(2.5)
Pakistan	(48)	(3.3)
Southeast Asia	49	2.9
Malaya	(41)	(2.9)
Philippines	(50)	(3.5)
Thailand	(46)	(3.2)
East Asia	35-37[3]	2.1-2.3[3]
China (mainland)	(37-40)	
Japan	(17)	(1.0)
Taiwan	(38)	(2.7)
Middle and South America	41	2.8
Middle America	45	3.0
Mexico	(46)	(3.1)
South America	40	2.7
Argentina	(22)	(1.4)
Brazil	(43)	(3.0)
Chile	(36)	(2.2)
Colombia	(44)	(2.9)
More Developed Regions	22	1.4
Northern America	24	1.8
Europe	19	1.3
Oceania	24	1.8
USSR	25	1.4

[1] Annual births per 1000 population.

[2] This is a more refined measure taking into account the age-specific birth rates to females in the reproductive age. Technically it is defined as the number of daughters that would be born to a hypothetical female cohort if she were subject to current age-specific fertility rates and zero mortality before the end of the reproductive age.

[3] Range of estimated values corresponding to alternative estimates for China (mainland).

3. As of 1960 the significant differentials between major regions of the less developed world related as much to *pre-modern cultural differences and affinities* as to rating on a scale of modern socioeconomic development.[6]

(a) Natality in tropical Latin America[7] is quite homogeneous, high but not the highest. Registered or estimated birth rates for all mainland countries fall in the range of 40-50. It is the region of most rapid population growth, thanks as much to its lower death rate as to its high natality.

(b) Natality in tropical Africa is mixed. Reports indicate very high fertility in some countries, close to the highest if not the highest in the world; in other areas natality is quite low, a factor which has given rise to some research, and much more conjecture, on causes of low birth rates among some tribal groups. There is no indication that these differences have any close relation to present levels of modern development.

(c) Natality in Moslem countries is universally high and generally higher than that of non-Moslem neighbors.

(d) India has rather lower fertility than most less developed countries.

(e) The Far East is today, and apparently was historically, a region of lower natality than the greater part of the presently underdeveloped world. There are analogies to western Europe, notably in Japan, where the birth rate seems to have been well below 40 before she entered the modern era. Estimates for mainland China are shaky; all one can say is that existing evidence suggests that it has and has had low or moderate fertility for a less developed country.

Trends Past and Present

Earlier estimates and data on birth rates in the presently less developed countries suggest, if anything, *lower* natality in the past than in 1960. There have been fluctuations related to war (effects of mobilization and demobilization), to economic cycles (in a small way mirroring those in the West), and to major catastrophes (famines, epidemics, etc.). But even more, there is a strong suggestion that "normal" natality may actually have risen in many countries. It is not clear whether this is a matter of (1) real trends, (2) better measures and estimates, or (3) changes in the climate of opinion of observers as to what level of natality may be regarded as "reasonable." In my judgment, all three are involved, and they are, of course, not unrelated.

In some cases, notably among West Indian populations, there are clear cases where the birth rates rose prior to 1960 (e.g. Jamaica,

Trinidad, and British Guiana). These are in areas where birth registration has been satisfactory for many years and therefore the rise cannot be attributed merely to more complete registration. Two possible explanations are reduction in venereal disease and some trend to regularization of mating and marriage.

Other cases are hard to document because of faulty data, but there has been a tendency to raise estimates of birth rates in the light of survey data (e.g., in Africa, in the Middle East, in Pakistan) over earlier figures.

In addition to factors mentioned above, a number of other changes accompanying modernization *could* tend to increase natality: reduction of mortality and morbidity, especially the reduction of widowhood[8]; increased vitality as a result of gains in nutrition and modest gains in level of living; reduction in prenatal mortality and stillbirths; changes in cultural practices that may accompany modernization such as shorter periods of breast-feeding following childbirth (i.e., a woman's chances of conceiving are diminished during lactation); less observance of ritual inhibitions on intercourse following childbirth and on certain ceremonial days; reduction of husband-wife separation as result of less observance of the traditional practice (e.g., in India) of a wife returning to her parental home for several months before and after childbirth; and possibly reduction in polygyny.[9]

There are, of course, other factors accompanying modernization which tend to *reduce* natality quite aside from the adoption of birth control. These include rising age at marriage; reductions in infant mortality (which lengthen average period of lactation); separation of married couples for seasonal work, for migration, etc.

In balance, the initial stages of modernization may well tend to *increase* rather than reduce natality. While the data are not so good as to give decisive evidence, it seems very likely that natality has risen over the past generation—certainly in the West Indies, very likely in tropical America, and probably in a number of countries of Africa and Asia.

On the other hand, as recently as 1960 very few of the less developed countries seemed firmly on the path to fertility declines. In only a handful—Taiwan, Singapore, Puerto Rico—had the trend been securely established.

Since 1960 the small list has grown. There are important harbingers of change.

The clearest of these are in East Asia, in the former Japanese territories and among the Chinese populations of Hong Kong, Singapore, and Malaysia (see Table 2).

Table 2. Birth rates in selected Asian countries, 1955-66

	Ryukyus	Taiwan	Hong Kong	Singapore	Malaya	Ceylon
1955	31.1	45.3	36.3	44.3	44.0	37.3
1956	31.1	44.8	37.0	44.4	46.7	36.4
1957	27.8	41.4	35.8	43.4	46.1	36.5
1958	28.7	41.7	37.4	42.0	43.3	35.8
1959	27.4	41.2	35.2	40.3	42.2	37.0
1960	25.0	39.5	36.0	38.7	40.9	36.6
1961	25.2	38.3	34.3	36.5	41.9	35.8
1962	23.4	37.4	33.3	35.1	40.4	35.5
1963	23.8	36.3	32.8	34.7	39.4	34.5
1964	22.2	34.5	30.1	33.2	39.1	33.1
1965	21.7	32.7	27.7	31.1	36.7	32.7
1966	18.5	32.5[1]	24.9	29.9	. . .	. . .

[1]Figure for 1966 is not comparable owing to more (i.e. earlier) registration of births in the latter part of the year in connection with the national census. This is reflected in very low birth rates reported for the first months of 1967.

Source: United Nations, *Demographic Yearbook, 1965 and 1966,* New York, 1966 and 1967; and United Nations, *Population and Vital Statistics Report,* 1 July 1967' Statistical Papers, Series A, Vol. XIX, No. 3. Korea is omitted because of lack of reliable vital statistics.

These reductions have been in the Western pattern with characteristic differential fertility, i.e., rural-urban, occupational, educational, etc. In Hong Kong and Singapore particularly, the *level* of the rates has been affected by anomalies in the age-sex structure arising from migration, but there is little question that there has been a real drop in fertility.[10]

Among these populations, at least, modernization is being accompanied by a rapid decline in the birth rate. The first two were decisively influenced by Japan. A crucial question is the extent to which the peripheral Chinese may represent what is happening or may happen in mainland China. Probably no one knows for sure, including the Chinese themselves.

Do the Chinese in Southeast Asia represent a beachhead for the spread of birth control in that region? In Singapore and Malaysia there has been some fertility decline in other major immigrant groups but probably not yet among indigenous Malays. Asian migrants have also shown declines in fertility in several other areas, including Hawaii, Mauritius, and Trinidad.

As yet there are no clear evidences of declining fertility in other parts of Southeast or South Asia, except in Ceylon. Ceylon is an interesting case, a sort of Ireland of Asia, in which late marriage has reduced natality. While conventional fertility differentials exist within the country and the national birth rate is low for Asia, the downward trend has been slower and less consistent than in East Asian countries.

There are no clear signs of lower birth rates in the Middle East and Africa aside from Israel, a highly developed country; Cyprus, which is more European than Asian; and the white populations of South and Central Africa.

In Latin America, the two most advanced countries, Argentina and Uruguay, have low birth rates and in Chile the birth rate is now falling fast. Despite rapid urbanization, other mainland Latin American countries have not achieved the social and economic conditions that have historically brought about smaller families. Several countries, such as Mexico and Costa Rica, are approaching this threshold and in the latter the reported birth rate has dropped rapidly in the last few years. But as yet there is no general downward trend of birth rates in tropical Latin America.

There does appear to be such a trend in several of the West Indies. Between 1960 and 1966 the reported birth rate in Puerto Rico fell steadily from 32.3 in 1960 to 28.3 in 1966; in Trinidad from 39.1 to 29.4; in Barbados from 33.6 to 25.2; and in Jamaica from 42.0 to 38.8. While the data are poor, the birth rate in Cuba is apparently low for a Latin American country, the United Nations estimate being 34-36 for the period 1960-66. Declines have been reported in a number of other islands, including St. Kitts-Nevis, St. Vincent, Dominica, Grenada, Bermuda, Guadeloupe, Martinique, and the Netherlands Antilles. Many of these are small territories in which out-migration, in particular of young adults, could produce a decline in natality. Such data must be interpreted with caution pending further analysis.

A striking feature of very recent reductions in natality since 1960 is that many of the areas concerned are *islands*, which are perhaps more readily susceptible to outside influence.

Fertility reduction has also appeared at points of *intersection of major cultures*, which often do not much affect national totals. Cases in point are Asians in Hawaii and the continental United States, Mexicans in the United States and Moslems in Eastern Europe, all of whom are now experiencing reductions in natality.

The last is perhaps the most significant in view of the impressive resistance of Moslem peasant culture to European influence in this as in other areas of behavior. Albania and neighboring Moslem areas in Yugoslavia are the last high fertility areas left in Europe. Now a reduction of the birth rate has appeared in Albania (from 43.4

in 1960 to 34.0 in 1966). Moslem birth rates in the Soviet Union have been about twice those of Slavs in recent years, but birth rates in the Soviet Central Asian republics (in majority of Moslem tradition) are now declining. It should be noted that these republics are now quite developed by some economic standards and have significant components of European Russians. It is not clear how much of the decline results from Slavic immigration and how much from fertility decline among the indigenous peoples. Otherwise in the Moslem world there is no clear sign of diminished fertility.

The Situation Today: The Broad View
Earlier experience had shown that the demographic transition could transcend (1) Communist ideology, as in the experience of Eastern Europe and the USSR; (2) cultural and ethnic barriers between Europe and the Orient, as in Japan and neighboring areas; and (3) religious interdiction, as in Catholic countries of Europe and temperate South America.

Recent experience has further confirmed (1) that major immigrant groups from the developing countries, living in areas of greater socioeconomic development, will reduce their birth rates, as have Asians in Hawaii, Chinese and Indians in Southeast Asia, and Mexicans in the United States; and (2) that life in the tropics is not an insuperable barrier to reductions in natality (as has been demonstrated in Singapore, Puerto Rico, and Trinidad).

But major barriers remain—cultural and socioeconomic—which are still strong today.

The latter phases of the demographic transition (i.e. definitive declines in birth rates to low or moderate fertility) have now reached almost all people of European ethnic background,[11] and are now washing against the walls separating European culture from the other major world cultures. A line from the Strait of Gibraltar across the Mediterranean and Black Seas and on through Central Asia to China divides Moslems and Europeans, on the one side with birth rates usually of 20 per thousand or less, on the other with birth rates of 40 or over. The division is sharp—Moslems vs. Europeans of Judeo-Christian tradition.[12] Elsewhere the Rio Grande and the Caribbean separate the United States, with a 1966 birth rate of 18, and Mexico (43 in 1966) and other Central and South American countries with current birth rates of 40 and more. The contrast between Argentina and Uruguay (largely European populations) and tropical America (mixed populations) is almost as great. Even in Asia the transition in fertility has been primarily among orientals (i.e., Japanese, Chinese, Koreans) and has not widely spread to the indigenous peoples of Southeast and South Asia. Important as the developments have been since 1960 there has not yet been a major breakthrough in the other major culture areas of the underdeveloped world (tropical America, tropical Africa, the Moslem world, India, and Southeast Asia). As noted above, there are beginnings, but only beginnings, of penetration of these cultural barriers. The barriers are not insurmountable, especially with the greater contacts derived from improved communication and transport. Some seem much more permeable than others. But they still exist.

Furthermore, it has not yet been demonstrated that major fertility reduction can be achieved in advance of, or without, parallel major economic and social advance. It is significant that the countries in which there has been a recent reduction are countries that are experiencing an economic take-off and otherwise relatively good socioeconomic conditions: Taiwan, South Korea, Malaysia, Singapore, and Puerto Rico are all cases in point. The tough, hard-core masses of the less developed world are not yet in this category. This is the great challenge to national population policies and programs: Can fertility reduction be initiated and accelerated ahead of its "normal" pace within the general framework of socioeconomic development?

Against these formidable traditional barriers to reduction of births there are now arrayed a series of very favorable developments which augur well for the future. In what follows I will discuss future prospects in terms of (1) the favorable setting, (2) the impact of national family planning programs, (3) projections made by the United Nations.

Future Prospects: The Favorable Setting

A number of factors favor a much more rapid transition than occurred in the West. Since these have been discussed elsewhere I will limit my discussion to what is more a listing than a discussion.[13]

(1) *Changed climate of opinion.* The reduction of natality in the West was accomplished by individual couples in the face of restrictive legislation, religious opposition (Protestant as well as Catholic), and public denunciation of birth control. The private decisions and actions of couples were made within a "conspiracy of silence" which deprived them of the psychological reinforcement that friends and neighbors with common views would normally give. The hitherto restrictive atmosphere in the less developed countries is rapidly giving way to free discussion and permissive attitudes and even outright social and government pressure to adopt birth control.

(2) *Religious doctrine,* except in Latin America, is not a serious obstacle. Buddhist, Hindu, and Moslem religions do not proscribe

most methods of birth control.[14] The rapid shift in the position of many Catholics and perhaps even of the Church itself may soon be reflected in less opposition to family planning in Latin America.

(3) *The rapid decline of infant mortality* in the developing countries has had a major impact on family size and on pressure to restrict family size. In most less developed countries the number of *living* children per family is higher than before. A survey of 35 less developed countries[15] for which inter-censal comparisons may be readily made indicates that the ratios of children at ages 0-4 to women at ages 15-44, compared in the last two censuses, have risen in 30.[16]

Whether this is due in part to a rise in the birth rate (as it may be in some cases) or to lower infant mortality, the effect is the same— to increase the number of living children physically present in the household. The pressure to control family size is increased as fears abate that the parents may be left without children, especially sons.

(4) *Modernization*, with its motivations and opportunities for family planning, is spreading. In addition to reductions in infant mortality most countries are making progress in many, sometimes all, of the usual indicators of economic and social development.

(5) *Fertility differentials* on the Western pattern suggest the beginnings of diffusion of the small family patterns. Studies almost universally show lower fertility among the better educated and modernized segments of the populations concerned, although these are often still only a small minority. The rapid increase in populations living in the modern sector predisposes them to a decline in fertility.

(6) Numerous studies evidence a *widespread grass roots concern and felt need* for family planning in the developing countries. Field surveys on knowledge, attitudes, and practices relating to family planning have been conducted in at least 28 such countries.[17] These universally show a stated desire by a majority or substantial minority to limit family size. Such verbalization is, of course, not the equivalent of action; often few have detailed information about birth control and only small proportions were actually practicing it. But the studies show approval of and interest in family planning. A potential "market" for birth control services is there.

(7) *Improvements in contraceptive technology* now provide a wider choice of methods, including some which seem more appropriate to the needs of the developing countries than those available even a few years ago. The two major developments, the oral contraceptives and the intrauterine devices, are gaining considerable acceptance, the first in the developed areas and in Latin America, the second as

promoted in family planning programs in the developing countries. Both have the great advantage that their use is independent of sexual intercourse. Better methods are on the way.[18]

In Western and Japanese experience the decline in the birth rate was brought about by a combination of (a) later age at marriage (in some cases); (b) male methods of contraception, especially coitus interruptus and the condom; and (c) the female method of abortion. These are still the prevailing methods of birth control in the world at large. The "conventional" chemical and mechanical methods formerly advanced by the planned parenthood movements have had some importance in the United States but not a great deal elsewhere. Whether introduced by governments or through private marketing channels, the new and forthcoming "easier" methods should accelerate the use of birth control.

The cumulative impact of these developments will surely be great, quite aside from government programs in family planning. They should give momentum to the already marked acceleration in the rapidity with which countries move through the demographic transition on the natality side. In other words, countries entering this phase are experiencing a much more rapid decline in the birth rate than their predecessors.

To test this generalization, a compilation was made measuring the length of time required for the country to drop from a birth rate of 35 to a birth rate of 20. Since 1875 some twenty-seven countries with usable data have passed or are passing through this transition.[19] The results are shown in Table 3.

While these data are rough there seems little question but that the speed of transition, once firmly begun, has accelerated over time. On the basis of past experience the average country beginning this phase of the transition now might be expected to complete it in some twenty years and very likely less in view of the continuing acceleration in the rates of decline.

Table 3. Years historically and presently required for countries to reduce annual crude birth rates from 35 to 20, 1875 to present

Period in which birth rate reached 35 or below	Number of countries	Number of years required to reach birth rate of 20		
		Mean	Median	Range
1875-1899	9	48	50	40-55
1900-1924	7	39	32	24-64
1925-1949	5	31	28	25-37
1950-	6	23	23	11-32

A parallel generalization is that the higher the birth rate at the time of entering the transition the more rapid the decline. The higher birth rates are, the faster they fall, *once they start to fall.*

Here is the rub—What is the take-off point? Is there evidence that the necessary threshold of socioeconomic development is lowering? The comprehensive United Nations survey of fertility levels as of 1960 points out that relatively few countries were then in the threshold zone, i.e., the level of development at which birth rates have empirically begun to decline.[20] After elimination of extreme observations for particular indices, less than 5 percent of the countries were in the threshold zone for four of the twelve items (life expectancy, hospital beds, newspaper circulation, radio receivers); 11-16 percent of the countries were in the threshold zone for four other indicators (female literacy, later marriage, income per head, and energy consumption); 20-26 percent for three indices (non-agricultural activities, infant mortality, cinema attendance); and 35 percent for one index (urbanization). These are, of course, individual items, and very few countries were in the threshold zone on over half the items.

Among these 12 indicators, gross reproduction rates were found to be most highly correlated with newspaper circulation. Information, health, and education items were found to be more closely correlated with fertility than were economic, industrial, and urban development. This, again, is encouraging in that these items have proved more tractable to improvement than changes in the economic system and achievement of higher per capita income.

Since the United Nations study was made, more countries are moving into this threshold zone and on the basis of past experience[21] may be expected to reach the take-off point in reduction of the birth rate. The socioeconomic context is becoming more favorable to fertility declines.

Future Prospects: The Impact of National Family Planning Programs
Some 18 countries in the developing regions now have an official family planning policy and/or a family planning program. Most of them were initiated in the last three years in a spectacular growth of government concern and interest in problems of population growth. Several programs have achieved most impressive success in recruiting "acceptors," especially of the intrauterine devices.[22] Here we are concerned with their present and potential impact on the birth rate.

In most countries it would be unfair at this stage to judge national programs by their immediate effects on the birth rate. Most national policies and programs are very new. Furthermore, there is an all-too-easy tendency to take the word for the deed. A *pronounce-*

ment favoring family planning by a high public official is not necessarily a government policy. An announced *policy* is not in itself a program; nor does the existence of a *program* guarantee *performance* or achievement. These things take time. India has had a population policy for 15 years but is still far short of providing services accessible to the majority of the population.

Caution is also called for in interpreting the effects of program success in reaching what seem like (and are indeed) very large numbers. All methods of contraception except sterilization have high rates of attrition in actual use. So there is always a substantial shrinkage from numbers of initial acceptors. Furthermore, what seem like large numbers of users may be small in relation to the country's population size. This is the case in India and Pakistan.

The major successes so far have been in countries already moving toward the small family pattern (e.g., Taiwan, Korea, Singapore). In such countries one must think in terms of *accelerated* decline of the birth rate. This apparently occurred in Taiwan and probably in Korea. In Taiwan the birth rate declined from 50.0 in 1951 to 36.3 in 1963. The average annual decline from 1951-63 was 2.6 percent and from 1959-63, 3.1 percent. The island-wide program was adopted in 1964, based on the IUD. In that year and in 1965 the declines in registered births were 5.0 percent and 5.2 percent, strongly suggesting an acceleration due to the program.[23]

However, the higher rate of decline in 1964 is curious in view of the nature of the program. IUD insertions after April could scarcely have affected births in 1964. Insertions prior to April 1 (about 2500) were far too few to have had such an effect. The reduction, if assignable to the program at all, must have come about through other means. Either the additional reduction was fortuitous, i.e., due to causes unrelated to the program, or the program must have stimulated greater use of methods that would terminate pregnancies in less than nine months, specifically abortion. This unanticipated consequence of the program may well have occurred, that is, the campaign for the IUD increased the salience of the problem and the greater use of a method already known and widely practiced.[24]

Evidence is gathering that in Taiwan, as in Japan, abortion has played a major role in the reduction of the birth rate. The interrelation of abortion and the IUD is shown by the data from a major follow-up study of IUD acceptors after 24 months.[25] Fifty-nine percent of the respondents stated that they then still had the IUD in place. The fertility of all IUD acceptors was reduced 56-80 percent from pre-insertion fertility, depending on assumptions made. However, the reduction in *pregnancies* was very much less. Over half of the pregnancies occurring among IUD acceptors were terminated by induced abortion, 51 percent or 62 percent, depending on whether current pregnancies are included.[26] If we take the lower of these two figures and if there had been no abortions among IUD acceptors, their fertility would have been reduced in the range of 10-60 percent of pre-insertion fertility, again depending on the assumptions made in the measurement of pre- and post-program fertility.[27]

This range is unrealistic and illustrates the great difficulties of measurement. But it is hard to escape the conclusion that abortion was an important silent partner, accounting for a substantial part of the fertility decline among IUD acceptors and in the general population.

Data for South Korea are much less complete than for Taiwan, but the evidence suggests somewhat parallel experience. Up to 1960 there was little indication of a secular decline in natality, but it must be remembered that the country was the scene of war, internal disorder, and economic disruption well into the 1950's. After 1960 there is clear evidence of a reduction in fertility. The census of 1966 shows a substantial drop in proportion of small children in the population as compared with 1960, indicating a lower birth rate in the period 1960-66. Owing to the mixture of oriental and Western methods of reporting age, it is very difficult to reconstruct annual birth rates from the census and registration data on young children. Furthermore official vital statistics are too incomplete and unreliable for this purpose. Indirect evidence on year-to-year changes is given by annual year-end registrations, which include data on age and sex. These show reductions in ratios of children to women in both urban and rural areas of every province during the period 1962-65, with some acceleration in 1964-65. Declines were twice as great in urban as opposed to rural areas.[28]

Did the national program generate the take-off in the reduction of the birth rate which occurred after 1960? If so, what were the mechanisms?

The initial drop in fertility could hardly be attributed to the direct effect of the national program. Though a population policy was stated in December 1961 and a preliminary education campaign was started in 1962 the national network of services was not established until 1963, when it recruited a monthly average of about 130,000 users of conventional contraceptives (i.e., received supplies). The IUD program did not get into high gear until June 1964, and in that year there were 112,000 IUD insertions. Government provision of services could not have reduced the birth rate much before 1964 and the intensified effort beginning in June 1964 could not have had much effect before late 1965. Nevertheless there appears to have been a substantial decrease in the birth rate before that time.

Again, an important mechanism was probably abortion, though, as in Taiwan, induced abortion was illegal and outside the national family planning program. The incidence of induced abortion was apparently rising rapidly. In his study of married women in Sung-Dong Gu, a district of Seoul, Hong found that the ratio of induced abortions to births was as follows: 1961, 21.1 percent; 1962, 37.6 percent; and 1963, 49.0 percent.[29] Comparable figures for a rural sample were: 1961, 2.0; 1962, 1.1; 1963, 3.5; 1964, 8.0; 1965, 9.6 (up to time of interview).[30]

As to be expected, abortions were much more common among urban women of Seoul, and the lower fertility of the city and of other urban areas is certainly in part explained by this factor. It is interesting to note that the reported ratio of abortions rose sharply in the rural study area coincidentally with the intensification of the national family planning program. Ninety percent of the abortions in the rural area were performed by physicians, and their inaccessibility must have been a major handicap for rural people in procuring abortions. Abortion is correlated with education of women, occupation of husband, economic status, and accessibility of physicians in the classic pattern of the demographic transition.

If Hong's data may be generalized, abortions alone could have accounted for a reduction of about 15 percent in the birth rate in Seoul in the two-year period 1961-63 and for a decrease of 6-7 percent from 1961-62 to 1964-65 in the rural areas.

We do not yet have a basis for fully evaluating the impact of the stepped-up program of IUD insertions after 1964. These rose spectacularly to 233,000 in 1965 and 342,000 in 1966.[31] The impact on the birth rate should be cumulative and substantial. One estimate is that some 547,000 IUD's were in place at the end of 1966 and that, depending on assumptions regarding losses, etc., these would prevent 110,000-160,000 births in 1967, or the equivalent of a reduction of 3.7 to 5.3 per thousand in the birth rate. This is an estimate of the *cumulative* effect of the IUD program on the birth rate in 1967 as compared with 1964, when the program began. This is not the additive effect of this program over the situation without the IUD, since on the basis of earlier experience a considerable drop in fertility could have been expected anyway. The IUD was to some degree substituting for other effective methods.[32] As the authors of the above estimate state, "We cannot, therefore, say that the use of IUDs has reduced birth rates *more than would have been the situation without IUDs* [italics theirs]."[33] This is a cautious statement. It is almost certain that the program has had an important *additive* as well as a *substitutionary* effect. But this additive or net effect is less than the *potential* total effect implied in the above estimates of births prevented by the IUD.

Attempts to measure the specific effect of a program are inevitably confounded by the question of what would have happened in the absence of a program (a) among the clients of the program and (b) among the general population. Births *prevented* is not the measure of the effect of a program on the birth rate, which is rather *net reduction* of births after allowing for the substitutionary factor and for secular trends in the absence of a program. In other words, there can be no precise measurement of the effects of a program on the birth rate—only general magnitudes.

Perhaps the question is irrelevant—the important thing is the total effect, not the cause. General socioeconomic progress and specific population programs will reinforce each other in many ways and they should be designed to do so.

The above discussion may suggest pessimism as to the prospective effects of population programs on the birth rate. That is not intended. The experience of Taiwan, for example, suggests that a well-designed program may accelerate the drop in the birth rate as much as 2 percent annually, i.e., increase the annual reduction from 3 percent to 5 percent; if continued this will greatly speed the transition from high to low fertility. In Korea the highly successful national programs doubtless accelerated the take-off in fertility reduction. As programs gain strength and momentum similar results may be expected elsewhere.

The above analysis does suggest, however, that family planning programs may have quite different results and by different means from those anticipated. Their success rests ultimately on motivation and the social change in which it is nurtured. In the continuing tradition of the family planning movement too much has sometimes been expected of technological innovation as over against earlier and often quite effective methods. In Taiwan and Korea a major part of initial program effect was indirect, i.e., the program increased the saliency of the problems and possible solutions, and the actual means of birth control were often other than those recommended.

Future Prospects: United Nations Projections of Birth Rates
In connection with its population projections to the year 2000 the United Nations made estimates of future trends taking into account some of the factors discussed above. These estimates are summarized for major regions of the underdeveloped world in Table 4. The projections have been done with great care, but in view of the hazards of

Table 4. Crude birth rates implied in "medium" estimates of world population by the United Nations

Area	1960-65	1980	1995-2000
World	34	31	26
(a) More Developed	20	19	18
(b) Less Developed	40	35	28
A. East Asia	33	26	20
China (mainland)	34	27	20
Other East Asia*	40	30	23
B. South Asia	43	37	27
Middle South (mainly India and Pakistan)	44	37	25
South East Asia	42	36	30
South West Asia	41	38	30
C. Africa	46	44	40
D. Latin America	40	36	30
Tropical South America	42	38	31
Middle America (mainland)	44	40	33
Caribbean	38	35	28
Temperate South America	26	23	21

*Excluding Japan.

Source: United Nations, *World Population Prospects as Assessed in 1963,* New York, 1966, p. 34. Rates are rounded to nearest whole number and interpolated for 1980 from data given for 1975-80 and 1980-85.

forecasting no one should regard these figures as more than illustrative.

These estimates postulate only modest declines in the birth rate of the less developed world before 1980 and a birth rate in the year 2000 that would still mean a population growth of close to 2 percent per annum. Noteworthy are the low birth rates forecast for mainland China; also the assumption that birth rates will fall more rapidly in India and Pakistan, because of their active population policies, than in other regions such as Southeast Asia and Latin America that might on other grounds (e.g., socioeconomic development) be expected to move faster. In the medium variant the total world population grows from 3.0 billion in 1960 to 4.3 billion in 1980 and 6.1 billion in the year 2000.

This projection has been attacked as much too conservative in the light of very recent developments in the adoption of family planning programs. According to one observer:

... Even conservative evaluation of the prospects for growth suggests that instead of a "population explosion" the world is on the threshold of a "contraception adoption explosion."

. . . From 1965 onward, therefore, the rate of world population growth may be expected to decline with each passing year. The rate of growth will slacken at such a pace that it will be zero or near zero at about the year 2000.[34]

There is as yet no empirical evidence to support the optimistic view that we did indeed reach the turning point in 1965. The United Nations medium variant would put this point about 1980. The implications for future population are enormous. Bogue pictures an increase of world population from 3.3 billion in 1965 to 4.1 billion in 1980 followed by modest increase and stabilization at 4.5 billion in the year 2000.[35]

Bogue's thesis that the spread of contraception will proceed with startling rapidity is tempting in view of the rush of countries to adopt family planning policies. But the magnitude of the task is sobering.

Outside of China there are about 1.6 billion people in the less developed countries among whom are perhaps 280 million couples in the reproductive ages. These will produce some 70 million births this year. In the order of 40 million of these would have to be eliminated to bring the birth rate down to the European level. So far there have been over 3 million acceptors of the IUD, with over 2 million in situ, in my judgment a remarkable achievement in so short a time. Oral contraceptives are also gaining ground; the estimated number of women in the less developed countries using oral tablets has increased from 795,000 in January 1965 to 2,883,000 in July 1967.[36] There are at least as many more users of older methods, such as sterilization, abortion, and the condom. All these numbers will continue to increase, but they have a long way to go to reach a large fraction of the population.

One does not see the growing use of the new contraceptives, even in combination with existing and foreseeable new methods, quickly closing the enormous gap. This will take time and major social change as well as technological innovation. Fortunately, both are occurring rapidly and are working together in the same direction. One can see as a reasonable possibility the achievement of present European and Japanese birth rates (i.e., 17-18) in many presently less developed countries by the end of the century. But this would still be far from zero rate of growth as postulated by Bogue.

Where do we come out? Planners would do well to plan for the UN projections or worse, hope for the Bogue estimates, and expect something in between, likely much nearer the former than the latter.[37] To make better estimates we need much better measures than we now have (a) of the threshold of socioeconomic progress necessary to generate and facilitate major fertility reduction in each of the several major regions and (b) of the potential effects of the new national family planning programs.

Conclusions

We are at a dynamic, perhaps decisive stage in the demographic transition. For two decades cultural barriers and laggard socioeconomic development have blocked the spread of fertility reduction into the developing regions. A sharp dichotomy has arisen between low fertility, developed countries and high fertility, underdeveloped countries, with very few countries in the transition from one to the other. There have been important harbingers of change, but, aside from East and Southeast Asia, as yet no decisive breakthrough in the major regions and countries of the developing world.

The setting for such a breakthrough is now favorable in many ways. More countries are approaching the threshold of social development at which birth rates have empirically begun to decline. The tempo of the transition, once begun, is faster than before.

And now national family planning programs, armed with better contraceptive methods, are reinforcing the "normal" diffusion of family planning practices. These programs have been most successful in countries where the transition was already under way, but are making some headway even in less tractable countries like India and Pakistan.

Often too much is expected of the programs; they are too new and the problems are much too great to be solved overnight. Definitive solutions will take many years, and there will be a need for the support of less glamorous but widely practiced methods such as induced abortion and surgical sterilization. The "new" methods will be replaced by still better ones. But the elements for success are gathering—government action, improved contraceptive technology, broad social development, and, to less extent, economic growth. With continuing progress in these elements, it is a reasonable prediction that by 1975 the downward trend in birth rates will have been firmly established in several major countries and in quite a few additional smaller ones, especially in Asia and Latin America. There are rational grounds for hope that by the end of the century most of the more important less developed countries will be well along the transition to lower fertility and relief from the problems of rapid population growth.[38] The problems are prodigious—especially those of meeting the needs of rapidly burgeoning populations in the next two decades —but there are now real prospects for a long-run solution.

Notes

1. The less developed regions are broadly defined as Africa, Latin America, and Asia, excluding Japan and the Asian parts of the Soviet Union. Also where convenient, Argentina and Uruguay are considered separately from the remainder of Latin America since these are more European than Latin American in level of development. Further refinements are possible but impractical for present purposes. Thus Albania is an underdeveloped country in Europe; Israel is a developed country in Asia; Melanesia, Micronesia, and Polynesia are underdeveloped sub-regions of Oceania.

2. United Nations, *Population Bulletin No. 7* (1963) p. 13.

3. *Ibid.,* for major regions, p. 1; for Africa, pp. 18-19; for Asia, p. 43; and for Latin America, p. 66.

4. Interestingly enough, the exceptions are islands (i.e., Puerto Rico and several of the former British West Indies; Cyprus; the Ryukyus; Singapore) and the political "islands" of Israel and Hong Kong.

5. Since 1960 birth rates in the USSR, the United States, Canada, and Australia have fallen rapidly, and by 1966 were all below 20.

6. The relationship is explored in the United Nations, *op. cit.,* chap. IX.

7. I.e., Latin America exclusive of Argentina, Uruguay, and Chile.

8. The complicated effects of general mortality reduction are discussed in Jeanne Clare Ridley, *et al.,* "The Effects of Changing Mortality on Natality," *Milbank Memorial Fund Quarterly:* XLV, 1 (Jan., 1967), 77-97.

9. There is controversy and differing evidence on the effect of polygyny on natality. On the average, polygynous husbands obviously have more children than they otherwise would, but the polygynous women have fewer than women mated singly.

10. Crude birth rates are used here because more specific measures of fertility are unavailable for recent years.

11. Exceptions are Costa Rica and, up to recently, Chile.

12. This sharp division also existed in North African countries before the exodus of Europeans and exists today as between Jew and Arab in Israel.

13. Dudley Kirk, "Prospects for Reducing Natality in the Underdeveloped World," *Annals* of the American Academy of Political and Social Science, 369 (Jan., 1967) 48-60.

14. On the other hand, specific practices and attitudes prevailing in the Moslem world and closely associated with the Moslem religion (for example) are a major barrier to the spread of family planning in that region. Cf. Dudley Kirk, "Factors Affecting Moslem Natality" in Bernard Berelson *et al.* (eds.) *Family Planning and Population Programs* (University of Chicago Press, 1966).

15. 14 Asian, 14 Latin American, and 7 Middle Eastern and North African countries.

16. Of the five exceptions, three are readily explainable; in Korea, the Ryukyus, and Taiwan the birth rate has been declining. Earlier intercensal comparisons in Korea and Taiwan show rising ratios of children to women. I have no ready explanation for the other two—Pakistan and Iraq. Such figures may, of course, be affected by improvement or changes in the accuracy of census enumeration. Data from United Nations, *Demographic Yearbook, 1965.*

17. A compilation of the results of such studies is given in W. Parker Mauldin, "Fertility Studies: Knowledge, Attitude and Practice," in Population Council, *Studies in Family Planning,* No. 7 (June 1965); and in Bernard Berelson, "KAP Studies on Fertility" in Berelson *et al.* (eds.), *op. cit.*

18. Cf. Sheldon J. Segal's paper in this volume: "Biological Aspects of Fertility Regulation."

19. Countries included are: 1875-1899: Austria, Australia, England and Wales, Finland, Italy, Netherlands, New Zealand, Scotland, United States; 1900-1924: Argentina, Czechoslovakia, Germany, Hungary, Japan, Portugal, Spain; 1925-1949: Bulgaria, Poland, Rumania, U.S.S.R., Yugoslavia; 1950-   : Ceylon, Chile, Hong Kong, Puerto Rico, Singapore, Taiwan.

Sources: Historical data for Europe, Robert R. Kucynski, *The Balance of Births and Deaths,* Vol. I, New York, Macmillan, 1928; and Vol. II, Washington, D.C., Brookings Institution, 1931; for Portugal and non-European countries, national statistical sources; for the United States (white population), Ansley J. Coale and Melvin Zelnik, *New Estimates of Fertility and Population in the United States,* Princeton, 1963, pp. 21-23; for later dates, generally United Nations, *Demographic Yearbook,* various years.

The initial and terminal dates were determined by 3-year averages rounded to 35 and 20 respectively. A crude birth rate of 35 was chosen to eliminate countries where there have been fluctuations in natality probably unrelated to the widespread adoption of family planning. In some countries, including all of those entering the transition since 1950, the reduction of the birth rate has not yet reached 20. In these cases, the decline in the birth rate after reaching the 35 level, or data for at least 7 years, was projected by linear extrapolation of the average annual rates of decline. Values determined by extrapolation vary considerably depending upon the specific assumptions; those used here are conservative in view of the acceleration of declines in the birth rate in very recent years. Two countries, namely Argentina and Portugal, have not yet reached a birth rate of 20 even though they entered the transition phase, as defined, in 1915 and 1912. The projected rates will not bring them to this level until 1970 and 1976 respectively.

In a number of countries (e.g., Australia, Canada, New Zealand, and the United States) the birth rate fell to 20 or below in the initial period of decline but later returned to somewhat higher levels in the post-war "baby boom." All of these countries, except New Zealand, now again have birth rates below 20, but the years in transition were computed only for the initial period of consecutive downward trend.

20. The socioeconomic indicators relate to various dates, chiefly in the late 1950's. United Nations, *Population Bulletin, No. 7,* p. 149.

21. Thus the 5 top-ranking countries in East and South Asia on a crude socioeconomic index are all countries that have experienced the take-off in decline of the birth rate: Japan, Singapore, Taiwan, Hong Kong, and South Korea. With the possible exception of Korea the take-off occurred before the adoption of government family planning programs or the widespread introduction of the new contraceptives. The next three countries in rank are Ceylon, the Philippines, and Malaya. Ceylon and Malaya are the only other 2 countries in Asia in which there has been a measurable reduction in the birth rate in recent years; for the Philippines no trend data are available. Other countries may be expected to follow these leaders when they attain a comparable level of development, as some may soon. The components of the index (unweighted) are: GNP per caput, expectation of life at birth, percent urban, percent of adult literacy, students enrolled in higher education per 100,000 population, inhabitants per physician, and radios per 1000 population. Data from United Nations publications and from Bruce M. Russett *et al., World Handbook of Political and Social Indicators* (New Haven: Yale University Press, 1964).

22. These remarkable achievements are described by Bernard Berelson in his paper on "National Family Planning Programs: Where We Stand" in this volume. No attempt is made here to review the very good group of studies evaluating various aspects of the programs (cf. Population Council, *Studies in Family Planning,* various issues, 1963-67) because very few deal directly with the impact of programs on the national birth rate.

23. Experience since 1965 is difficult to assess. The reported birth rate for 1966 (32.5) was only slightly lower than for 1965 (32.7) but there clearly was some earlier than usual registration of births in connection with the national census of December 1966. Some births were "borrowed" from 1967 (i.e., registered earlier than normally) thus depressing the reported birth rate in the early part of 1967. The actual reduction of the birth rate in 1966 was certainly larger than reported. More definitive evaluation of the program effects will require analysis with the help of more refined measures of fertility. Cf. Ronald Freedman, "The Continuing Fertility Decline in Taiwan: 1965," *Population Index,* 33, 1 (Jan.-March 1967) 3-17.

24. It may be remembered that Yoshio Koya's several successful experiments in introducing family planning in Japan encountered this effect. Thus reduction in the fertility of his study populations was at first due as much to the heightened practice of abortion as to the recommended methods of contraception. Cf. Yoshio Koya, *Pioneering in Family Planning: A Collection of Papers on the Family Planning Program and Research Conducted in Japan* (Tokyo, Japan. Medical Publishers, 1963).

25. "Taiwan: Births Averted by the IUD Program" in Population Council, *Studies in Family Planning,* No. 20 (June 1967). This analysis draws upon the outstanding research on the Taiwan program being conducted by L. P. Chow, Ronald Freedman, and their colleagues at the Taiwan and the University of Michigan Population Studies Centers.

26. These estimates are presumably minimal since they are based on the voluntary responses of women in a country where abortion is illegal.

27. Even this is an oversimplification: Some 40 percent of the original

acceptors not wearing the IUD at the time of interview were using other contraceptive methods or had been sterilized. Some reduction of fertility among original IUD acceptors is assignable to these other methods as well as to abortion.

28. In the period 1962-65 the computed ratios of children 0-4 to women 15-44 fell 22 percent for urban areas, 11 percent for rural areas and 14 percent in the country as a whole. The annual percent reductions for Korea were successively 3.9, 4.2 and 6.4. This ratio is in effect a five-year moving average affected both by births and by deaths to this age group and therefore is a very rough indicator of changes of natality in any given year. The registration for 1962 also indicates a drop of 10.2 percent from the corresponding ratio of children to women in the 1960 census, but these two sources are of dubious comparability. Registration data are from communications from the Bureau of Statistics, Korea.

29. Sung-Bong Hong, *Induced Abortion in Seoul, Korea* (Seoul: Dong-A Publishing Co., 1966), p. 19. This report is based on a survey of a random probability sample of 3204 eligible married women in a total population of 370,000, of somewhat lower economic status than Seoul as a whole. Other studies cited by Hong, p. 18, also suggest a high incidence of abortion in that city for various years ranging from 1958-62. However, unlike his study, these are based on clinic and hospital samples.

30. Sung-Bong Hong, "Induced Abortion in Rural Korea," in *Korean Journal of Obstetrics and Gynecology* 10(6):275-95 (June 1967). This study surveyed a sample of 2084 wives in a rural district. The 1965 and 1966 National Family Planning Surveys reported similar and rising frequencies of induced abortion for rural Korea as a whole, 5.4 percent of women in 1965 and 7.3 percent in 1966 reporting that they had *ever* had an abortion, as compared with Hong's figures of 4.9 percent for his study area. (Ministry of Health, Korea, *The Findings of the National Survey on Family Planning*, 1966, p. 183). Unfortunately the latter studies do not ask the year of occurrence and therefore cannot be compared with Hong's results on an annual basis.

31. S. M. Keeny, "Korea and Taiwan: The Score for 1966" in Population Council, *Studies in Family Planning*, No. 19 (May 1967).

32. Thus Hong found that 45.3 percent of 1000 women patients of family planning clinics at a major health center in Seoul had had a previous record of abortion. These patients came to the clinics in June-August 1964, the first three months of the intensified national program. (Hong, *op. cit.* p. 18.) This substitution may be regarded as eminently desirable on humanitarian grounds but it does reduce the effectiveness of the program in cutting the birth rate.

33. Parker Mauldin, Dorothy Nortman, and Frederick F. Stephan, "Retention of IUDs: An International Comparison," in Population Council, *Studies in Family Planning*, No. 18 (April, 1967) p. 11.

34. Donald J. Bogue, "The Prospects for World Population Control," in *Alternatives for Balancing World Food Production Needs* (Ames, Iowa: Iowa State University Press, 1967), pp. 82-83.

35. *Op. cit.* p. 84.

36. Gavin W. Jones and W. Parker Mauldin, "Use of Oral Contraceptives with Special Reference to Developing Countries," Population Council, *Studies in Family Planning*, No. 24 (December, 1967).

37. In another publication the author has ventured guesses on the probable development in the several major regions. Dudley Kirk, "Prospects for Reducing Natality in the Underdeveloped World," *Annals* of the American Academy of Political and Social Science 369 (Jan., 1967) 48-60.

38. I.e., these countries will have reached or will be approaching present levels of population growth in Europe, North America, Australasia, Japan, and Argentina. These now range from ½ to 1½ percent per annum with an average of about 1 percent. There is some concern that even a low rate of growth (say 1 percent) will ultimately lead to disastrous crowding and that the world population will in some remote future outrun any conceivable means of subsistence. This is certainly true, but not immediately relevant; *any* unidirectional geometric rate of growth, no matter how minuscule, ultimately leads to astronomical absurdities, in population or anything else. This ultimate problem is not the present world population problem, which is much more urgent: to bring birth rates and population growth down as soon as possible to manageable levels, not to eliminate population growth altogether.

THE EMERGENCE OF A MODERN
FERTILITY PATTERN:
UNITED STATES, 1917-66 *

Norman B. Ryder
The University of Wisconsin

Introduction

THIS IS AN ESSAY in demographic measurement. My intention has been to describe the changing reproductive behavior of American women by exploiting the resources of an extraordinary times series of vital statistics covering a 50-year span of time. Specifically, the data I propose to analyze are the age-specific order-specific birth rates, and the age-specific (first) marriage rates, for the cohorts of women born 1891-1945.

The Federal Government has published the requisite birth data for the years 1917-64, and it is possible on the basis of less detailed information for 1965 and 1966 to extend this series up to the beginning of the present year, without risk of grave error. This represents 50 years worth of information (1917-66) but not in the form in which I intend to present my results, i.e., for successive cohorts. Indeed if no projection or retrojection were attempted, the only cohorts which could be studied over the entire reproductive age span (arbitrarily fixed at ages 14-49 inclusive) would be c.1903-17 (the cohorts of years 1903 through 1917)—the limits being set by the cohort which was 14 in 1917 and that which was 49 in 1966. I have considered it not unreasonable to undertake an extension of the basic data back in time to encompass the early childbearing of the cohorts of 1891-1902 and forward in time to encompass the late childbearing of the cohorts of 1918-45.

* A conventional acknowledgment of thanks to my research assistant, Mr. Bohdan Czarnocki, would be quite inadequate. He displayed extraordinary devotion and tenacity in programming the calculations for this paper, all the while bedeviled by my experiments with new measures, none of which proved adaptable to routinized procedures.

The assumptions, and the procedural details, are explained in Appendix I. The most questionable aspect is the projection beyond the beginning of 1967, for the younger cohorts. In essence, I have assumed a graduated movement over the next ten years toward the levels of cohort fertility implicit in the behavior of the early 1950's. I do not regard this as a realistic forecast, but merely as a simple and plausible way of completing the reproductive histories of cohorts now in the middle of the childbearing period. One implication of this admission is that information reported for cohorts at the extremes of each time series must be regarded with due skepticism.[1] I want to emphasize that my intent is not to forecast fertility but to describe what has happened.[2] In the main, the analysis is restricted to those cohorts which have probably completed more than half of their childbearing within the time span of observation, c.1891-1940, although I have included parenthetically measurements for c.1941-45, despite their speculative character, as a concession to the high interest in current behavior and in recognition of the important changes now under way. Compromises of this sort are unavoidable for a person who regards cohort behavior as the primary descriptive target of the demographer.

A special note is necessary for the measures of nuptiality reported here, because the data required for accurate calculation of marriage rates are not available. I have taken advantage of a new tabulation published in the 1960 Census, and supplementary data for 1960-66 from the Current Population Reports. It will be evident at several points below that my efforts to produce cohort nuptiality tables in parallel with the cohort fertility tables have not been entirely successful. The defense for publishing these imperfect data is that movements of nuptiality are too important for fertility behavior to be ignored and I know of no better estimates at present of the parameters employed.[3]

There are three parts to the body of this paper. The first of these contains observations concerning the quantity of fertility, and the second concerning the tempo of fertility.[4] In the third section, I introduce a new procedure for assessing the relative importance of the quantity and tempo of nuptiality and marital parity for changes in the level of period fertility. This essay is long on measurement and short on analysis. The former is a demanding and humiliating task which most demographers seem to undertake reluctantly but necessarily—because it provides the raw materials for their interpretation. Since I judge my capacities to be less inadequate in the former than in the latter task, I have chosen to concentrate on measurement, in confidence or at least in hope that others will provide explanations for the variations described. This posture is coordinate with my belief that the growth of social science will be accelerated by a greater division of labor than now exists between method and analysis, as well as between theory and policy.

The Quantity of Fertility

Three measures relevant to the question of the quantity of fertility are displayed in Table 1 for c.1891-1945.

Table 1. Quantity of Fertility: Total Fertility Rate (TFR); Total Nuptiality Rate (TNR); Mean Marital Parity (MMP); c.1891-1945

Cohort	TFR	TNR	MMP
1891-95	2.96	0.91	3.27
1896-00	2.68	0.91	2.93
1901-05	2.42	0.91	2.66
1906-10	2.27	0.92	2.47
1911-15	2.32	0.94	2.47
1916-20	2.55	0.95	2.70
1921-25	2.86	0.96	3.00
1926-30	3.11	0.96	3.24
1931-35	3.36	0.98	3.42
1936-40	3.31	0.98	3.40
(1941-45)	(2.98)	(0.95)	(3.13)

The total fertility rate (TFR) is the sum over all ages of the birth rates for all orders. It may be interpreted as the mean number of births per woman if the cohort were mortality-free. The TFR declined to a minimum of 2.27 for c.1906-10, and then rose to a maximum of 3.36 for c.1931-35, 50 percent higher in 25 cohort years; the most recent cohort group has retreated somewhat below that peak.

The total fertility rate is the product of the total nuptiality rate (TNR) and the mean marital parity. The TNR can be interpreted as the proportion of women married (at least once) by exact age 50,[5] again under mortality-free conditions. Throughout the whole era the TNR has been rising; in the process it has contributed to the upward movement of the TFR. It would be difficult to defend the accuracy of the estimate that 98 percent of the women of cohorts of 1931-40 marry (by age 50); nevertheless I am confident that the TNR has risen, and to a very high level. A further important circumstance is that, unlike the other series in Table 1, TNR shows no depression-associated trough.

The mean marital parity (MMP) is operationally defined as the ratio TFR/TNR. It may be interpreted as the mean number of births per ever-married woman—more familiarly, if less accurately, called "average family size."[6] The source of the trough in TFR is clearly the trough in MMP. The latter parameter fell 24 percent to a minimum for c.1906-15, and then rose 38 percent to a maximum of 3.42 for c.1931-35; it has since subsided a little.

For interpretation of the movements of the total fertility rate, as in Table 1, the problem of a proper time perspective must be faced. From the cohort fertility tables we know that the TFR declined monotonically from 3.74 for c.1876 to the beginning of the series in Table 1; from other sources it seems highly likely that, transitory fluctuations aside, the decline began at least as far back as the start of the nineteenth century, from a level several times as large as that for c.1891-95. One reading of Table 1 would be that the long-term secular decline continued until c.1906-10 and was then reversed. In my opinion, a more plausible interpretation would be that the minimum was predominantly a depression-induced trough, appreciably below what would otherwise have occurred, and that, although there has indeed been a rise in TFR, its dimensions are much more modest than generally suggested.

Underlying and to some extent concealed by the movements of mean marital parity are important changes in the parity distributions summarized by the means. To illustrate these changes, Table 2 has been prepared.

Table 2. Proportions (per thousand) of (Married) Women in Each (Completed) Parity, Selected Cohorts

Parity	c.1897	c.1909	c.1921	c.1933
0	116	165	65	39
1	218	236	175	98
2	206	238	270	220
3	146	141	200	232
4	103	83	122	172
5	62	47	66	98
6	46	30	39	58
7	35	20	23	32
8+	67	40	40	50

The cohorts in Table 2 have been selected for the following reasons: c.1909 had the minimum (2.42) and c.1933 the maximum (3.46) in mean marital parity. These cohorts were age 24 in 1933 and 1957 respectively, representing the trough of the depression and the peak of postwar prosperity. C.1921 is midway between these two; it also can be taken to represent the cohorts of World War II, since it was 20 in

1941. Similarly c.1897 was 20 in 1917, the beginning (for the United States) of World War I. Conveniently, and coincidentally (unless one has a fatalistic theory of cycles of war and depression) the four cohorts are equidistant in time, and c.1897 happens to have the same mean marital parity (2.98) as c.1921. (It is, however, apparent from Table 2 that they achieved this same mean in very different ways: c.1897 had higher proportions below 2 and higher proportions above 5 than did c.1921.)

Between the World War I cohort of 1897 and the depression cohort of 1909, the proportions with fewer than three children swelled from 54 percent to 64 percent, and the proportion in every parity above 2 declined. Between the depression cohort of 1909 and the prosperity cohort of 1933 there was a comprehensive upward transformation of the parity distribution. Not only did the mean increase by 1.04, the whole distribution was displaced upward by approximately one parity step, and the mode shifted from 1 or 2 to 2 or 3. Although c.1921 has a parity distribution which lies approximately midway between those of c.1909 and c.1933, there is one interesting difference of detail: a very low proportion infertile had already been achieved, but the proportions in the highest parities were virtually unchanged. This is a reflection of the elementary circumstance that higher order births occur later in time to a cohort than do lower order births.

One of the more interesting and important changes that have been occurring in American fertility is the diminution in the dispersion of women among the various parities. This phenomenon may be directly measured by parity variance. This parameter has declined from 7.89 for c.1891-95 to 4.25 for c.1936-40, a decline interrupted only momentarily by the recent upsurge in fertility.[7] To compensate for the direct relationship which ordinarily exists between the variance and the mean, I have calculated the coefficient of variation (the ratio of the standard deviation to the mean); it declined from 95 percent for c.1906-10, at the bottom of the depression, to 61 percent for c.1936-40. This bespeaks the extraordinary extent to which the population is becoming progressively more homogeneous in the numbers of births per marriage.

Although parity distributions provide important raw materials for the analysis of the consequences of changing reproductive behavior, they are unsatisfactory for causal analysis because they represent the net compounded consequences of different behavior in the successive birth intervals. To obviate this difficulty, I devised the measure known as the parity progression ratio—the proportion of women with at least N births who go on to have at least N+1 births. The parity progression ratios for a cohort represent a series of conditional probabilities of more fertility. These are presented in Table 3.

In Table 3, different cohort ranges are shown for different parities in keeping with the principle that no measures should be presented unless they are based on data for at least half the experience summarized. Thus the range is more recent for events occurring earlier in the reproductive age span.

I have attempted to summarize the time series for each parity with the aid of two measures, shown at the foot of the table. The first of these, total change, is the percent by which the last observation is higher or lower than the first observation in each column. This crude indication of trend indicates that the series fall into 2 categories: the lower 3 parities, for which there has been increase—substantial only for progression from parity 1 to parity 2; and the upper 5 parities, for which there has been decrease—substantial for all but the highest. In other words there has been a large increase in the conditional probability of having a second child once the first has been born, and a large decrease in the conditional probability of having another child for those arriving at parities 3 and higher.

The second summary measure for each time series, labeled "trough," is the percent by which the observations fall below a

Table 3. Parity Progression Ratios (per thousand) Parities 0-7, Selected Cohorts*

Cohort	Initial Parity							
	0	1	2	3	4	5	6	7
1881-85								673
1886-90				743	720	730	714	674
1891-95		784	720	706	691	718	705	664
1896-00	876	752	682	678	671	705	687	661
1901-05	867	719	639	647	653	687	667	667
1906-10	845	715	609	618	630	662	663	665
1911-15	849	743	605	589	601	640	646	659
1916-20	892	789	626	584	581	610	630	645
1921-25	933	832	663	597	580	605	612	632
1926-30	935	871	713	623	587	599	603	625
1931-35	952	895	745	637	580	587	590	
1936-40	971	892	740					
1941-45	932							
Total								
Change (%)	+ 6	+14	+ 3	−14	−20	−20	−17	− 7
Trough (%)	− 5	−13	−17	−14	− 7	− 4	− 1	0

*For method of calculating the ratio for the highest parity PPR, see Appendix III.

straight line drawn from the first to the last entry; in each case the trough value indicates the maximum relative departure. This is a simpleminded way of indicating the magnitude of response in each parity to fertility-depressant factors which were prevalent in the first half of each series. The maximum response is for parity 2, and adjacent parities; all other troughs are small. In a sense this measure identifies the discretionary span of parities: the most likely change during a depression is for couples to stop at two children rather than proceed to a third. The progressively smaller responses in the higher reaches of the parity sequence are probably attributable to progressive selectivity—partly for fecundity, but partly and probably principally for inability (or reluctance) to control fertility.

The series in Table 3 provides the basis for some important inferences about the future of fertility. The sources of increase in the total fertility rate are clearly identified as increases in the earlier parity progression ratios which more than compensated for decreases in the later ratios. It can safely be asserted that the ratios for parities 0 and 1 are highly unlikely to increase further because they are very close to their maxima. Even if the only women who remained in parities 0 and 1 were those who were physiologically unable to proceed further, the maximum would be of the order of 950 per thousand—and it seems unlikely that there would be no voluntary termination.[8]

As for the proportion proceeding from two to three children, it is now not much different from what it was before the depression; its recent rise is impressive only if measured from the trough in fertility. (The value of this ratio for c.1886-90 was 761.) The parity progression ratios above parity 2 have all declined, when viewed in 50-year perspective. An appropriately substantial base is essential for a long range projection: to project upward the ratio for parity 3, for example, on the ground that it has been rising over a few recent cohorts, would be tantamount to treating the experience of the depression as "normal."

Since these observations are somewhat novel, and, if valid, of considerable importance, it seems worthwhile to restate the argument in another way. Between the beginning of our series, with c.1891-95, and the group with the maximum fertility, c.1931-35, the TFR rose from 2.96 to 3.36. The composition of this impressive increase by birth order reveals the necessity for caution in contemplating what may happen next. Births of the first three orders rose from 1.91 to 2.39, while those of higher orders declined from 1.05 to 0.97. Stated in this way the latter decline looks quite modest, but not when it is considered that those 1.05 were produced by only 46 percent of the women of c.1891-95, (each having 2.28 additional births), while the 0.97 were produced by 62 percent of the women of c.1931-35 (each having only 1.55 additional births). In terms of average parity progression ratios, the ratios producing the first three orders of birth rose from 86 percent to 92 percent, while those producing the higher orders fell from 70 percent to 61 percent. The position is compelling that the former trend can continue very little farther—that 2.39 is close to the maximum number of births of orders 1-3 that women can be expected to produce—whereas it is not at all unlikely that the latter trend will continue downward. To exemplify the implication, a drop to 50 percent in the ratios for parities 3+ would yield a 10 percent decline in the total fertility rate—provided the same high proportion continued to progress as far as a third birth.[9]

The conclusion I come to is that the most likely direction of long-run movement of the total fertility rate for cohorts, on the basis of continuation of those trends which can continue, is downward, although the pace of decline will not be rapid unless the progression ratios in the lowest parities slacken from their currently very high levels.

The Tempo of Fertility

The preponderance of analytic attention in the literature has been directed at the quantity of fertility. Three complementary reasons for this may be suggested: (1) the major secular change over the past century has been in quantity; (2) almost all measurements of fertility have been period-specific, a circumstance which inhibits consideration of intrinsically cohort parameters like time of occurrence of vital events; (3) the influence of changes in tempo on the quantity of births from year to year is subtle, and still frequently misapprehended.

In consequence, publications reporting tempo parameters are hard to find. This is regrettable because changes in tempo have always been substantial, they now rival changes in quantity in their impact on annual fertility, and they are likely to carry the predominant responsibility for future variations. Since we know so little about the determinants of reproductive tempo, in contrast to the mountain of information concerning completed parity, my measurement program has incorporated a strong emphasis on the subject. Table 4 presents a set of summary measures of tempo for the quinquennial cohort groups in our series.

Between c.1891-95 and c.1921-25, the movements of the mean age of fertility were irregular; since then there has been an abrupt decline. This is a puzzling observation because one would expect, before the fact, that the depression would have pushed the mean up

Table 4. Moment Measures of Fertility Tempo: Mean Age of Fertility (MAF);
Standard Deviation (DAF); Skew (SAF); and Kurtosis (KAF)—Cohorts
1891-1945

Cohort	MAF	DAF	SAF	KAF
1891-95	27.54	6.27	+0.46	−0.43
1896-00	27.12	6.14	+0.55	−0.26
1901-05	26.89	6.29	+0.61	−0.29
1906-10	27.29	6.51	+0.46	−0.59
1911-15	27.79	6.39	+0.33	−0.61
1916-20	27.78	6.17	+0.36	−0.52
1921-25	27.49	5.95	+0.40	−0.41
1926-30	26.86	5.74	+0.54	−0.16
1931-35	26.19	5.72	+0.69	+0.14
1936-40	25.94	5.94	+0.76	+0.05
(1941-45)	(26.42)	(6.20)	(+0.58)	(−0.35)

sharply, as a reflection of the postponement of births. Resolution of
this quandary is postponed to the next part of this section because it
requires a different calculation.

The standard deviation of fertility by age (DAF) has the same
pattern of movements as the mean. In fact, the coefficient of variation (ratio of standard deviation to mean) has been of the order of 22
or 23 percent throughout virtually the entire series, a remarkable constancy given the large changes observed in other parameters. There
is good reason for more than idle interest in the movements of DAF.
Every irregularity in the number of births from year to year, and thus
in the size of the cohorts then initiated, tends to be repeated in each
subsequent generation, as those cohorts, and then their descendants,
have their children. What causes the irregularity to be dampened
through time is the dispersion of a cohort's childbearing throughout
its reproductive age span. The smaller the value of DAF, the sharper
the fidelity of reproduction of the irregularity in subsequent generations. Accordingly one cost of a tendency toward greater conformity
with respect to norms concerning the appropriate age pattern of
childbearing is a reduction of the dampening effect and therefore
more persistent irregularity than would otherwise be the case.

For the record, and without discussion, we note that there is a
small positive skew in the fertility-age distribution (SAF), slightly
more pronounced recently, and that the distribution has been slightly
platykurtic but recently became slightly leptokurtic.[10]

As mentioned, there is something peculiar about the movements
of MAF. One difficulty is that it is not a pure measure of timing because it tends to vary directly with the total fertility rate—since more

births take more time. To cope with this difficulty we have devised a standardized mean age of fertility (MAX). This is the weighted mean of the mean ages for each birth order of a cohort, the weights being the mean proportion of births of that order for all cohorts (1891-1940). A comparable procedure yields a standardized standard deviation (DAX). These are shown in Table 5, together with the total fertility rate for purpose of convenient comparison.

This table shows us that some large changes in the mean age had been masked in Table 4 by compensatory quantity-associated changes. The standardized mean rose by more than 1 year and then declined by more than 2 years. Yet, despite the precaution of standardization, something still seems peculiar: there is no one-to-one correspondence between the movements of MAX and the movements of TFR. The former reaches a maximum for c.1911-20; the latter reaches a minimum for c.1906-10. The explanation for this is that a period-specific phenomenon, like the depression, affects earlier cohorts at older ages and later cohorts at younger ages. The postponements by the former are more likely to become terminations than the postponements by the latter, because there is less time to recoup losses (and perhaps less inclination to do so) as age advances. The cohorts who were beyond thirty by 1935 (c.1891-1905) show little change in their standardized mean age of fertility despite the fact that their TFR has declined. But the younger cohorts experiencing the depression had sufficient time subsequently to have their postponed children, and this raised their MAX. (Likewise the DAX rises, as another manifestation of the same phenomenon.) The same pattern is apparent later in the time series. C.1921-25 had 23 percent more fertility than c.1911-15, but only a slightly lower MAX. The reason is that c.1921-25

Table 5. Standardized Mean and Standard Deviation (MAX and DAX) of Fertility by Age, and the Total Fertility Rate, c.1891-1945

Cohort	MAX	DAX	TFR
1891-95	26.90	6.05	2.96
1896-00	26.78	5.98	2.68
1901-05	26.84	6.20	2.42
1906-10	27.47	6.47	2.27
1911-15	28.09	6.41	2.32
1916-20	28.08	6.24	2.55
1921-25	27.67	6.04	2.86
1926-30	26.83	5.81	3.11
1931-35	26.11	5.81	3.36
1936-40	26.01	6.07	3.31
(1941-45)	(26.61)	(6.34)	(2.98)

encountered prosperity at a relatively late age; higher birth rates mean a higher mean age of fertility. Movements of MAX since then have been more as one would expect.

The most important determinant of the tempo of fertility is the tempo of nuptiality. Accordingly we have prepared Table 6 as a parallel to Table 4 above. This table must be used with caution— as should any American marriage data—because the sources are perhaps inadequate to bear the burdens on reliability required for refined analysis. The justification for its presentation is the paucity of information on this important subject.

The mean age of nuptiality (MAN) has tended to decline throughout the whole series, at first slowly—presumably because of the depression—and then much more rapidly (by almost two years over a twenty-cohort span of time). The downward trend appears to have recently been reversed. The nuptiality-age function has a small standard deviation (DAN), a strong positive skew and a pronounced and increasing leptokurtosis. Such distributional characteristics are not unexpected with a function which has a mean declining toward a relatively fixed lower bound. The strong and growing concentration of nuptiality within a narrow age span is suggested by the statistic that, for c.1910, 40 percent of marriages occurred in ages 17-21, while for c.1930 it was 60 percent.

More detailed inquiry into the time pattern of marital reproductivity really requires data that are not collected in the United States, such as the answers which would be forthcoming to a question on the birth certificate concerning the time elapsed since the woman's previous birth. I have calculated the moment measures separately

Table 6. Moment Measures of Nuptiality Tempo: Mean Age of Nuptiality (MAN); Standard Deviation (DAN); Skew (SAN); and Kurtosis (KAN). Cohorts 1891-1945

Cohort	MAN	DAN	SAN	KAN
(1891-95)	(23.33)	(5.80)	(+1.34)	(+2.37)
1896-00	23.10	5.90	+1.56	+3.17
1901-05	23.21	6.27	+1.49	+2.45
1906-10	23.18	6.13	+1.34	+1.96
1911-15	23.16	5.73	+1.29	+2.21
1916-20	22.73	5.31	+1.50	+3.40
1921-25	22.10	4.85	+1.79	+5.45
1926-30	21.56	4.79	+2.19	+7.53
1931-35	21.35	5.00	+2.32	+7.62
1936-40	21.32	5.21	+2.32	+6.94
1941-45	21.55	5.32	+2.47	+6.15

for the birth rates of each successive order, and compared the differences between successive means. This is an unsatisfactory approach to birth intervals because the mean for the higher order in each pair applies only to the women who have a birth of that order, whereas the mean for the lower order applies also to women who have terminated their childbearing with that birth, and these terminators are likely to have a different (higher) mean age than those who do progress to the next parity. I did develop an estimating procedure designed to obviate this difficulty, but the results were sufficiently flawed that I decided to relegate them to the appendix.[11]

Components of Period Fertility
One question predominates in analyses of time series of fertility: To what extent are temporal variations in period fertility attributable to changes in the quantity of cohort fertility, on the one hand, and to changes in its tempo, on the other hand? Subsidiary to this, but of independent interest, is a second question: To what extent do these changes reflect modifications of nuptiality, on the one hand, and of marital parity, on the other hand?

The principal stumbling-block in the way of answers is that there is no obvious way to compare a number of births with a number of years. I have devised a new procedure which I think overcomes this difficulty. The relative importance of quantity and tempo can be judged in terms of the extent of their contribution to the explanation of fertility movements from year to year. These are now known to be a composite of variations produced by increase or decrease in the quantity of cohort fertility and variations which are responses to the acceleration or deceleration of the tempo of cohort fertility. To describe this process in a simple way, I devised the formula:

$$PTFR(T + CMAF(T)) = CTFR(T) \times (1 - CMAF'(T)),$$

where PTFR is the period total fertility rate for year $T + CMAF(T)$, CMAF(T) the mean age of fertility for the cohort born in year T (and CMAF'(T) its annual change), and CTFR(T) the cohort total fertility rate. This is an exact formula when there is linear change of the fertility rates in each individual age. It can be shown that PTFR is estimated quite well from knowledge of CTFR and CMAF even when there is considerable departure from the specified assumption. Nevertheless the validity of the approach used below rests not on the quality of this estimate but rather on the position that this formula provides an appropriate kind of measurement structure, in terms of dimensionality, for comparing the consequences of variations in quantity with those of variations in tempo.

The type of procedure to be followed can be exemplified as follows: For each cohort we obtain, by moving average techniques, smoothed values of TFR and MAF. Each TFR is then expressed as a proportion of the mean TFR for c.1891-1940. The deviation of the period TFR from the all-cohort mean is the product of this proportion and the term $(1 - CMAF'(T))$. To simplify comparisons and permit further subdivision of components, we convert the calculation to additive form by the use of (natural) logarithms. Thus we compare $\ln (TFR/ \text{ mean } TFR)$ with $\ln (1 - MAF')$.

This procedure is readily adaptable to a subdivision of fertility into the part contributed by nuptiality and that contributed by marital parity, in the manner already adopted. On the quantity side, $TFR = TNR \times MMP$; on the tempo side, $MAF = MAN + MDF$ (where MDF, the mean duration of marital fertility, is obtained by subtracting MAN, the mean age of nuptiality, from MAF, the mean age of fertility).

One further refinement is appropriate. In the preceding section we characterized MAF as a defective measure of tempo (because it reflects variations in the quantity of fertility) and therefore employed a standardized mean, MAX, to solve that problem. In assessing the consequences for period fertility of changes in quantity, we should include those changes in the tempo of cohort fertility which are caused by changes in the quantity of cohort fertility, i.e. changes in MAF-MAX, and allocate to the tempo side of the ledger only the consequences of changes in MAX.[12]

Table 7 shows the consequences of this procedure for the ten cohort groups with firmly-based data: the first and last groups are truncated as a consequence of the smoothing operation employed. In addition, because of the high degree of interest in contemporary behavior, I have appended the results for c.1939-43, to be used with caution. Each two-by-two table shows, in the row marginals, the relative influence of nuptiality (N) and marital parity (P); in the column marginals, the relative influence of quantity (Q) and tempo (T); and in the internal cells, the four cross-classified components. The summary numbers in the lower right-hand corner of each sub-table constitute the simultaneous effects of all components. The natural antilogarithms of these numbers represent an estimate of the relative level of period fertility for that period when the cohort was at its mean age of fertility. The average error of this estimate is 2 percent. As a basis for comparison, the average error, if cohort total

Table 7. Components of Change in Fertility: Quantity (Q) and Tempo (T) of Nuptiality (N) and Marital Parity (P), expressed in natural logarithms of ratios, x 10,000, c.1893-1943

1893-95	*Q*	*T*	*Q+T*	*1916-20*	*Q*	*T*	*Q+T*
N	− 355	+ 678	+ 323	N	+ 69	+1135	+1204
P	+1426	− 455	+ 971	P	−1116	− 646	−1762
N+P	+1071	+ 223	+1294	N+P	−1047	+ 489	− 558
1896-00	*Q*	*T*	*Q+T*	*1921-25*	*Q*	*T*	*Q+T*
N	− 310	− 277	− 587	N	+ 158	+1127	+1285
P	+ 398	+ 360	+ 758	P	− 242	+ 89	+ 153
N+P	+ 88	+ 83	+ 171	N+P	− 84	+1216	+1132
1901-05	*Q*	*T*	*Q+T*	*1926-30*	*Q*	*T*	*Q+T*
N	− 326	+ 205	− 121	N	+ 224	+ 743	+ 967
P	− 455	− 802	−1257	P	+ 547	+ 957	+1504
N+P	− 781	− 597	−1378	N+P	+ 771	+1700	+2471
1906-10	*Q*	*T*	*Q+T*	*1931-35*	*Q*	*T*	*Q+T*
N	− 211	− 157	− 368	N	+ 399	+ 247	+ 646
P	−1457	−1482	−2939	P	+1563	+ 597	+2160
N+P	−1668	−1639	−3309	N+P	+1962	+ 844	+2806
1911-15	*Q*	*T*	*Q+T*	*1936-38*	*Q*	*T*	*Q+T*
N	− 42	+ 435	+ 393	N	+ 421	− 20	+ 401
P	−1594	−1075	−2669	P	+1774	− 184	+1590
N+P	−1636	− 640	−2276	N+P	+2195	− 204	+1991
				1939-43	*Q*	*T*	*Q+T*
				N	+ 201	− 564	− 363
				P	+1136	− 882	+ 254
				N+P	+1337	−1446	− 109

fertility rates had been used without an adjustment for the consequences of tempo change, would have been 8 percent. The estimates are extraordinarily good for c.1916-43, for which the error is less than one-half of 1 percent. This is a most encouraging finding because it provides some support for the admittedly hazardous estimates for c.1939-43 and therefore for assertions about the contemporary situation.

The first observations about the results of Table 7 are directed at the four time series for the individual components: QN, TN, TP and QP. The first of these, QN (consequences of changes in the quantity of nuptiality) follows an almost linear path from small negative values for the earlier cohort groups to small positive values for the latter. The other three components, on the contrary, have a cyclical character. TN (consequences of changes in the tempo of nuptiality) declines from +678 to −277, then rises to +1135, and finally declines to −564. TP (consequences of changes in the tempo of marital parity) declines from −455 to −1482, then rises to +957, and finally declines to −882. QP (consequences of changes in the quantity of marital parity) declines from +1426 to −1594, then rises to +1774, and finally declines to +1136. The amplitude of the fluctuation is least for TN and greatest for QP. Furthermore the cycles for these three components, TN, TP and QP, are arranged in staggered fashion. The early troughs for TN, TP and QP respectively are located in c.1896-1900, c.1906-10, and c.1911-15 respectively; the later peaks are located in c.1916-20, c.1926-30 and c.1936-38 respectively.

Observations comparable to those in the preceding paragraph I have not seen elsewhere; they prompt some speculation. It would appear that the succession of depression and then prosperity, which has so noticeably marked the events of this era, produced a response first in the tempo of nuptiality, then in the tempo of marital parity and finally in the quantity of marital parity, and each response was larger than the one before it. This sequence is suggestive of a decision strategy for meeting a new situation: the response with the least consequences, a change in the time of marriage, is the first undertaken; that with the greatest consequences, a change in the number of children, is the last undertaken. Also a postponement of birth, if extended long enough, becomes a termination; and a preponement of birth is likely to lead to an increase in eventual quantity.

The form of Table 7 makes it possible to evaluate the relative importance of the components cohort by cohort. The sub-table for c.1893-95 is dominated by a large positive QP. For c.1896-1900 the components are small and counterbalancing. TP exerts a strong negative influence over c.1901-15; QP exerts a strong negative influence over c.1906-20; TN exerts a strong positive influence over c.1916-30. The minimum cohort group is that for c.1906-10: all of the components are negative, and both QP and TP are very large. Similarly the cohorts which are the highest in net overall assessment, c.1926-35, are those for which all components are positive, particularly TP for the former and QP for the latter.

Table 7 is particularly interesting for the light it may shed on the recent decline in fertility. The sources of moderate decline from c.1931-35 to c.1936-38 are TN and TP, both of which changed from moderate positive to small negative values, and counterbalanced a continuing high positive QP. For the contemporary cohort group, c.1939-43, there has been an easing of the quantity components but the principal reason for the overall component sum becoming negative once again is the change in tempo, for both nuptiality and marital parity. Thus we would assert on the basis of Table 7 that the reason for the decline of the birth rate from 1957 to 1966 has been a reversal of tempo (rising in place of falling mean ages) both for marriages and for births within marriage, followed by a small decline in the quantity of nuptiality and marital parity.

It is evident from the above that any assertions about the relative importance, for temporal variations in period fertility, of movements of quantity and tempo (or of nuptiality and marital parity) would depend very much on which phase of the history was being discussed. Nevertheless, to provide a kind of average assessment for the era under observation, I have calculated the mean absolute deviation for each component, for c.1893-1938. Of the absolute deviations contributed by quantity and by tempo respectively, 57 percent are quantity and 43 percent are tempo. For nuptiality separately the split is 19 percent quantity and 81 percent tempo; for marital parity separately, the split is 58 percent quantity and 42 percent tempo. Thus quantity is only a little more important than tempo in terms of influence on the level of period fertility, both overall and with respect to marital parity in particular. For nuptiality alone, changes in tempo are much more significant than changes in quantity.

Looking at the system of data from the opposite direction, of the absolute deviations contributed by nuptiality and by marital parity, 29 percent derive from nuptiality and 71 percent from marital parity. For timing separately, nuptiality contributes 44 percent of the deviations; for quantity separately it contributes only 19 percent of the deviations.

It would seem unlikely that a future balance sheet of components of period fertility would show a similar distribution of influence. In particular, the advance of effective fertility regulation is likely to emphasize in general the role of tempo variations relative to quantity variations, and in particular the role of the tempo of marital parity relative to that of nuptiality.

Concluding Comments

Although most of the measurements presented in the foregoing have a satisfying basis in reality, those which are of the most immediate interest because they pertain to the state of contemporary fertility are the data of the most dubious validity. Without denying the possibility of further improvement in measurement techniques, it seems clear that the essential requirement for confidence in the analysis of the behavior of the present is the continuing infusion of new data made possible by the passage of time. No methodological trickery can permit escape from the circumstance that women may bear children over a long span of time. It seems useful, nevertheless, to suggest what the shape of the future would look like if present patterns of change were to persist.

The interpretation of the trend in the cohort total fertility rate depends in the first instance on the time perspective with which the series is viewed and on the perceived depth of the trough associated with the depression. It is true that, even with a long view, the TFR for c.1936-40 exceeds that for c.1891-95 by 10 percent. Nevertheless a substantial part of that margin is attributable to an increase in the total nuptiality rate—and further increase in that component is highly unlikely. The small residual rise in mean marital parity is revealed by further decomposition to have been based on an unrepeatable development—the virtual disappearance of those remaining in parities 0 and 1 by choice. Examination of the progression ratios for parities 3+ reveals a persistent downward drift; indeed it is not implausible that our anachronistic large families might gradually vanish altogether. Accordingly, unless there is an increase in the progression ratio for parity 2—a development not suggested by the available data—the clear implication is that the cohort total fertility rate will experience secular decline, although there are no data suggesting that this would proceed to a sub-replacement level.

We appear to have arrived close to the end of an era of quantitative adjustment of the parity distribution to the exigencies of the modern world. Although there may be no overriding reason for anticipating a cessation of normative innovation, either in reproductive ends or in the means to achieve them, there appears to be no evidence on hand to suggest anything but a consolidation of the already clearly defined outlines of the modern fertility pattern.

With regard to the tempo of cohort fertility, we have observed a downward movement of the (standardized) mean age of fertility— the kind of change which buoys up the birth level from year to year. Although there is no intrinsic foundation for predicting a cessation of the decline in the age at marriage, it certainly seems to be a likely accompaniment of a rising age of leaving school, as well as of the increasing protection against premarital conception which is provided by modern contraceptives. The latter should also permit more success in the planned delay of marital fertility. In sum, the expectation is that the mean age of nuptiality will stop declining, the mean duration of marital fertility will begin to rise, and thus that the mean age of fertility will experience a trend reversal and rise. The consequence for period fertility will be a downward distortion, so long as the upward direction of the mean age is maintained.

Thus, from a standpoint of perceptible trends in quantity and in tempo—with the aid of component analysis—it seems likely that there will be downward pressure on period fertility. But I think it improbable that these forces will be as consequential as unforeseen transitory phenomena. The future of fertility is likely to be increasingly bound up with questions of fluctuation rather than of trend. The history of the past 50 years is a demonstration of the considerable capacity for response to temporarily unfavorable or favorable economic conditions; such responsiveness should be markedly enhanced in the future. Although some part of the recent drop in the birth rate seems attributable to the observed long-run trends in quantity and tempo, my impression is that most of it has transitory origins. If my diagnosis of a future characterized by predominance of fluctuation over trend is a correct one, the implication for research is that we should devote a large part of our attention to the determinants and consequences of the changing tempo of cohort fertility.

NOTES

1. The parameters for the earliest cohorts are more substantially based than those for the latest cohorts, because estimates of their cumulative fertility up to the beginning of 1917, based on census fertility data, are provided in the cohort fertility tables.

2. I hope to pursue the question of optimal forecasting strategies in a subsequent article.

3. See Appendix II. I have a research project under way which should permit some improvement over the measurements used here.

4. Despite its unfamiliarity, I have settled on the word "tempo" as a terse designation of the observed time pattern of marriage rates or birth rates. The words "spacing" and "timing" are more common, but they are unsatisfactory because they imply rather more volition than is appropriate for most couples.

5. This is more commonly known as the proportion ever-married by age 50. Such a definition is awkward because it is self-contradictory. I have provided the new name, total nuptiality rate, because of its precise parallelism with the now-familiar total fertility rate. Even though many of the marriages which occur in the later years of the reproductive age

span will not be fertile, it is convenient to use the same age limits for TNR as for TFR.

6. The definition of mean marital parity contains an inference that all women who bear children marry at least once. It is obvious from illegitimacy data that many bear children before they marry—if they marry. Given the circumstance that the data summarized in the TNR are self-reports, the assumption is that all women who have borne a child report that they have been married.

7. Calculation of parity variance requires an assumption about the distribution of births in orders eighth and higher; the procedure is described in Appendix III.

8. The highest values in the column for parity zero, 952 and 971, are considered to be implausibly high. The source of the error may be a tendency for women to report higher order births as first births, perhaps partly because of the death of their firstborn.

9. Note, however, that, even if the PPRs for parities 3+ were to vanish—meaning no births of higher than third order—the consequent TFR of 2.39 would still be sufficient to guarantee population replacement.

10. The normal distribution has a kurtosis of zero. For successively higher orders of birth, skewness declines from somewhat larger to somewhat smaller positive values and the distributions shift from moderately leptokurtic to moderately platykurtic. Both of these are reflections of the tendency for birth rates at each higher order to display the consequences of a progressively greater overlapping of family life cycles.

11. The details are presented in Appendix IV. I am currently experimenting with a different approach which attempts to make maximum use of the data on the age distributions of birth rates by order.

12. See Appendix IV.

Appendices

I. Sources of Birth Data

The first step in the computation program was production of a three-dimensional table, R(I,J,K), the age-specific order-specific cohort-specific central birth rates for 36 ages (I = 14, 49), for 8 orders (J = 1, 8+), for 55 cohorts (K = 1891, 1945). These are fiscal cohorts: their birth dates are centered on January 1 of the year used to identify the cohort. The rate for age x for the cohort born in year t-x is assumed to be identical with the rate for age x in year t.

The principal source of birth rates is the following: Pascal K. Whelpton and Arthur A. Campbell, "Fertility Tables for Birth Cohorts of American Women, Part 1," National Office of Vital Statistics, *Vital Statistics—Special Reports*, Vol. 51, No. 1, January 29, 1960. This covers the experience of years 1917-57 inclusive; an extension of these tables for years 1958-64 inclusive is contained in the 1964 edition of *Vital Statistics*. For that part of the experience of c.1891-1902 which preceded the beginning of 1917, the former source provides cumulative birth rates by order by cohort as of the age reached by 1917. I distributed these sums by age on the assumption that the distribution was the same, order by order, as that for c.1903-07 (the first five cohorts for which a complete age-specific record exists).

To extend the series forward through 1965 and 1966 I used quinquennial age-specific birth rates for 1965, and a provisional estimate of total births for 1966, supplied by Arthur A. Campbell, National Center for Health Statistics. Rates for single ages for all births in 1965 were estimated by comparing birth rates for quinquennial age groups in 1964 and 1965, and adjusting for changing size of birth cohort—a currently important factor with respect to the youngest fertile ages. I assumed that the proportional change in the birth rates based on provisional totals for 1965 and 1966 was the same as that for the final birth rates. The total fertility rate for 1966 was estimated by assuming that the decline in the ratio of the total fertility rate to the crude birth rate over 1962-65 continued through 1966. Single-age birth rates for 1966 were obtained by assuming that the ratio of the total fertility rates for 1965 and 1966 applied to each individual age. To convert the all-order birth rates in each age in 1965 and 1966 respectively into order-specific rates, I assumed that the proportion in each order of the birth rate for each age changed linearly over 1963-64-65 and 1962-64-66 respectively.

The final task was to estimate the experience of the younger cohorts subsequent to the beginning of 1967 (and prior to exact age 50). I assumed that the rate for each age and order would move from its 1966 value to a value for 1976 which corresponded with the mean corrected value for the cohorts in the same age and order in the period 1950-57, and would remain constant beyond 1976. For the path of change I fitted a cubic, on the additional assumptions that the time slope in 1966 was that of the period 1962-66 and that the time slope in 1976 was zero. The 1950-57 period was chosen as a standard because it was the most recent period during which there was monotonic change in the birth rates by age within each order. The correction mentioned was designed to remove the upward distortion occasioned by changes in the tempo of fertility; the method was a straightforward adaptation of the formula presented in the second paragraph of Section III above.

II. Sources of Marriage Data

My aim was to construct a table of rates of (first) marriage, for ages 14-49, and for cohorts 1891-1945, i.e., comparable in form with those for order-specific birth rates. The basic source was Volume PC(2) 4D, *Age at First Marriage, 1960 Census*, Table 2. This gives the numbers of women ever-married, by age at first marriage and age at census date. Given the proportions of all women ever-married, by age, production of a table of first marriage rates by age for each cohort was straightforward. Interpolation provided the required estimates for fiscal cohorts on the basis of the cohorts which were ages 15-69 at census date. In cases where the census table did not provide single ages, interpolation across age groups was accomplished by using estimates of the age distribution of cohort marriages, prepared by Arthur A. Campbell while at Scripps Foundation.

To extend the table beyond 1960 I used the *Current Population Reports*, P-20 Series; these provided the proportions ever-married, by age groups for March, 1960-66. In the younger age groups the proportions ever-married change rapidly from age to age, and the cohort size has been changing rapidly recently. I corrected for this by using routine standardization procedures. In the higher ages I smoothed the data for each age group for successive years, to eliminate what was presumably sampling variability. To extrapolate marriage rates beyond 1966 I used the same procedure as for birth rates.

These marriage data are imperfect in several ways. The census tabulation could provide information only for survivors, and these would presumably be selected in ways relevant for age at marriage. I think that error from this source is small, because survivorship is high over the relevant ages and for the relevant time period. Nevertheless my table should be revised when better data become available. A good source of information about necessary corrections would be a duplicate for 1970 of the census table used. This would also yield some information relevant to a second difficulty: relative recall by age. A third problem with the data is that some women reported as ever-married have not experienced a marriage ceremony, while some reported as never-married have done so. Thus the data used are self-definitions, although not for that reason alone less valuable in analysis than records restricted to legal marriage.

III. Measures for the Highest Orders

Given birth rates for orders 1, 2, . . . , 7, 8+, the highest progression ratio which can be calculated in the conventional way is that for parity 6 (the ratio of the 7th to the 6th birth rate). Since this would leave unexploited some relevant information (the combined birth rate for orders 8+), I have devised the following procedure:

Assume that the parity progression ratios for parities 7, 8, . . . , $= R$. Then the rate for orders 8+, $B(8+) = B(7) \times R + B(7) \times R^2 + \ldots = B(7) \times R/(1 - R)$, and $R = B(8+)/(B(7)+B(8+))$. Thus R is the (geometric) mean of parity progression ratios for parities 7+. This is the value reported in the right-hand column of Table 3, and used in calculating parity variance, and so forth.

Following a similar logic, I assumed that the differences between the mean ages of 7th and 8th births, of 8th and 9th births, and so forth, were equal to d. Then the mean age for 8th births, $A(8) = A(7) +d$, and so forth. Since the mean age for 8+ births, $A(8+)$, is the sum over $J = 8, \ldots,$ of $B(J) \times A(J)/B(8+)$, and we have assumed values for $B(J)$ and $A(J)$, we solve for $d = (A(8+) - A(7)) \times (1 - R)$. The estimates for $A(8)$, $A(9)$, and so forth, follow.

IV. Estimation of Birth Intervals

It is obvious that the mean interval between a Jth and a J+1th birth is not $A(J+1) - A(J)$, because some of those who have a Jth birth do not have a J+1th birth, and their age at the time of their Jth birth is likely to differ from that of those who do. Suppose $A'(J)$ and $A''(J)$ are the ages at Jth birth for those who do and those who do not have a J+1th birth. Then:

$$A(J+1) - A'(J) = A(J+1) - A(J) + (1 - R) \times (A''(J) - A'(J))$$

where R is the relevant parity progression ratio. If we assume that $A''(J) = A(J+1)$ then the required birth interval is $(A(J+1) - A(J))/R$.

The estimated birth intervals are presented in Table 8.

Table 8. Estimated birth intervals, Orders 1-8*, c.1881-1945

Cohort	1	2	3	4	5	6	7	8
1881-85								1.50
1886-90				2.33	2.28	2.08	1.92	1.44
1891-95		3.13	2.76	2.39	2.35	2.06	1.78	1.51
1896-00	−0.02	3.31	2.74	2.30	2.44	2.00	1.89	1.55
1901-05	−0.08	3.52	2.89	2.39	2.43	2.06	2.09	1.51
1906-10	0.63	3.90	3.06	2.24	2.11	1.84	1.96	1.43
1911-15	1.26	4.03	3.30	2.22	1.89	1.62	1.63	1.35
1916-20	1.46	3.87	3.62	2.61	1.95	1.62	1.48	1.27
1921-25	1.51	3.56	3.77	2.93	2.18	1.72	1.29	1.28
1926-30	1.41	3.01	3.46	2.86	2.25	1.83	1.47	1.40
1931-35	1.11	2.62	3.14	2.73	2.16	1.86	1.73	
1936-40	0.98	2.69	3.15					
1941-45	1.07							
Total								
Change	+1.08	−0.45	+0.40	+0.40	−0.12	−0.23	−0.19	−0.11
Peak	+1.00	+1.10	+0.75	+0.28	+0.19	+0.05	+0.23	+0.09

*For method of calculating highest interval, see Appendix III.

Table 8 has the same staggered character as Table 3, and for the same reason. The first observation about the table is a disconcerting one: two of the entries in the left-hand column are negative. These are suspect data: the component parts for this column come from different sources, one of which (marriages) might very well be unreliable, particularly for earlier cohorts; furthermore, the estimating procedure may be less valid for the first interval than for the others. But the negative intervals are not inherently false. Marriage is neither a necessary nor a sufficient predecessor of a first birth. Many first births are illegitimate (and many more arrive an embarrassingly short time after the wedding). We are prepared to defend the indication that the interval between marriage and first birth rose sharply between c.1896-00 and c.1921-25, without saying how sharply.

The pattern of intervals by order within each cohort has plausibility to it: the longest intervals are those preceding the second birth (in the earlier cohorts) and the third birth (in the later cohorts); with successively higher orders the intervals decrease, sharply at first and then more gradually. Some such variation would be expected as a consequence of the progressive selection with each higher order—

selection both for fecundity and for non-regulation of fertility. This patterning gives us a little confidence in our estimating procedure.

As in Table 3 above we have provided two summary rows: "Total change," a comparison of the first and last values in each column; and "Peak," the maximum deviation of the observations in the column above the straight line drawn from the first to the last observation. (It is presumed that a peak in the interval series is the equivalent of a trough in the parity progression ratio series.) In an approximate way the set of change values for the various orders are patterned: positive for the lower intervals and negative for the higher intervals. This would be a reasonable eventuality from a pattern of increasing dissemination of fertility control: those who confine their childbearing to the lower orders are also likely to be the most able to postpone their births, and vice versa. Likewise there is pattern to the order structure of the peaks: major delays are evident in the lower but not in the higher orders.

For one of the intervals, that preceding the second birth, the total change shows a negative slope, in contrast to positive slopes for its neighbors. My first inclination was to take this observation at face value and devise a post factum interpretation. Thus a shorter interval between first and second may have come to be considered desirable, as part of a plan for the age structure of the children. For earlier cohorts the longer interval may be associated with the lower parity progression ratios, noted in Table 3 above; perhaps in addition to those who did succeed in preventing a second birth were those who tried, lengthened their interval in the process, but failed eventually.

But reproductive phenomena are so neatly structured in so many ways that I suspect that the negative "change" for the interval between first and second is an artifact, and that it has the same roots as the problem which led to the negative intervals in the first column. These two column share one piece of information—the mean age at first birth—and it is this datum that I am now inclined to suspect. Notice that the sum of the first two columns (bypassing the dating of first births) would give a combined interval of 3.29 for c.1896-00 and of 3.73 for c.1931-35, and thus an increase of 0.44, in comparison with an increase of 0.40 for the next interval and of 0.34 for the next after that (for the same pair of cohort groups). And we already know that there is something wrong with first birth data: for some cohort groups the progression ratio for parity zero is impossibly high. (See Table 3.) Accordingly I conclude that there is a problem with the second as well as the first column of Table 8, and that it is more likely to lie with the cohort fertility data for first births (used in both columns) than with either the nuptiality data or the estimating procedure.

One further reservation is necessary concerning Table 8. The three highest intervals have shown a recent tendency to increase, contrary to the expectation that progressive selection would continue to force them down. This is an artifactual result. I adopted the same mode of projection for birth rates of all orders, viz., constancy at the 1950-57 cohort level. For the higher orders a much more realistic assumption would be decline; this would give lower mean ages for these orders with successively later cohorts, and consequently shorter intervals than those displayed in Table 8.

V. Components of Period Fertility

The basic equation for the period total fertility rate (the period being the time at which the cohort in question is at its mean age of fertility) is $(TFR) \times (1 - MAF')$. Now $TFR = TNR \times MMP$, to separate quantity of nuptiality and quantity of marital parity. Also TFR/MU $(TFR) = TNR/MU(TNR) \times MMP/MU(MMP)$, where MU for each parameter is the all-cohort mean. Also $(1 - MAF') = (1 - MAN') \times$ $(1 - MAF')/(1 - MAN')$ to separate tempo of nuptiality and tempo of marital parity. Furthermore $(1 - MAF') = (1 - (MAF - MAX)')$ $\times (1 - MAF')/(1 - (MAF - MAX)')$ to separate movements of MAF attributable to changes of TFR from those attributable to changes of MAX. Thus the ratio of the period TFR to the all-cohort mean is: $(TNR/MU(TNR)) \times (MMP/MU(MMP)) \times (1 - (MAF - MAX)') \times (1 - MAN') \times ((1 - MAF')/((1 - (MAF - MAX)') \times (1 - MAN'))$. By taking natural logarithms we obtain the following: $QN = \ln(TNR/MU(TNR))$; $QP = \ln(MMP/MU(MMP)) + \ln(1 - (MAF - MAX)')$; $TN = \ln(1 - MAN')$; and $TP = \ln(1 - MAF') - \ln(1 - (MAF - MAX)') - \ln(1 - MAN')$, where QN, QP, TN, and TP are the effects on period fertility of the quantity (Q) and tempo (T) of nuptiality (N) and marital parity (P).

II. CAUSES AND CONSEQUENCES OF FERTILITY TRENDS

TOWARDS A SOCIOECONOMIC THEORY OF FERTILITY: A SURVEY OF RECENT RESEARCH ON ECONOMIC FACTORS IN AMERICAN FERTILITY[*]

Richard A. Easterlin

University of Pennsylvania

Economics is all about how people make choices. Sociology is all about why they don't have any choices to make.[1]

THE ORIGINAL AIM of this paper is denoted by the subtitle. As the paper progressed, however, it became increasingly clear that economists and sociologists engaged in demographic research were largely talking past each other. Too often, sociologists view the economic theory of fertility as simply an argument for the effect of income on behavior. On the other hand, economists have substantially ignored factors emphasized in sociology, such as education, religion, farm background, and so on. The reason for this lack of communication seems to be the absence of a commonly accepted analytical framework embracing the variety of factors considered in both disciplines and making clear their interrelations. Hence, Part I of this paper is concerned with this task.

The key to Part I is the epigraph. The basic organizing framework is the economic theory of household choice. Economics is given this central role, not I hope out of undue disciplinary loyalty on my part, but because historically, the systematic study of choice has been one of the foremost concerns of economic theory. In principle, this theory has room under the topic of "tastes" for the constraints on choice emphasized in sociology, but it must be admitted that in prac-

[*] I am indebted to conversations with my colleagues William M. Evan and Ralph Ginsburg in sociology, and Edwin Burmeister and David M. O'Neill in economics. I am grateful too for comments by Gary S. Becker, David M. Heer, Edgar M. Hoover, Jacob Mincer, and Julian L. Simon. Work on this paper was supported in part by National Science Foundation Grant GS-1563.

tice, little recognition has been given to such factors. Hence, the first requisite for a "socioeconomic" theory of fertility would seem to be the elevation of "taste" considerations bearing on choice to a position equal to that of other factors. This is a central thesis of the first part.

Until some reasonably common grounds for discourse can be established, a survey and appraisal of the type for which this paper was commissioned is likely to be largely futile. Hence the theoretical discussion in Part I is rather extended, perhaps unduly so to some. Of the various needs for research, however, such discussion is, in my view, the foremost one, though that offered here is at best only a step in this direction.

Part II then proceeds to the original aim of the paper, a review of postwar research on economic factors in American fertility. It is guided by the framework developed in Part I, and the emphasis reflects the views expressed there. It is suggested that there are developments pointing to the evolution of a more unified approach, and these are therefore given special attention.

I. Theory

The basic view adopted here is that fertility behavior is the result of household choices, in which resources are weighed against preferences. In the economic theory of household behavior, consumers with given tastes are viewed as maximizing utility subject to the constraints of income and prices. Thus three factors—income, tastes, and prices—are the basic building blocks for study of household behavior.

The pioneering application of this framework to fertility behavior is Gary S. Becker's well-known article[2] which provides the point of departure for the present discussion. As in Becker's treatment, household choices on fertility matters are seen as arising from the interaction between preferences on the one hand and income and price constraints on the other. However, as a result of theoretical developments since this article, developments to which Becker himself has made fundamental contributions, the relevant concepts of income and prices call for further discussion. In addition, more explicit attention is needed to taste phenomena. Finally, fertility control behavior, which occupies a rather anomalous position in Becker's theory, needs to be assimilated to the theory of consumer choice.[3]

Income—There has been growing recognition in recent years that observed income at a point in time may not be a valid representation of the income concept relevant to household decisions. Particularly on items involving substantial outlays, decisions are geared to the longer term income prospects of the household, to its "permanent income" level, as it has been termed by Milton Friedman.[4] The relation of observed to permanent income varies with the shape of the prospective income stream and because cyclical or irregular factors occasion deviations from the prospective path.

The permanent income concept can be viewed as emphasizing that it is the *potential* income flow *through time* that is pertinent to household decision-making, and that observed income may be an unreliable proxy for this. To minimize multiplication of concepts, I propose to embrace the permanent income notion in that of "potential" income. There is a second dimension to potential income, however. Even if there were no difference between prospective annual income and that currently observed, the potential income of a household would exceed its observed income, for the simple reason that typically money income is foregone in order to have time for other pursuits. Observed income may be an unreliable index of potential income because it inadequately reflects not only prospective earnings through time, but foregone earnings at a point in time as well.

The income concept relevant to the decision-making process is potential income. Moreover, this magnitude together with the relevant price and taste variables, determines not only fertility, but also the amount of market labor done by the household members and even observed income itself. Demographers have often expressed doubts about attributing cause-effect significance, one way or the other, to the observed inverse association between fertility and wife's labor force participation. Similar reservations may attach to that between fertility and observed income, except where the latter is a valid index of potential income. To illustrate the point, consider two examples:

> *Case 1* (tastes differ, potential incomes and relative prices identical): Households A and B have equal possibilities for earning money income in the market place. A, however, is interested only in money income; B, in other sources of satisfaction as well, among them, children and leisure. The first household devotes all its time to earning income.[5] For this household, observed income equals potential income. The second household sacrifices some money income because the utility of increments of leisure and/or children exceeds that of the money income foregone. How much it sacrifices depends on the strength of its desires for leisure and/or children relative to goods, and the relative price of the latter. Compared with the first household, the second has traded money income for leisure and/or children. The equilibrium value of observed income of the household is as much a product of the basic determinants—potential income, relative desires, and relative prices—as are leisure (alternatively, the amount worked in the market place) and the number of children. From the inverse

association between *observed* income and fertility for the two households, one might infer that higher income caused lower fertility; actually, the cause of both the fertility and income differences was different tastes.

Case 2 (potential incomes differ, tastes and prices identical): In households C and D, the earnings possibilities of husbands are identical but that of the wife in household C much exceeds that of the wife in household D. (The wife in C, say, is a remedial reading tutor who can earn in 8 hours work on Saturday what the wife in D earns in 40 hours.) Hence the potential income of household C exceeds that of D. In household D, the wife works 40 hours and has no children; in household C, the wife works 8 hours in the market place and raises a family. Money incomes are the same, but fertility differs because potential income differs.[6]

These examples make clear that cross-section associations between fertility and current income may be of dubious causal significance.[7] The income concept for which an estimate is needed should take account of the potentials represented by the earnings capacity of the wife (and other household members) and prospective changes in the income stream over time. However, in time series analysis, current income observations, though defective with regard to level, may be indicative of changes in potential income. Thus, use of current income may be more justifiable in time series, though even here its appropriateness needs to be carefully examined.

Relative Prices—The first issue to be considered under this head is whether the prices pertinent to decisions regarding children are properly approximated by actual expenditures per child. It is sometimes argued, for example, that the fact that the rich spend more per child than the poor is indicative of the operation of a differential, higher price constraint, adverse to fertility.[8] This argument has been effectively countered by Becker,[9] and I can do little more than amplify his argument by some illustrations.

Clearly, differences in observed *expenditures* per child do not necessarily reflect differences in the set of prices constraining household choices, because expenditures contain both price and quantity components. If household incomes or tastes differ, then expenditures per child can vary even if the price tag attached to each potentially relevant quantity is the same for all households, simply because different quantities may be purchased. Consider the following:

Case 3 (tastes and *prices* identical, incomes differ): Households E and F have identical tastes and are confronted with the same set of prices, but the potential income of household E is much higher. (For example, E and F are former college roommates following identical careers, but E unexpectedly falls heir to a large financial estate.) Household E not only has more children than F, but also spends more money per child, educating each, for example, in private schools rather than in the tuition-free public schools to which F sends its children. From observed expenditures per child, one would infer that E had more children *despite* the pressure of a severer price constraint. Actually, in making their decisions, both households were confronted with the same prices, but household E chose to have more children and spend more per child because its income was considerably higher than that of F.

Case 4 (income and prices identical, tastes differ): Households G and H have the same potential income and are faced with the same prices. Both households desire both children and education for their children. However, household G is, say, Jewish, and places a greater premium on education, while household H is Catholic and places relatively more emphasis on having a large family. Household G, therefore, has fewer children and spends more per child than household H. From observed expenditures per child, one might infer that G had fewer children because it was confronted with a relatively higher price for children. Actually, both households were faced with the same prices, but household G behaved differently because of different tastes.

These examples suffice to show that while variations among households in expenditures per child could conceivably reflect differences in the prices households face, they could also be due to differences in incomes or tastes, prices remaining constant. Actually, it seems that there has been a tendency to infer that expenditure differences imply price differences, when they really reflect variations in tastes. Thus, defending Leibenstein against Becker, Duesenberry observes:

> Becker has taken the occasion to correct the simple-minded who fail to distinguish between the cost of children of given quality and expenditure per child. . . . But not all of those who say that the cost of children rises with income are so simple-minded as Becker suggests. . . . What Leibenstein, for example, appears to mean is that the expenditure per child *which the parents consider to be necessary* rises with income.
>
> .   .   .   .
>
> Becker assumes that any couple considers itself free to choose any combination it wishes of numbers of children and expenditure per child (*prices of particular goods and services being given*). I submit that a sociologist would take the view that given

the education level, occupation, region, and a few other factors, most couples would consider that they have a very narrow range of choice [italicizing added].[10]

As the last paragraph makes abundantly clear, Duesenberry is here arguing about the influence on behavior not of prices but of taste-shaping factors such as education and occupation. This is not a mere theoretical quibble, for confusion about the proper concept of price can result in a mistaken representation in empirical research of the price variable relevant to fertility decisions. For example, from the upward trend in expenditures per child in the U.S. since 1940, one might infer that there has been a steady downward pressure on fertility. This trend, however, may reflect largely the influence of rising income. Whether the relative prices of the items potentially relevant to children have moved in a manner adverse to fertility is far from clear.

Recently a quite different argument, one not involving the above confusion, has been advanced to suggest that the prices relevant to fertility do vary cross-sectionally directly with income. This view, put forward by Jacob Mincer,[11] stresses that the appropriate prices include not only those of goods and services directly required for childbearing and rearing, but also the imputed price of the time required in this activity.[12] Mincer argues that the appropriate price to impute to this time is the opportunity cost of the wife, that is, her potential earnings in the market place. The higher the wife's potential earnings, the higher the price of a child. An important corollary of this reasoning is that a change in a wife's potential earnings tends to affect fertility decisions through two different channels and in opposite directions. On the one hand, a rise in the wife's earnings possibilities raises the potential income of the family and thereby tends to affect fertility positively; on the other, it increases the price of children, by raising the opportunity cost of child care, and thus tends to discourage fertility. Mincer attempts to estimate the relative strength of the two effects, termed in economic analysis, respectively, income and substitution effects, and concludes that the adverse substitution effect tends to outweigh the favorable income effect. He suggests also that since wife's and husband's earning possibilities tend to be positively correlated, failure to allow for this price influence biases downward estimates based on cross-section data of the effect of income on fertility, more so when the family's than when the husband's income is used.

The time that will be required in childbearing and raising is obviously relevant to fertility decisions, but it is not clear that the best price to attach to this time is the potential earnings of the wife, for some, perhaps a substantial proportion of the work of child care may be performed by domestic help. A wife with a high earning potential who is contemplating a child would not necessarily assess the cost of child care in terms of earnings she must forego, but at least in part at the price of pertinent service. In a situation where another family member is available for this work, it is his opportunity cost that is relevant. Conceivably, this might approach zero, as, for example, in the case of an elderly relative. The same would be true of public provision of free day nurseries. Assessing the bearing of these considerations on higher versus lower income households, one might infer that they would probably yield an association between price and income of the same (positive) direction, though not magnitude, as Mincer had found when valuing the time required for child care at the wife's opportunity cost. Thus his conclusion would still be relevant regarding the biased nature of inferences regarding the cross-section association between income and fertility that fail to allow for this, even though his proxy for the price variable does not seem wholly defensible.

Tastes—Perhaps the greatest obstacle so far to development of a unified socioeconomic theory of fertility, and, correspondingly, the most promising opportunity for advance, lies in the subject of tastes. To most economists, explanation of behavior in terms of tastes is anathema.[13] In contrast, the principal emphasis of sociology is on the tendency of behavior to conform to "social norms," the conceptual embodiment of preferences. Each discipline can benefit from the other's approach. The economist has much to learn from the sociologist regarding the *formation* of tastes. At the same time, the sociologist may benefit from the economist's conception of the *nature* of tastes. Let me develop these points with reference to fertility analysis.

With regard to the nature of tastes, the economist conceives of a preference field or map, embracing all possible combinations of goods, i.e. satisfaction-yielding objects. Attached to each combination is a subjective evaluation of its worth in terms of satisfaction to the household. Ideally, empirical inquiry would seek to map such preference fields, though little research has yet been done along these lines, partly because of the cost, and partly the general neglect of this area by economists.[14] Nevertheless, the conception itself has some useful implications for current fertility research on preferences.[15]

First, with regard to any given good, households do not necessarily desire a single fixed amount; rather, they consider a variety of alternatives ordered in terms of prospective satisfaction. A survey question oriented toward a single-valued answer, such as "housing preference" or "desired family size" would presumably elicit a response relating to some point on this continuum, but exactly where is hard to say. Such a response would undoubtedly be colored to some extent by subjective consideration of resource constraints. For example, an individual might specify a $20,000 suburban home as his housing preference and subsequently purchase a $60,000 one because of an unexpected inheritance. Nevertheless, given limited resources for eliciting preference information, responses to a single valued question may be useful as indicating differences or changes in preference fields, though such responses clearly are not necessarily statements of quantity compatible with maximum possible satisfaction.[16]

The other important implication of the economist's conception of tastes is that they are relative not absolute in nature. Tastes are not "either-or," but "more or less." Typically, households do not want either A or B. Rather they desire both A and B, and a certain combination of less A and more B may leave them just as satisfied as an alternative of more A and less B. The subjective rate at which a household is willing to "trade-off" A for B (technically, the marginal rate of substitution) is variable, but the important point is that such subjective trade-offs do exist, and hence even a household with a strong B-bias may, if the terms of trade are favorable, give up some B for A and consider itself better off.[17]

It follows that the strength of a household's desire for any given good, say, children, must be evaluated in the context of its attitudes toward other goods. Consider two households each of which reports the same desired family size. Does it follow that their preferences are the same? Suppose attitudes of the two households are explored with regard to objects of expenditure which compete with children—a new home or additions to the present one, recreation (foreign travel, purchase of a summer home or boat), purchase of a business, education of children, leisure, and so on—and that the first household evinces desires in this regard consistently in excess of those of the second. Clearly, then, the *relative* preference for children is less for the first than the second household. Given the same income constraint and price configuration, one would expect a difference in fertility behavior despite identical statements as to family size desires. Similarly, over time, one cannot infer from constancy of responses on desired family size that preferences have not changed. If the strength of preferences for other goods has grown, then the relative desire for children has diminished, and this would make for lower fertility, given the same income and price constraints. It follows that empirical research on family size preferences, even if based on a single-valued concept, should not be confined to a fertility dimension alone, but should include, in addition, attitudes toward goods competing with children for the household's resources.

To turn to the formation of tastes, it is here that many of the fertility variables emphasized by the sociologist come to the fore. While it is attitudes toward goods such as those above, conceptualized in terms of a preference map, which together with resource and price constraints immediately determine fertility decisions, a host of other variables lie behind these attitudes. In general, one's preference system at any given time may be viewed as molded by heredity and past and current environment.[18] The process starts with birth and continues through the life cycle. Religion, color, nativity, place of residence, and education enter into the shaping of tastes. So, too, does one's childhood and adolescent experience in one's own home with material affluence and family size. One reaches family-building age with preferences already molded by this heritage, but these preferences are subsequently modified by ongoing occupational, income, and family building experiences, among others. Exposure to various information media influences tastes throughout the life cycle.

Because of the important role of cumulative experience in the formation of tastes, it is probably correct that typically tastes change rather slowly over time. For some analytical purposes, this may justify the economist's usual assumption of constant tastes. But in areas of behavior such as fertility, which involve a substantial time period or where cross-section differences among classes are of interest, such an assumption seems dubious. Nor can the economist dismiss taste phenomena as non-economic in nature, for it is clear that economic variables enter into the shaping of tastes and affect behavior through this channel as well as via the resource and price constraints traditionally emphasized. Hence, an adequate framework for fertility analysis calls for explicit attention to preference phenomena and the factors entering into their formation.[19]

Fertility Control—Another area in which the economic analysis of fertility seems in need of improvement is the subject of birth control. Becker's treatment of this subject keeps uneasy company with the rest of his analysis, for in turning to it, he shifts from a framework based on the theory of consumer choice to one which he labels "supply." The main point he develops is that children are by and large a home-produced good, and because of lack of birth control knowledge, the actual number of children produced may exceed that desired.

Hence, cross-section or temporal variations in birth control knowledge (and techniques) may lead to differences in fertility over and beyond that attributable to consumer choice.

While the occurrence of unwanted pregnancies is a well-established fact, it is questionable on both theoretical and empirical grounds whether the above argument provides a sufficient explanation. The most obvious analytical objection is, if children are the *only* good in question, why would a household even engage in the production process once the desired number is reached? On the empirical side, there is ample evidence that attitudes toward (or "tastes for") fertility control differ among segments of the population (the Westoff-Ryder paper[20] in this volume provides a valuable survey). This difference in tastes for fertility control would be expected to cause variation in its use, even if knowledge were uniform. Again, the effectiveness of a *given* method of fertility control tends to increase as desired family size is approached. This is even true of supposedly "inefficient" methods, such as rhythm. Moreover, the most efficient method of all, abstinence, is universally known, and other highly effective pre-modern techniques such as withdrawal, abortion, and infanticide are widely known. Indeed, the fertility decline in Western Europe appears to have involved a substantial growth in the practice of withdrawal, a technique whose adoption can hardly be explained in terms of changing knowledge.[21] Clearly, the explanation of changes or differences in fertility control behavior and, consequently, in "unwanted" births, requires more variables than the state of knowledge or technique alone.

The approach proposed here is self-evident. It is simply to apply the theory of consumer choice to decisions regarding fertility control as well as desired family size, thus providing a more unified treatment. For this purpose a new good must explicitly be recognized, coition. It is obviously this good that explains how more children may be produced than are desired, for associated with its consumption is the possibility of an unwanted outcome, the conception of a child. Fertility control measures enter as possible forms of insurance, of varying effectiveness and cost, against the unwanted outcome. But the employment of any given insurance measure itself involves certain costs, pecuniary and psychological. Thus, in considering the use of a fertility control measure, the household weighs the loss of utility attributable to the possibility of an unwanted birth against that arising from the cost of fertility control, including subjective costs.

For the population as a whole, this decision-making process results in a certain level and distribution of fertility control practices, and a corresponding incidence of unwanted pregnancies. The factors responsible for more extensive use of these practices may be grouped under two heads—those lowering the cost of contraception and those raising the cost of an unwanted pregnancy. Under the former head, progress in contraceptive techniques is an obvious factor. The principal advantage of modern over pre-modern methods would seem to lie, not in their effectiveness, but in their lower subjective costs. The objection to abstinence is clearly that it entails giving up coition altogether, while practices such as abortion and infanticide also involve high subjective costs. The latest techniques—the IUD and the oral pill—by separating the act of contraception from that of coition have doubtless served to lower subjective costs further than previous modern methods. A second factor would be diffusion of knowledge of given techniques. This would lower the cost of contraception by reducing the search costs of information. A third would be a favorable shift in attitudes toward contraception, as might occur, for example, as a result of a weaker stand of the Catholic church on artificial birth control practices. Finally, the standard economic considerations of price and income would fall under this head. Lower pecuniary prices of given techniques or higher household incomes both would make for more extensive use of contraception.

Among the factors raising the cost of an unwanted pregnancy would be first the degree to which satiation regarding family size is approached. This is an obvious reason why the effectiveness of a technique rises as desired size is reached. A second reason would be a decrease in the *relative* desire for children, perhaps reflecting, for example, greater aspirations for material goods. Still another would be a lengthening of time horizons, which might lead to greater weight being attached to the possibility of a future unwanted outcome.

This list of factors is scarcely exhaustive, but it is sufficient to indicate that the framework proposed here is capable of application to a wide variety of experience. It also helps clarify the issue of knowledge and technique versus motivation in the adoption of fertility control practices. Thus advances in knowledge and technique by reducing the cost of contraception increase the likelihood of its adoption, holding motivation constant. On the other hand, holding knowledge and technique constant, an increase in the desire for goods relative to children raises the cost of unexpected pregnancy, and increases the motivation to adopt fertility control practices. The relative importance of these influences in adoption of contraception is a major research question.

This framework has implications too for the touchy issue of rationality. It should be clear that the balance of considerations for a given household may lead to a decision not to employ contraception and consequent acceptance of the risk of an unwanted pregnancy. Such behavior is no more irrational than that of the businessman who may forego getting the maximum profit possible because he feels the extra gain is not worth the effort attendant upon it.

Finally, this framework helps to highlight the fact that a given causal factor may work through several different channels. For example, in Becker's framework, an increase in income tends to raise fertility by relaxing the budget constraint. The present scheme suggests that there is also a negative influence on fertility because the rise in income brings contraception more within reach financially and thus makes for a reduction in unwanted pregnancies. Or, consider the effect of education, which by widening horizons, may raise the preference for goods relative to children. Given income and prices this would tend to reduce fertility. Further, by increasing the subjective cost of an unwanted pregnancy, this tendency is enhanced because of the spur given to contraception and the consequent reduction in unwanted pregnancies. Finally, education may directly affect knowledge of contraceptive technique or significantly reduce the search costs of information, and through this channel as well make for a reduction in unwanted pregnancies.

Synthesis—How does all this add up? At any given time, a household (or a couple contemplating union) has, on the one hand, a structure of preferences relating to goods, children, leisure, and fertility control practices, shaped largely by prior experience. The household has also certain income potentials, taking account of the earnings possibilities of husband, wife, and other family members as well as any non-labor income. There are, in addition, various price constraints, such as the prices of child care and of various fertility control methods relative to those of goods in general. Out of the balancing of preferences and constraints, decisions are reached on marriage, fertility control practices, fertility, wife's labor force participation, and perhaps even husband's hours of work. In the course of the reproductive years preferences are modified by ongoing experience, and income potentials, prices, and available fertility control methods may change with consequent appropriate changes in these decisions. The fertility record of a given household reflects this balancing of preferences against constraints over the course of the full reproductive age span.

The question may be asked whether these considerations determine the timing or total number of births a household has during the course of the reproductive years. The distinction between timing and completed family size has come into prominence as a result of the development of cohort fertility measures and attempts to clarify the relation between cohort and period fertility.[22] Recently, it has been hypothesized that certain economic factors affect only the timing of births, though others may affect completed size as well.[23]

While the present theoretical framework does not supply a clear-cut answer, it leads to the expectation that timing and number changes would usually be mutually reinforcing. Thus, if the balance of preferences and constraints for cohort A versus cohort B were consistently more favorable for fertility throughout the entire reproductive age span, one would expect cohort A to have its children earlier and to end up with a larger completed family size. Circumstances are conceivable, of course, in which timing differences might occur although total numbers were the same. For example, if the underlying factors were more favorable to fertility for cohort A during the early childbearing years, but less favorable during the later, then both cohorts might produce the same number but cohort A's births would be concentrated more in the earlier years. Again, it is conceivable that a new contraceptive with lower subjective costs might be adopted by households earlier in the reproductive years in order to space children more satisfactorily with no effect on total number. But it seems likely that such a development would at the same time reduce the proportion of unplanned births and thus completed family size as well.

Actually, experience in the U.S. since 1917 shows that timing and number changes have, in fact, been reinforcing.[24] Thus it accords with the view that the same pressures typically induce similar responses in both.

II. Postwar Research on Economic Factors in American Fertility
The previous discussion provides a background for surveying postwar research and considering prospective needs. The present treatment is selective. It touches first on the main findings in the principal areas of fertility research, and then focuses on a few lines of inquiry that seem especially promising.

Preliminary Survey
To turn first to fertility movements through time, the principal development has been methodological, the introduction of cohort analysis.[25] To date, however, little has been published on the factors underlying cohort fertility differences. Campbell reports on the basis of an ongoing study that "there is as yet no evidence that the total number of children couples have is influenced by economic conditions per se. This conclusion is based on a study of the relationship between

the completed fertility of cohorts and measures of the economic conditions prevailing while those cohorts were in the most fertile years of the childbearing period."[26] He goes on to note that "it is possible, however, that some aspect of our changing economy affected couples' *desires* for children"[27] [italicizing added]. This observation ties in with the viewpoint adopted here, in which fertility decisions involve a balancing of resources and desires. A multivariate analysis of the cohort data, taking account not only of income experience, but factors which enter into the formation of tastes, and also price phenomena, would seem an attractive possibility.[28]

As in the past, the most favorable results on the influence of economic factors have been obtained in analyses of fluctuations in fertility. In business cycle studies, Kirk,[29] Kirk and Nortman,[30] and, more recently, Silver[31] have obtained results highly consistent with the earlier findings of Dorothy S. Thomas and others.[32] These studies are commonly interpreted as showing a positive response by fertility to income fluctuations, presumably associated with movements in unemployment.[33] My own work has focused on longer-term variations in fertility, "Kuznets cycles," in which the postwar baby boom and recent fertility decline are seen as the most recent in a succession of long swings.[34] It is argued that the current swing reflects the shifting balance between preferences and resources of successive cohorts. Economic conditions are seen as working in part via the income effect and in part via preferences by shaping material aspirations during adolescence.

The principal focus of demographic research on American fertility in the postwar period has been, not on time series, but on cross-section studies, especially special surveys, such as the Princeton Fertility Studies[35] and Growth of American Families Studies.[36] These investigations, following in the tradition of the Indianapolis Fertility Study,[37] have vastly expanded factual knowledge of fertility behavior. Their results on the causal influence of economic factors have been, on the whole, disappointing, though perhaps no more so than for social and psychological factors. On the one hand, these studies frequently turn up responses indicating that households consider economic or financial considerations important in fertility behavior.[38] One striking finding is that when housewives were asked what they considered the ideal number of children for families of "low," "average," and "high" incomes—the number was more than twice as large for the high income as for the low income family.[39] It appears, therefore, that many wives think that income should influence fertility positively and to a substantial extent. Nevertheless, cross-section associations between income and actual fertility consistently show little or no evidence of a positive association. It is possible, of course, that the cross-section differentials reflect the influence of a larger number of factors than time series fluctuations. For example, religion, a "taste" factor which appears to play a prominent part in cross-section differentials, is invariant in the ordinary business cycle. But allowing as best as possible for such additional influences in cross-section analysis, the lack of association between income and fertility typically persists. This result has been a major stumbling block in acceptance of economic factors as important determinants of fertility.

Thus, viewing postwar research in the broad, one finds much the same paradoxical situation as prevailed before the war. Economic factors appear to play a prominent part in fertility fluctuations, a conclusion which has been strengthened by extension to longer-term Kuznets cycles as well as shorter-term business cycles. On the other hand, in cross-section studies, where the largest amount of new evidence has been amassed, the results have been largely negative. The same is true of the effect of economic factors on secular trends, though relatively little work has been done on this. Thus the central problem remains of reconciling seemingly conflicting results on the importance of economic factors.

Promising Lines of Inquiry

The puzzle of the true nature of the income-fertility relation has plagued and perplexed fertility research down through the years, and continues to do so. This problem, it would seem, should constitute a central focus of research, not only because of its inherent interest and importance, but also because its solution is likely to lead to a broader and deeper understanding of the various factors determining fertility. The subsequent discussion accordingly centers on this issue. Fortunately, in recent years several studies have explored new and promising lines of inquiry. One deserving special mention is that by R. Freedman and Coombs.[40] In the present brief review these studies will be discussed in terms of the analytical framework set out earlier, since this framework itself suggests additional possibilities.

Cross-section Income/Fertility Relation

A number of reasons come to mind why the expected positive relation between income and fertility does not emerge in a simple cross-section association. These are as follows:

1. Differential bias by income level in current income as a proxy for potential income.
2. Differential prevalence of fertility control by income level.
3. Differential price of child care by income level.
4. Differential relative desire for children by income level.

With the exception of the first one, these are, in general, factors making for lower fertility which are positively correlated with income. While each will be taken up separately below, an actual empirical inquiry would, of course, need to consider them simultaneously.

Bias in Current Income as a Proxy for Potential Income—The income measure usually used in correlations with fertility is current income, either husband's income or family income. In different ways, two recent studies have experimented with income concepts more in keeping with the present framework.

R. Freedman and Coombs found no consistent relationship between family income in 1961 and expected family size.[41] In an effort to get at "permanent income" expectations, "all respondents were asked how much change they expected in their income in the next ten years, and how much difference they expected this change to make in their standard of living." Their results "lend support to the hypothesis that a positive correlation between expectations and income may be obscured temporarily by using present rather than the respondent's evaluation of her 'permanent income' as the economic measure. For the relationship to hold, however, two conditions must be present; the anticipated change in income must be perceived as large and one that will make a substantial difference in the family's standard of living."[42]

Mincer's analysis[43] is of interest in the present connection, too. Mincer performs several regression analyses of fertility in relation to income and price variables, the latter relating to the opportunity cost of child care. He finds, as expected, that the pure price effect on fertility is negative and that the influence of "potential family income," as he terms it, is positive. The latter, in this connection, is estimated as the sum of the husband's income and the wife's *potential* full-time earnings, a treatment consistent with the present framework.

Further exploration with an income concept more relevant to household decision-making seems desirable. The aim should be to obtain a measure which will order households in terms of their evaluations of the resources potentially available, taking account of all income sources and prospective changes through time. It should be recognized, of course, that even a more meaningful concept than current income will not necessarily show a positive association with fertility in a simple cross-section, since factors such as those discussed below may still obscure the true relationship.[44]

Differential Prevalence of Fertility Control—It is this factor which Becker emphasized in reconciling actual experience with his theoretical expectation of a positive income/fertility relation. He reasoned that contraceptive knowledge was positively correlated with income. Low income households consequently produced a disproportionate number of unplanned births, obscuring the positive income/fertility relationship that consumer choice alone would otherwise have produced. In support of this he gave prominence to the Indianapolis study results which showed a positive relation between fertility and income for couples using contraception to plan the number and spacing of children.[45]

The present analytical framework supports the view that the income/fertility relation may be distorted by variations in fertility control, though it suggests that such variations may arise from factors other than contraceptive knowledge alone. However, it is not certain that this factor can bear as much weight as Becker gives to it. Recent surveys do not fully confirm the Indianapolis results.[46] More importantly, the survey evidence—even with reasonable allowance for possible biases—does not support the view implicit in his argument that lower income households *want* fewer children than higher income households.[47] Hence, while variation in fertility control practices may be one factor upsetting the a priori expectation, and clearly should be included in the analysis, other factors must be at work as well.

Differential Price of Child Care—Reference has already been made to Jacob Mincer's study, which suggests that the wife's opportunity cost, and hence the price of child care, varies directly with income, and tends to offset the positive effect of the latter on fertility.[48] Although doubts were expressed earlier about the appropriateness of Mincer's use of the wife's full-time earnings as a basis for estimating the price of child care, nevertheless, it seems likely that the appropriate prices do vary positively with income, and thus tend to have the effect suggested by him. Clearly, there is need for more research on the manner in which the price of child care (as distinct from expenditures thereon) varies by income level.

Differential Tastes—Two levels of research may be distinguished in this respect, that directly on tastes, obtained from attitudinal surveys, and that on factors entering into the formation of tastes, which may be used as proxy variables where direct attitudinal data are not obtainable.

Under the former head would be included recent demographic research on family size preferences and contraceptive attitudes.[49] As has been indicated, however, there is need to obtain from the respondents additional information on desires relating to material goods that compete with children for the household's scarce resources, so that the *relative* strength of the desire for children may be assessed. The work of Katona and his associates on material aspirations provides relevant guidance in this respect, although because it has been primarily oriented toward business cycle research, somewhat longer time horizons may be needed.[50] The AIPO data which Judith Blake has been studying[51] might also yield possibilities along these lines. In their recent study, Freedman and Coombs take a step in this direction by exploring parents' aspirations for their children. "Respondents were asked a number of questions about how important they thought it was for their children to have such items as: a separate bedroom, a good allowance, private lessons, membership in clubs or scouts, and summer camp experience. Their replies were combined in an Index of Aspirations for their children."[52] While the index was not highly correlated with (current) income, they found an inverse association with family size expectations, suggesting the type of quantity-quality trade-off in the structure of tastes which one would expect. Other standard of living items were also explored, relating more to the family as a whole or of a non-family oriented nature, especially housing and cars, but with disappointing results. This may be due, however, to the fact that the analysis shifted in this case to data on actual expenditures rather than aspirations.

The second level of work involves the use of variables underlying attitude formation, in lieu of direct data on tastes. (Ideally, such variables would ultimately be derived from empirically tested models of attitude formation.) One factor brought out by the work of Goldberg and others is the influence of farm background.[53] For the non-farm population as a whole, it appears that the inverse association between income and fertility is partly produced by differences among the various income levels in the composition of the population according to farm background. At lower income levels, a higher proportion of couples with farm background, those with higher fertility "tastes," are included thus making for an inverse income/fertility relation for the group as a whole. If one controls for farm background, the negative association is reduced, and, with allowance for degree of fertility control, transformed into a positive relation.[54] In an interesting extension of this work, Duncan[55] has found that attainment of high levels of schooling may have the same effect as two generations of non-farm residence. His statement is of special interest in emphasizing the importance of pre-adult experience in the formation of tastes. "It is as though a committment to the 'modern' fertility pattern could be made either by non-farm rearing or by prolonged contact with the educational system. In either event, the relevant experience is one that occurred early in the life cycle, before the period of family growth was well under way."[56]

A second and particularly promising line of work that may be noted under this head is that on the "relative income" hypothesis. Actually, as will be discussed more fully, the relative income hypothesis may best be viewed as combining a resource variable, actual income, and a taste variable, an empirical proxy for the living aspirations of the household. Deborah Freedman pioneered in the application of the relative income hypothesis to cross-section data.[57] More recently, R. Freedman and Coombs have experimented with a somewhat different formulation.[58] The present discussion will focus on Mrs. Freedman's analysis.

Mrs. Freedman compares the association with fertility of two income variables: (1) actual income of the husband, and (2) husband's income as a relative of that which might be expected on the basis of that typical for his occupation, education, age, and residence (South or non-South). Her results are as follows:

> There is evidence that husband's income does make a difference over the longer childbearing period if it is considered in relation to the average income for the husband's occupational status and age. An income which is above the average for one's status is associated with more children, but being in a higher absolute income class means fewer children if the higher income is only what is usual for the husband's age and occupational status.[59]

The relative income interpretation has an interesting implication for the prospective trend in fertility differentials by income status. The typical relation suggested by the data tended to shift after 1940 from a generally negative to less negative or non-significant association. This led, in turn, to predictions that a positive relation might appear in the future, presumably reflecting the gradual emergence of the "true" effect of income as class differences in fertility control disappeared. If the relative income interpretation is correct, however, it is not at all clear that the simple association between income and fertility would be positive even if all births were wanted.

Time Series Income/Fertility Relation

As has been noted, the association observed over time between income and fertility has been varied in nature. While the relation during the business cycle has been of the expected positive sign, the secular relation has been inverse. Moreover it seems that absolute income movements alone are not sufficient to account for Kuznets cycles in the level of fertility.

The same factors just reviewed with regard to the cross-section association may in principal account for the varied time series experience. There is little point to repeating the previous discussion, however, because actual analysis of time series experience has been quite limited. Clearly, the main conclusion is the need for new research along these lines.

One investigation, however, has yielded findings paralleling rather closely those obtained in cross-section analysis, and the implications of this call for further discussion. A little reflection will show that there is a close similarity between Mrs. Freedman's cross-section analysis and the interpretation I have advanced for the recent fertility decline.[60] In both cases, actual income is compared with a hypothetical income which may be viewed as a crude proxy for living level aspirations. (The time series analysis uses as an indicator for young adults' desired living level the income situation which they experienced in their parents' households when they were teenagers.) Both analyses arrive at the conclusion that higher fertility is associated with situations in which actual income is highest in relation to the desired living level.

Because the two studies together provide the most consistent interpretation yet offered of time series and cross-section experience, it is of interest to consider the implications of the relative income view for the secular trend in fertility. This was outlined in a previous paper:

> Young persons currently in the childbearing ages were a few years back dependent members in their parents' households. It seems plausible to argue that the consumption levels experienced in the parents' households served, among other things, to shape their current preferences [for material goods] . . . Moreover, the situation in the parents' household when the children were in their teens would seem more relevant than when the children were quite young . . . In a developing economy the second generation's income at ages 20-24 is typically greater than the first generation's was at that age. The second generation could achieve the consumption level the first generation had at age 20-24 and have something left over for other purposes, such as saving or increased family size. But if the *desired* consumption level inherited from their parents by children relates to the parents' situation not at ages 20-24, but at, say, 35-44, then it is less certain that the second generation's income at ages 20-24 will suffice to achieve the desired consumption level. In other words, there is an intergeneration effect tending to increase consumption at a given income level. Clearly by varying the parameters involved, one could develop alternative models in which secular growth in absolute income was accompanied by increasing, decreasing, or constant fertility.[61]

Contrast this view with the predominant one. It is typically assumed that if the effect of income (viewed in the sense of resource constraint) on fertility is positive, that secular growth in real per capita income tends to increase fertility. The failure for this to occur presumably reflects the influence of other factors such as spread of fertility control, whose influence diminishes as growth proceeds. Eventually, however, an upward fertility trend may set in as the income influence starts to prevail. In the relative income view, however, per capita income growth operates through two channels. On the one hand, it has the effect usually emphasized of tending to increase fertility by giving the second generation more resources. On the other, it tends to lower fertility through the side of tastes, by increasing the relative desire for material goods. Since these two influences may be more or less offsetting, it no longer follows that per capita income growth tends to increase fertility secularly. If, in historical experience, these influences have in fact been offsetting, then the cause of the secular decline in fertility must be sought in factors other than per capita income change, factors which may have shifted preferences even more strongly against children, changed the relative price of children, or encourage wider adoption of fertility control practices.

It should be noted that even if the effects of per capita income growth are offsetting secularly, this is not necessarily the case over shorter periods. This is because the effect via the resource constraint relates to ongoing experience, while that via preferences is primarily a lagged one, deriving from the previous course of income change. Thus, if there are long swings in the secular growth of per capita income, it is possible that a cohort brought up in a "boom" period may go through the prime family-building years during a "bust." In this case, it would have acquired strong desires for material goods which would be difficult to realize because of the adverse labor market situation, and hence would be under pressure to curtail fertility.

In concluding this section, I wish to make clear what I consider the real significance of the relative income hypothesis, namely, that it provides a *crude* embodiment of the view that fertility behavior reflects a balancing of preferences against certain resource constraints. Thus, "relative income" is seen here as a composite of two variables, one representing available resources, and one representing preferences. But in terms of the present framework this is far from a perfect embodiment of the relevant variables. Current income is not necessarily the best measure of the resource constraint. And the reference income measure used as a proxy for tastes is, at best, one of the "second level" factors shaping the formation of tastes, rather than a direct taste variable. Moreover, it is not cast in a form relating to the *relative* strength of desires. For example, in my time series analysis, it would seem preferable, at a minimum, to consider the heritage of those in family-building age, not only with regard to parents' income experience, but also size of family from which they came (though a check suggests the results would not be seriously altered). Nor is parents' income necessarily the measure most relevant to the formation of material desires—during 1941-45, for example, income experience was relatively good, but the visible manifestations of it slight. Hence the relative income approach is a start along the right path of inquiry, but the more general aim should be to develop better measures of both preferences and the resource constraints.[62]

Summary

Although the following is oversimplified, it may convey by way of summary the flavor of the analytical viewpoint suggested in this part:

Hypothesized Influence of Specified Factor in Observed Fertility Variations

	Fertility Determinant			
Nature of Observations	*Income*	*Tastes*	*Prices*	*Fertility Control Practices*
Cross-section	Positive	Negative	Negative	Negative
Secular	Positive	Negative	Negative?	Negative
Long swings	Positive	Negative	Negligible?	Negligible?
Business cycle	Positive	Negligible	Negligible	Negligible

The cross-section fertility-income pattern at a point in time reflects the differential balance between preferences and constraints at successive income levels. On the one hand, the influence of available resources makes for higher fertility at higher income levels. But operating to counter this are a number of other factors. For one thing, the desire for children relative to goods is probably stronger at lower income levels, because, for example, education is less, farm background more predominant, and pre-adult exposure to large families greater and to material affluence less. In addition, the price of child care is probably less at lower income levels, because of the more frequent presence of older relatives. Finally, fertility control attitudes and knowledge are such as to make for a larger proportion of unplanned births at low income levels. Clearly, there is no a priori expectation that fertility and income will be positively correlated in a simple cross-section analysis. Neither is it necessary that the observed relation, whatever its nature, remain stable from one cohort to the next, for the relative weight of the various factors may shift.

In secular observations on fertility (in the sense of surviving children) again all four sets of factors are operative. Available resources of the household are increasing, thus making for a larger number of children. Offsetting this are developments in various factors affecting tastes such as rising material aspirations inherited from parents' households or stimulated by new goods, and rising education. Price factors may perhaps be a negative influence because offsets to child costs arising from children's contributions to household income and to the support of parents in old age diminish in importance. Under the head of fertility control practices, secular improvement in techniques and availability of contraceptive knowledge reduces the relative magnitude of unplanned births by lowering the cost of contraception.

During long swings, prices and fertility control practices drop out as regular influences, though of course any single swing might reflect new developments in these conditions. A systematic inverse variation in tastes tends to be produced by a long swing in income operating with a lagged effect. To illustrate very simply, assume the desired living level of those aged 20-24 equals the actual living level of those aged 35-44 ten years ago (their parents). Assume also that initially income is growing steadily at a rate such that the growth in resources of young adults just balances their rising desires, with no net influence on fertility. Suppose now that the economy undergoes a 20 year swing, experiencing a retardation in growth for 10 years followed by accelerated growth in the next decade. Then the balance between desired and actual income of young adults will shift in a way first adverse, and then favorable, to fertility. In the first decade inherited desires would continue to rise at the average secular growth rate, but resources would grow at a lower rate, generating a net negative pressure on fertility. In the second decade, inherited desires of young adults would grow at a below average rate while resources would grow faster than average, thus making for a net positive effect on fertility. The observed fertility movement would thus reflect the dual role of income growth—directly via resources and indirectly via a lagged effect on tastes.

Because of the shorter duration of business cycle fluctuations, the influence of tastes drops out along with prices and fertility control practices as a systematic source of fertility variation, leaving income as the factor typically dominating the observed fluctuation. In the other sets of observations, however, any simple correlation between income and fertility obscures the pure effect of income because of systematic variation in one or more of the other sets of factors.

III. Summary Assessment

The current state of knowledge on the role of economic factors in American fertility can perhaps best be characterized as generally cloudy, but with some promising glimmerings of light. The greatest need is for a theoretical framework which will enable economists and sociologists each to see the relevance of the other discipline's work. Such a framework can be developed from the economic theory of household choice, if it is expanded to give explicit scope to the influence of "taste" factors, those emphasized in sociology. Fertility behavior, then, becomes a matter of constrained choice; fertility variations in time and space reflect variations in the relevant preferences and/or constraints.

Guided by such a framework, empirical inquiry is needed along several lines. On the side of constraints, experimentation is needed with income concepts more pertinent to long run decision-making. With regard to prices, fuller information is needed to establish the relevant prices of childbearing and rearing. Both of these subjects fall within the traditional purview of economics. Perhaps even more promising is research on preferences. Attitudinal research needs expansion to permit assessment of the *relative* strength of the desire for children. There is need too for the development of models of the formation of attitudes, in which preferences are related to background variables entering into the shaping of tastes. In addition to its inherent sociological interest, this work would facilitate research on topics where no direct preference data are obtainable, as in the case of secular trends.

In all of these areas, promising ideas have been explored in recent years, among them, the permanent income concept, the opportunity cost of a wife's time, parents' aspirations for their children, the effect of farm background, the relative income hypothesis. It is perhaps not too optimistic to view these as signs pointing towards the development of a more integrated socioeconomic framework of fertility analysis. But more research is clearly needed, research in which there is ample scope for a mutually beneficial association of both economists and sociologists. This attractive prospect should pay off, not only in the understanding of fertility, but in contributing more generally to the evolution of social science theory built on the work of both disciplines.

Notes

1. James S. Duesenberry, "Comment," in Universities-National Bureau Committee for Economic Research, *Demographic and Economic Change in Developed Countries* (Princeton: Princeton University Press, 1960), p. 233.

2. Gary S. Becker, "An Economic Analysis of Fertility," in *ibid.*, pp. 209-31. For the later work referred to later in this paragraph, cf. Gary S. Becker, "A Theory of the Allocation of Time," *Economic Journal*, LXXV, 229 (Sept., 1965), 493-517. This paper, together with Jacob Mincer's "Market Prices, Opportunity Costs, and Income Effects," in *Measurement in Economics: Studies in Mathematical Economics and Econometrics in Memory of Yehuda Grunfeld* (Stanford: Stanford University Press, 1963), has had an important influence on the treatment here of income and prices.

3. Although the framework developed here is applicable both to developed and less developed countries, several considerations are omitted from the present discussion whose inclusion would be necessary if the focus were on the latter. These are infant mortality, and the consequent difference between births and completed family size, the contribution to household income which children may make and also to the support of parents when they become old. Also omitted are fecundity considerations which may keep fertility below the desired level in a given household.

4. Milton Friedman, *A Theory of the Consumption Function* (Princeton: Princeton University Press, 1957).

5. The meaning of "all its time" can be clarified by quoting Becker's description of the "maximum money income achievable":

> This income could in general be obtained by devoting all the time and other resources of a household to earning income, with no regard for consumption. Of course, all the time would not usually be spent "at" a job: sleep, food, even leisure are required for efficiency, and some time (and other resources) would have to be spent on these activities in order to maximize money income. The amount spent would, however, be determined solely by the effect on income and not by any effect on utility. Slaves, for example, might be permitted time "off" from work only in so far as that maximized their output, or free persons in poor environments might have to maximize money income simply to survive. Becker, *op. cit.*, p. 498.

It may also be noted that Becker proposes as an alternative to the usual distinction between goods and leisure a classification of commodities on the basis of their time-intensiveness and goods-intensiveness. This treatment has certain advantages, but for simplicity, the present analysis retains the traditional classification.

6. For the present it is assumed that the relative price of children is unaffected by the wife's earning capacity. This assumption will be taken up in the next section.

7. The same applies to associations between fertility and an index of socioeconomic status, which incorporates in part a current income measure. The averaging in this index of current income with factors such as

education and occupation further complicates interpretation by confusing the analytical distinction between preferences and resources.

8. Cf. Duesenberry, *op. cit.;* Bernard Okun, "Comment," in Universities-National Bureau Committee for Economic Research, *Demographic and Economic Change in Developed Countries* (Princeton: Princeton University Press, 1960); and Harvey Leibenstein, *Economic Backwardness and Economic Growth* (New York: John Wiley, 1957). Empirical studies of the cost of children typically relate to expenditures, not prices. Cf. United Nations, *Foetal, Infant and Early Childhood Mortality. Vol.* II *Biological, Social and Economic Factors,* Population Studies No. 13 (New York: United Nations, 1954) chapter IV, which provides a valuable survey of the pertinent literature.

9. Gary S. Becker, "An Economic Analysis of Fertility," in Universities-National Bureau Committee for Economic Research, *Demographic and Economic Change in Developed Countries* (Princeton: Princeton University Press, 1960) pp. 214-15.

10. Duesenberry, *op. cit.,* p. 233.

11. Mincer, *op. cit.*

12. This consideration is also noted in United Nations, *op. cit.,* p. 35.

13. An illustrative discussion, exceptional for its forthright attention to the problem is that of Glen G. Cain, *Married Women in the Labor Force* (Chicago: University of Chicago Press, 1966), Appendix C. James S. Duesenberry's work, *Income, Saving, and the Theory of Consumer Behavior* (Cambridge, Mass.: Harvard University Press, 1952) is still one of the most pertinent. On both the conceptual and empirical level, George Katona and his associates have made pioneering contributions: *Psychological Analysis of Economic Behavior* (New York: McGraw-Hill, 1951); *The Mass Consumption Society* (New York: McGraw-Hill, 1964); *The Powerful Consumer: Psychological Studies of the American Economy* (New York: McGraw-Hill, 1960). Useful general discussions appear in Alfred Kuhn, *The Study of Society: A Unified Approach* (Homewood, Illinois: Richard D. Irwin, 1963); and Bernard Berelson and Gary A. Steiner, *Human Behavior: An Inventory of Scientific Findings* (New York: Harcourt, Brace, and World, 1964). Joseph J. Spengler, "Values and Fertility Analysis," *Demography,* 3, 1 (1966) 109-30, provides a recent survey of the literature as it bears on fertility.

There appear to be two sources of economists' resistance to "tastes" as an explanatory variable. One is the issue of measurability. Explanations based on tastes often seem unverifiable. However, it seems possible to quantify taste variables through attitudinal data or models of the formation of tastes employing observable magnitudes. The other is the determinacy problems that arise, if, e.g., tastes are assumed to vary with income.

14. A recent paper which applies the economist's conception of tastes to anthropological research, and derives empirical preference maps, is John M. Roberts, Edwin Burmeister, and Richard F. Strand, "Preferential Pattern Analysis," in Paul Kay, ed., *Explorations in Mathematical Anthropology* (Cambridge: Massachusetts Institute of Technology Press, forthcoming).

15. An article emphasizing the relevance to sociological theory of the preference map conception of tastes is Eugene B. Schneider and Sherman

Krupp, "An Illustration of the Use of Analytical Theory in Sociology: The Application of the Economic Theory of Choice to non-Economic Variables," *American Journal of Sociology*, LXX, 6 (May 1965) 695-703.

16. Field studies of family size preferences have experimented with a number of single valued concepts. (Actual responses sometimes are in the form of a range.) The tendency for "ideal" size to exceed "desired," and for the latter to exceed "expected," may be viewed as reflecting the increasing extent to which respondents take implicit account of personal resource constraints. As Judith Blake has emphasized in "Ideal Family Size among White Americans: A Quarter of a Century's Evidence," *Demography*, 3, 1 (1966) 154-73, statements regarding ideals or desires are probably better indexes of preferences than those regarding "expected" size, since in the latter concept an economic projection on the part of the respondent is most obviously implied. (This is shown in survey data by the predominant importance of economic reasons among those given for expecting fewer children than were wanted—see p. 55 of Whelpton, Campbell, and Patterson study cited in note 36.) In principle, it would seem preferable to project fertility by combining preference responses with independent projections of the relevant economic variables, rather than relying on the respondents' own economic projections.

17. Schneider and Krupp, *op. cit.*, provide an illustration in the industrial relations area. Management desires both authority and peace, and these are substitutable goals. Given the constraints, management may choose to sacrifice some authority to assure more peace, thereby maximizing its level of satisfaction with regard to both goals.

18. An interesting attempt to use cohort analysis to explore the relative importance in attitude formation of what are termed "aging" and "historical situation" is that of William M. Evan, "Cohort Analysis of Attitude Data," in James M. Beshers, ed., *Computer Methods in the Analysis of Large-Scale Social Systems* (Cambridge: Joint Center for Urban Studies of M.I.T. and Harvard University, 1965), though the conception of attitudes, judged from the viewpoint adopted here, seems unduly dichotomous.

19. An unpublished paper by Julian L. Simon, "The Effect of Income on Fertility," advances a similar view.

20. Charles F. Westoff and Norman B. Ryder, "Recent Trends in Attitudes Toward Fertility Control and in the Practice of Contraception in the United States," paper published in Part IV of this volume.

21. As is clear from Becker's footnote 11 ("An Economic Analysis of Fertility," p. 216), he is aware of some of these difficulties with his analysis.

22. Pascal K. Whelpton, *Cohort Fertility: Native White Women in the United States* (Princeton: Princeton University Press, 1954); Norman B. Ryder, "The Structure and Tempo of Current Fertility," in Universities-National Bureau Committee for Economic Research, *Demographic and Economic Change in Developed Countries* (Princeton: Princeton University Press, 1960). While the distinction is a useful one, there seems at times to be a suggestion in the literature that timing changes are somehow less important than those in completed fertility size. As Ryder and Westoff (Norman B. Ryder and Charles F. Westoff, "The Trend of Expected Parity in the United States: 1955, 1960, 1965," unpublished manuscript) have recently emphasized, for forecasting purposes—and, one may add, for any

study of time series experience—timing changes call for just as much attention as those in completed family size.

23. Ronald Freedman and Lolagene Coombs, "Economic Considerations in Family Growth Decisions," *Population Studies*, xx, 2 (November, 1966) 197-222.

24. Arthur A. Campbell, "Introduction to the Measurement of Fertility," unpublished manuscript.

25. Whelpton, *Cohort Fertility: Native White Women in the United States*.

26. Arthur A. Campbell, "Recent Fertility Trends in the United States and Canada," in United Nations *Proceedings of the World Population Conference, 1965, vol.* ii: *Selected Papers and Summaries, Fertility, Family Planning, Mortality* (New York: United Nations, 1967) p. 203.

27. *Ibid.*

28. Under the heading of secular investigations, mention should also be made of studies by Bernard Okun, *Trends in Birth Rates in the United States since 1870* (Baltimore: Johns Hopkins Press, 1958); Yasukichi Yasuba, *Birth Rates of the White Population in the United States, 1800-1860: An Economic Study* (Baltimore: Johns Hopkins Press, 1962); and Ansley J. Coale and Melvin Zelnik, *New Estimates of Fertility and Population in the United States* (Princeton: Princeton University Press, 1963). These, by contributing valuable new factual information on secular fertility movements, have further widened the opportunities for fresh inquiry in this area. Okuns study also has an extensive theoretical discussion.

29. Dudley Kirk, "The Influence of Business Cycles on Marriage and Birth Rates," in Universities-National Bureau Committee for Economic Research, *Demographic and Economic Change in Developed Countries* (Princeton: Princeton University Press, 1960).

30. Dudley Kirk and Dorothy L. Nortman, "Business and Babies: The Influence of the Business Cycle on Birth Rates," *Proceedings of the Social Sciences Section, American Statistical Association*, December 1958, pp. 151-60.

31. Morris Silver, "Births, Marriages, and Business Cycles in the United States," *Journal of Political Economy*, lxxiii, 3 (June 1965) 237-55.

32. Dorothy S. Thomas and V. L. Galbraith, "Birth Rates and the Interwar Business Cycles," in J. J. Spengler and O. D. Duncan, eds., *Demographic Analysis* (Glencoe, Ill.: Free Press, 1956).

33. Seemingly inconsistent results regarding unemployment have occurred in some of the sample surveys: Freedman and Coombs, *op. cit.*, p. 208; Charles F. Westoff, Robert G. Potter, Jr., and Philip C. Sagi, *The Third Child: A Study in the Prediction of Fertility* (Princeton: Princeton University Press, 1963) pp. 150-51. This may be partly explicable on grounds that the cyclical results mainly reflect movements in marriage and first parity births, influences largely or wholly omitted from these surveys.

34. Richard A. Easterlin, "On the Relation of Economic Factors to Recent and Projected Fertility Changes," *Demography*, 3, 1 (1966) 131-53. Richard A. Easterlin, *The American Baby Boom in Historical Perspective* (New York: National Bureau of Economic Research, Occasional Paper 79, 1962).

35. Charles F. Westoff, Robert G. Potter, Jr., and Philip C. Sagi, *The Third Child*. Charles F. Westoff, Robert G. Potter, Jr, Philip C. Sagi, and Elliot G. Mishler, *Family Growth in Metropolitan America* (Princeton: Princeton University Press, 1961).

36. Ronald Freedman, Pascal K. Whelpton, and Arthur A. Campbell, *Family Planning, Sterility, and Population Growth* (New York: McGraw-Hill, 1959); Pascal K. Whelpton, Arthur A. Campbell, and John E. Patterson, *Fertility and Family Planning in the United States* (Princeton: Princeton University Press, 1966). Ronald Freedman, "American Studies of Factors Affecting Fertility," in Union Internationale pour l'Etude Scientifique de la Population, *Congres International de la Population: New York, 1961, Tome I* (London, 1963) provides a concise and still pertinent summary of some of the principal results of both the special field studies and those based on official statistics. For examples of the latter, cf. Wilson H. Grabill, Clyde V. Kiser, and Pascal K. Whelpton, *The Fertility of American Women* (New York: John Wiley, 1958) and Richard and Nancy Ruggles, "Differential Fertility in United States Census Data," in Universities-National Bureau Committee for Economic Research, *Demographic and Economic Change in Developed Countries* (Princeton: Princeton University Press, 1960).

37. Pascal K. Whelpton and Clyde V. Kiser, ed., *Social and Psychological Factors Affecting Fertility*, 5 vols. (New York: Milbank Fund, 1946-58).

38. E.g., Westoff *et al.*, *Family Growth in Metropolitan America*, pp. 232 ff.

39. Whelpton *et al.*, *Fertility and Family Planning in the United States*, p. 35.

40. Freedman and Coombs, *op. cit.*, p. 170.

41. *Ibid.*, p. 200.

42. *Ibid.*, pp. 209-10.

43. Mincer, *op. cit.*, pp. 75-79.

44. If only current income data are available, how can one minimize the likelihood of bias? With regard to the time dimension of potential income, it seems likely that the current income rank of households at ages 35-44 is less likely to be biased than one at an early stage of the working career, say 20-24. With regard to income sources, current husband's income is likely to be less biased than current family income. This is because (1) actual husband's income is more likely to approximate potential than in the case of the wife, and (2) since wife's and husband's education tend to be positively correlated, the potential income of the wife is likely to vary directly with that of the husband. The wife's *actual* income is not likely to be a good index of her potential income, for a high actual income may reflect, not a high potential, but a strong desire for goods relative to children. (This is, in somewhat different words, the point made in Whelpton *et al.*, *Fertility and Family Planning in the United States*, p. 106, in comparing the association of fertility with husband's versus family income.)

45. Becker, "An Economic Analysis of Fertility," pp. 218-19.

46. Whelpton *et al.*, *Fertility and Family Planning in the United States*, pp 239-40, but cf. Westoff *et al.*, *The Third Child*, pp. 118-19.

47. In a paper just published, Judith Blake, "Income and Reproductive Motivation," *Population Studies*, xxi, 3 (Nov., 1967) 185-206, provides new evidence in support of this statement. However, her inference that such "results cast doubt on the notion that the economic theory of demand for consumer durables is relevant to reproductive motivation" (*ibid.*, p. 181) is incorrect. Her statement underscores the value of the analytical framework advocated here, for it provides an apt illustration of confusing the effect on fertility of income with that of tastes, the factor to which her evidence really relates. It is unfortunate that the Blake paper became available only after the present analysis was completed, for it merits fuller discussion.

48. Mincer, *op. cit.*

49. Freedman *et al.*, *Family Planning, Sterility, and Population Growth*, pp. 42-44, 46.

50. Katona, *Psychological Analysis of Economic Behavior; The Mass Consumption Society;* and *The Powerful Consumer*.

51. Blake, "Ideal Family Size Among White Americans."

52. Freedman and Coombs, *op. cit.*, p. 213.

53. David Goldberg, "Another Look at the Indianapolis Fertility Data," *Milbank Memorial Fund Quarterly*, xxxviii, 1 (January 1960) 23-36; David Goldberg, "The Fertility of Two-Generation Urbanites," *Population Studies*, xii, 3 (March 1959) 214-22.

54. Goldberg, "Another Look at the Indianapolis Fertility Data," p. 27.

55. Otis Dudley Duncan, "Farm Background and Differential Fertility," *Demography*, 2 (1965) 240-49.

56. *Ibid.*, p. 249.

57. Deborah Freedman, "The Relation of Economic Status to Fertility," *American Economic Review*, liii, 3 (June 1963) 414-26.

58. R. Freedman and Coombs, *op. cit*, pp. 211-12.

59. D. Freedman, *op. cit.*, p. 422.

60. Easterlin, "On the Relation of Economic Factors to Recent and Projected Fertility Changes."

61. *Ibid.*, p. 140.

62. This interpretation of the relative income approach differs from that usual in economic analysis. In the latter, relative income is quite specifically a ratio of two *incomes*, whereas here, the preference component of the ratio may be better represented by a non-income magnitude. Also the present treatment, by emphasizing that "relative income" really combines two distinctive components, implies that it is redundant to add absolute income to an explanatory model containing relative income, as, for example, in D. Freedman, *op. cit.*, pp. 418-19.

ECONOMIC ASPECTS OF FERTILITY TRENDS IN THE LESS DEVELOPED COUNTRIES

Simon Kuznets
Harvard University

Fertility Patterns

LESS DEVELOPED COUNTRIES (LD) are defined here as those with a per capita or per worker economic product that is distinctly below some low limit, an indication of substantial failure to exploit the potentials of modern material and social technology. To call these countries "developing" is to mask their problems; and is, moreover, confusing since all countries are (or try to be) developing. Nor would it be fruitful to spend much effort on setting the low limit that separates the LD from the developed or, precisely, more developed countries (MD). While there is a continuum with respect to per capita or per worker product, students in the field are in general agreement regarding the identity of the LD group. It includes Asia, except Japan (and Israel with its high per capita income); Africa, except possibly South Africa (and for certain purposes South Rhodesia); Latin America, except possibly Argentina, Uruguay, Venezuela, and Puerto Rico; and Oceania, other than Australia and New Zealand. There is some question concerning a few countries in Southern Europe (Greece, Albania, Portugal, Spain) and in Eastern Europe (Bulgaria and Romania); but for the present purposes we exclude them from the LD group. The MD group includes Northern and Western Europe, the U.S.S.R., a few countries in Eastern Europe (East Germany, Czechoslovakia, Hungary), Japan, North America, Australia and New Zealand, and some smaller units.

Given this broad classification, the differences in current fertility levels between the LD and the MD countries are marked. The average crude birth rate for 1960-64 for the LD countries is about 40 per thousand; for the MD group, about half that, over 20 per thousand.[1] And the contrast is even greater for some major subregions within the

157

two groups: thus, for Northern and Western Europe and Japan, the crude birth rate for the quinquennium was between 17 and 18 per thousand; for Africa it was 47 per thousand. Moreover these differences in fertility levels are neither recent nor short-term. United Nations sources reveal that in the late 1930's crude birth rates in Asia (including Japan), Africa, and Latin America (including all countries) ranged well above 40 per thousand, whereas those in North America, Europe including the U.S.S.R., and Oceania (which is dominated by Australia and New Zealand) ranged from 17 to 24 per thousand; and similar differences are found in the 1940's and the 1950's.[2]

These wide differences in level are not the only aspect of the fertility patterns in the LD and MD countries that should be of interest in an attempt to discern their economic causes and consequences. Several others, for which the underlying evidence, relating to the 1950's and early 1960's can be found in the United Nations demographic publications, are stated summarily here.

First, the differences in crude birth rates between the two groups of countries are *not* due to differences in the age structure of women within the childbearing ages, or in the shares of these women in total population. Adjustments for proportions of women and for their age structure have only minor effects: the gross reproduction rates are above 2.0 for almost all the LD countries, and are below 2.0 for all the MD countries.[3]

Second, the difference in incidence of marriage (including consensual) is significant only for women under 25 years of age. In these early ages the proportions of married women to all women are distinctly higher in the LD than in the MD countries, but the differences disappear in the older groups. With a rough allowance for disparities in intramarital fertility (for the 15-19 age class of women assumed to be zero, and for the 20-24 age class assumed to be about half-way between zero and the relative difference in the 25-29 age class), the difference in marriage incidence accounts for about a quarter of the total disparity in crude birth rates between the LD and MD groups— an estimate that is perhaps on the high side.

Third, there are wide differences in intramarital fertility in the two age classes of women that markedly affect the total birth rates— 25-29 and 30-34. The differences for these two age classes contribute about one-half of the total difference in crude birth rates between the LD and MD groups.

Fourth, the relative, though not the absolute, differences in intramarital fertility continue and rise for older women still in their childbearing period, 35 and over. As much as a quarter of the total difference in crude birth rates between the LD and MD groups is accounted for by the continuation of fairly high fertility beyond female age 35 in the LD group and by the rapid decline of fertility of the older women in the MD countries.

Finally, this prevalence of higher fertility in the LD group—associated with earlier marriages, with much higher intramarital fertility in the major childbearing ages below 35, and with the continuation of childbearing to more advanced ages beyond 35—results in distinctive characteristics of both births and parents in the LD, compared with the MD, countries. First, the share of higher order births in total births is larger in the LD than in the MD countries. Indeed, over one-half of the difference in the crude birth rates between the two groups of countries is accounted for by births of fifth or higher order. Second, parents, particularly fathers, of a substantial proportion of new-born children are older in the LD countries. Thus in countries with per capita product below $200 (in 1958), one-fourth of the children born had fathers 38 years old or older, and the birth rate specific to this age group was 120 per thousand; whereas in the high income countries, one-fourth of total births had fathers only 35.7 years old or older, and the specific birth rate was 30 per thousand.[4]

This persistence of higher fertility for a long time span within the family life cycle, which means large household units and many families with young children and fathers advanced in age, is one set of characteristics of the fertility pattern of the LD group relevant to any explanation of economic causes and effects. The second, only barely touched upon, is the clustering of fertility measures around a high average in the many LD countries, matched by a similar though less concentrated clustering of fertility measures around a low mean in the MD countries. Crude birth rates in the LD countries range from the high 30's upward, are mostly above 40 per thousand, and rise to the high 40's, whereas those for the MD countries cluster between 16 and 20 for the "older" countries of Europe and Japan, and between the lower and upper 20's for the "young" and open countries like the United States, Canada, and the U.S.S.R. In only a few countries in the world is the crude birth rate between the upper 20's and upper 30's, and the world distribution is distinctly bimodal, with the two modes representing the MD and LD groups. Gross reproduction rates show the same double clustering.[5]

The contrast between this bimodal distribution of fertility measures and the relatively unimodal distribution of per capita income and other economic and social characteristics is clearly pertinent to our theme. It immediately suggests that the relations between fertility as an effect and social factors as causes are neither simple nor continuous. It reflects the insensitivity of fertility levels to wide differences in economic and social factors despite the marked contrast between the LD and MD groups, each taken as a whole, with respect to both social factors and fertility.

Causes, Economic and Other

An economic explanation of the differences in fertility rates between the LD and MD countries would presumably identify the differences in material and social conditions associated with different per capita products and show how, given these differences, an economic calculus designed to optimize the contribution of children—as consumer and as producer "goods"—to the long-term economic welfare of the deciding unit (presumably the parent family) would yield different estimates of the number of children to be brought into the world. Questions would arise in identifying the relevant economic characteristics associated with different per capita incomes or other indexes of economic performance; in modifying the economic calculus to include responses that have been codified into social customs and prescribed patterns; and in considering the possible gap between decision and execution.

But important as these questions are, we can ignore them in the present connection and observe a variety of economic causes of the high fertility rates of the LD countries. If our comparison is limited to the LD and MD groups, each taken as a whole and distinguished initially by per capita product, the variety of associated differences in economic structure, institutions, and practices is wide-ranging from differences in relative shares of productive sectors (agriculture, manufacturing, etc.) to those in size and structure of economic units (large, small, individually managed, under corporation ownership, etc.), to differences in structure of the economically active population (by employment status, occupation, industrial attachment, education, etc.), to differences in use structure of product (between consumption and capital investment), to those in importance and structure of foreign trade, and so on. All of these reflect different conditions of life under which participation in economic activity—probably the most time-consuming activity of man—and the distribution of its product take place. If we assume that the social unit that decides on births makes such decisions after considering their consequences and if the consequences of births impinge upon the economics of the deciding unit, we may reasonably conclude that the differences in the structure of economic life associated with different per capita products exert a variety of influences on birth decisions. And we could easily prepare a lengthy list of economic causes to "explain" the higher birth rates of the LD countries: the use of young children's labor in agriculture and handicrafts; the reliance on offspring for old age security; the greater value of children in a traditional than in a market-oriented economy; the lack of productive outlets for the female members of the household, most of whose time is spent in bearing and rearing children, etc. And while these hypotheses cannot be proved, neither can they be denied in the simple associations and regressions in the cross-section comparisons that include both LD and MD countries.[6]

But although the economic factors obviously exert *some* influence on birth rates and make *some* contribution to the explanation of the higher fertility levels in the LD countries, they should not be unduly emphasized—for two reasons. First, even when we deal with the LD and MD groups as wholes, many other diverse social and demographic factors—most of them *loosely* associated with, but distinct from, the economic—may be equally, and perhaps even more, important. The most conspicuous of these other factors is the death rate— which for the LD group averaged, on a crude basis, about 20 per thousand for 1960-64, compared with less than 9 per thousand for the MD countries. If it is the surviving children that are planned for, the difference in death rates alone would account for more than half of the observed difference in crude birth rates.[7] Furthermore, many political and social variables, despite their economic implications, cannot be treated as economic factors. Thus, if the political structure is weak; or if the structure of the economically active population is determined by the extended family, the tribe, the caste, or the clan, rather than by each individual's capacity objectively tested in the market place, the whole economic and social calculus of childbearing is affected. The high fertility levels in the LD countries may therefore be associated more closely with these political and social characteristics than with economic variables (like the share of agriculture or level of per capita income). How do we distinguish the effects of each of these groups of variables—political, social, economic, and even demographic? We have ignored this question by dealing with economic causes alone, but it is clearly most significant for both analysis and policy-making. The answer to it may explain the failure of birth rates to decline in many LD countries despite a substantial long-term rise in per capita income, and may indicate the need for modifications in social institutions and practices before birth rates can be lowered.

We have no basis for assigning proper weights to the specific effects of economic and other variables on the high birth rates in the LD countries; and, in fact, we may not even have adequate tools for the purpose.[8] My inclination, not too firmly based, would be to assign rather limited weight to the purely economic variables, for several reasons: the decisions on birth rates are long-term; knowledge needed for the economic calculus is limited; and in the less developed countries the effects of different social institutions and life patterns minimize economic weights relative to sheer survival.

The statement that economic factors, in their possible effects on fertility, are part and parcel of a wider social and technological framework, and may be overshadowed by other components, is supported when we turn to the distinctions within the LD group. Four subregions are suggested by historical and geographical considerations: Asia, excluding Japan and the Southwest; the Near East, comprising Southwest Asia and Northern Africa; sub-Saharan Africa, including or excluding South Africa (and possibly South Rhodesia); and Latin America, including or excluding Argentina, Uruguay, Venezuela, and Puerto Rico. These four regions differ substantially in population density, historical heritage, per capita income, and related socioeconomic characteristics like industrialization, urbanization, etc. Per capita GDP in 1958 was $70 for sub-Saharan Africa, excluding South Africa and South Rhodesia; about $75 for Asia; about $150 for the Middle East excluding Israel; and about $210 for Latin America, excluding the four high-income countries. Yet the crude birth rates for 1960-64 averaged about 49 per thousand for Africa, 39 for Asia, 42 for the Middle East, and 43 for Latin America.[9] The range in economic and social variables among the four regions is wide, and would be much wider for individual countries in view of the range in their per capita GDP from more than $400 to below $50. The range in birth rates is much narrower, and is not clearly related to per capita product levels. If countries with per capita product as much as 8 times as high as that of other countries nevertheless have much the same birth rate, some aspects of society, presumably unrelated to per capita product and other characteristics of economic performance, must account for these fertility levels.

This implication is reinforced by the absence of significant statistical association between fertility and many economic and social variables when the high fertility (closely identified with the LD) and low fertility (closely associated with the MD) groups are studied separately. Table 9.8, p. 148 of *Population Bulletin No. 7* shows the correlations between GRR and 12 indexes (some economic, like per capita income; others social, like urbanization and newspaper circulation; still others demographic, like life expectancy). Only two of these (the correlations with shares of non-agricultural activities in labor force, and with urbanization) are barely significant within the high fertility group; and they are so low that they account for minor fractions of total variance. For the low fertility group not a single association is statistically significant. In other words, the differences among countries in per capita income and the other 11 variables within the LD group (or within the MD group) do not account for the differences in fertility; and the causes of the latter must be sought elsewhere.

What this means for movement over time is suggested in a recent study of birth rates for Latin America—the region with the highest per capita income in the LD group—which assembles and adjusts a significant body of demographic data.[10] According to this study, standardized (for age structure of women within the childbearing ages) birth rates hover around high levels or rise in all countries except Argentina, which is outside the LD group, and Chile, which shows a slight decline (to the high 30's). The period covered goes back to the 1910's or 1920's, when in several countries (e.g. Colombia and Venezuela) death rates and infant mortality declined (even though the decline was most precipitous after World War II) and product per capita was rising, at least since the 1920's, at a rate of 2 or more percent per year (so that in a country like Colombia, where standardized birth rates rose to the mid-40's in 1955-59, product per worker more than doubled between 1925 and 1953).[11] Similar combinations of constant or rising high birth rates, declining death rates, and sustained and substantial growth in per capita product can be found for several other countries in Latin America.

The use of the "threshold hypothesis"[12] to explain this insensitivity of fertility levels to wide differences in economic and social variables may be suggestive, but as indicated in *Population Bulletin No. 7* it is only that (even though some "threshold" values for several variables are given in Table 9.9, p. 149, implying some analytical and policy significance). The danger is that the hypothesis, by giving the puzzle a suggestive name, will divert our attention from the main question posed by the evidence. Why should there be a threshold and what determines its value? Theoretically, a threshold could be found in the response of a given process to variables a, b, c, d . . . only because the process actually responds to variables x, y, and z, which remain constant while a, b, c, etc., change within a wide range. The threshold hypothesis, in and of itself, is merely a reformulation of the insensitivity of a given dependent variable to a given set of independent variables within a given range, rather than an attempt to *identify* the independent factors that are in fact contributing to the level and range of the "insensitive" dependent variable. It may well be that when these relevant independent variables are identified, they will explain much or all of the change beyond the threshold level also— and thus replace the old set of explanatory variables for which a threshold hypothesis had been formulated.

Thus, further analysis of the factors that make for constant or rising birth rates in Latin America, or in the Near East, despite the high and rising incomes and declining death rates, may show that the key determinants (other than the declining but still high death rates) lie in the system of economic and social rewards to the younger generation—a system that may not change despite rising per capita income, and one that will change only under circumstances which will also necessarily mean a higher per capita income beyond a certain threshold value (which may shift significantly with technological or social changes). The important aspects of this reward system, or of alternative determinants, are still to be identified; and they may even turn out to be economic variables, although not the easily available and conventional ones included now. But once identified, they may also help to explain the differences in fertility rates between the LD and MD groups taken as wholes; so that the contrast between the inter- and intragroup association will disappear and with it the need for the threshold hypothesis as a crutch. Obviously, whatever the possibility, existing evidence reveals major gaps in our analysis; and the conventional indexes of economic (and possibly other) factors do not cover an important aspect of the social and economic determinants of fertility levels in the LD countries.

Economic Effects
In discussing the economic effects of higher fertility rates in the LD countries, we begin with four limitations. First, we shall deal with economic effects of high fertility only when the latter results in a high rate of natural increase of population. In setting this limitation, we are *not* implying that high birth rates combined with high death rates—and therefore, a low rate of population increase—do not produce undesirable economic effects. Obviously they represent not only a huge waste of human resources, but also conditions of life that inhibit the rational long-term planning requisite for economic growth. We are ignoring the economic effects of this demographic pattern precisely because they are negative and no discussion is needed. Naturally, reduction of high death rates is a matter of high priority—for many reasons, among which economic growth prospects are not necessarily the most important. Our problem here is with high fertility rates associated with moderate death rates—in other words, with the economic effects of high rates of population growth.

This stated, we should note that in many LD countries, particularly in Africa, both birth and death rates are high, and the rates of natural increase are as moderate as those in the older developed countries. It is difficult to estimate the size of the population with this pre-modern pattern of high birth and death rates, because the vital statistics, particularly for LD countries, are most unreliable.[13] But the number may be large; and we stress its existence as another indication of the diversity of demographic patterns within the LD group that is so relevant to any analysis of economic effects. Although we omit this pre-modern pattern from discussion for the reason indicated, we should bear in mind that the pattern is likely to change in the near future into the one with which we deal, i.e. a combination of high birth and moderate death rates.

Second, we shall consider the economic effects of high rates of population growth for some moderate span of time—say over the next three to four decades—rather than extrapolate population growth further into the future. Much of our concern with population growth, in both LD and MD countries, stems from the confrontation of the cumulative effect of fixed percentage rates of growth, at observed levels, with the limits, perceived or reasonably extended, of natural resource supplies or of other non-reproducible natural conditions of our universe. We could not deal effectively with this problem if it were projected far into the future—if only because we cannot forecast either technological or social capacity as easily as we can extrapolate simple growth rates (of population). If we confine our view to the period ending in the year 2000, it can be argued that for the present and prospective population growth (with rates as high as those now shown, or in prospect, for the LD countries), an increasing per capita supply of natural resources or their substitutes is technologically and economically feasible—in the sense that we know how to produce it (technological feasibility) and can do so without absorbing so much of capital and other productive resources as to inhibit the growth of total product per capita (economic feasibility).[14] If this argument is accepted, the economic effects of high rates of population growth can be discussed without concern that technological constraints, arising from shortages of natural resources, may overshadow the question of economic advantages and disadvantages. But even though we put the problem aside here, it should be noted that pressures of population on natural resources can be overcome only at some cost; and that techno-economic feasibility does not mean social feasibility, i.e. the likelihood that the necessary social innovations will be made—a point to which we return in our concluding comments.

Third, if we assume an adequate supply of natural resources, the economic effects of higher rates of population growth should be related to some criteria of adequate economic performance. It will facilitate discussion if only one criterion—sustained increase in product per capita—is used. This is a major limitation because other and quite different criteria—less inequity in distributon, greater freedom for consumers, a more meaningful connection between economic performance of individuals and the material conditions of their life, and so on—may be equally, if not more, important. Any attempt to trace the effects of a high rate of growth of population on all these aspects of economic growth is almost impossible. Yet we must emphasize that this limitation qualifies our conclusions severely. While a high rate of population growth may prove to have limited effects on growth of per capita product, it may well have more significant consequences for various structural aspects, the "quality" aspects, of economic and social growth.

The economic effects of a high rate of population increase are presumably those on the supply of productive factors, relative to a growing population. But what are the productive factors? The concept of capital may be limited to material investment, or may also include education, etc. The quality of labor may also be emphasized in diverse ways. Consequently we set a fourth limitation on our discussion, and confine our analysis, in the initial stages, to the effects of a high rate of population increase on the supply of productive factors conventionally and narrowly refined, i.e. on material capital formation and on labor supply without regard for quality changes resulting from investment in education, training, and other elements now conventionally included under consumption.

Within the four limitations set, a high rate of population increase has two types of economic effects: (a) on the age structure of the population, and hence on the relation of dependents to active members of the labor force (the dependency ratio); and (b) on the demand for capital equipment to supply the additions to the labor force (which are large because of the high rate of natural increase) with the average capital per worker of the original labor force, and hence on the possibility of *increasing* the average capital and thus the average product per worker (and possibly per capita).

(a) The effect on age structure can be seen easily from recent data on vital rates and the age distribution of the population of countries grouped by per capita product. For some forty countries with per capita GDP of less that $200 in 1958, which clearly belong to the LD group, the average crude birth rate in 1957-59 was 42.8 per thousand, the crude death rate was 17.6, and the crude rate of natural increase was 25.2, whereas the corresponding rates were 19.8, 9.8, and 10.0 for the twenty countries, with per capita GDP of over $575, in the MD group. The age composition of population around 1960 for a somewhat smaller sample shows that in thirty-four LD countries, the average share of the ages under 15 was 43.3 percent, of those 15 through 59, 51.3 percent, and of those 60 and over, 5.4 percent; the corresponding percentages for nineteen MD countries were 27.4, 58.2, and 14.4.[15] The dependency ratio, calculated as the ratio of total population (all population is dependent upon the product) to the population in working ages (defined here as those from 15 through 59), is 1.95 for the LD countries and 1.72 for the MD countries. Thus, the former had about 13 percent more dependents per member of the working age classes than the latter; and on the assumption of the same product per member of the working age classes, the product per capita would be 12 percent less in the LD than in the MD countries. Presumably, a shift toward a higher rate of natural increase would, via its effect on age structure, reduce any growth in the per capita product otherwise secured; and a lowering of the per capita product *level* would in turn have constraining effects on further growth of per capita product.

The ratios just calculated both under- and overestimate the effects on a more meaningful ratio of dependents to possible workers. They underestimate them because they disregard the greater proportional engagement of females, ages 15 through 59, in bearing and rearing children in the LD than in MD countries. If we assume that this proportion is about half in the LD countries but only a quarter in the MD countries, and also assume rough equality of sexes, the dependency ratios become 2.60 for the LD countries and 1.96 for the MD countries, with a relative differential of almost one-quarter (of the larger ratio). But these are overestimates because the consumption requirements of the young and the old are not as high (per unit) as those of the adult working ages; and if we set them at 0.6 of those of the adult working ages, the ratios become 2.09 for the LD group and 1.64 for the MD group. If in the two groups of countries, product *per working member of the adult age group* is assumed the same, the product *per consuming unit* would, according to the last pair of ratios, be 47.8 units for the LD countries and 61.1 units for the MD countries, a differential of over a fifth of the latter.

Granted the validity of the orders of magnitude suggested above, we can conclude that, under the conditions assumed and because of differences in age structure, per unit product associated with a high rate of population increase would be about 20 percent lower than that associated with a low rate of population increase. But what are the consequences, not for the level, but for the *rate of growth* of per capita product? Two may be suggested. First, during the period of *transition* from low to high rates of population increase, the rise in the dependency ratio would, ceteris paribus, lower the rate of growth of per consuming unit product (and the effects are assigned to changes

in age structure alone, *not* to the rise in the rate of population increase). The magnitude of this transitional effect depends upon the
length of the period of rising rates of population increase and upon
the lag in adjustment of the age structure. Thus, if the shift and its
age-structure effects take place over 20 years, a 20 percent differential
in per capita product can reduce the rate of growth in per unit product
over those two decades markedly. But this is purely a transitional
effect, and would cease the moment the age structure completed its
response to the rise in the rate of population increase. Second, ceteris
paribus, a per consuming unit product that is *persistently* lower (because of age-structure effects) than a relevant alternative, since at any
given time another age structure could have yielded a higher per
unit product, has an effect on savings, or investment, and consequently on the rate of growth of total product. This effect is persisting if the age-structure implications of a high rate of population
increase are compared with those that would have been obtained if
the specific age structure associated with a high rate of population
increase could have been avoided. The magnitude of this persisting
effect can be suggested, at least illustratively. Data for the 1950's indicate that the net savings proportion (net national capital formation
as a percentage of net national product) in the LD countries (those
with 1958 per capita GDP below $200) was roughly about 8.5 percent;
whereas that for the MD countries (with per capita GDP over $575)
was about 15.5 percent—say in the ratio of 1 to 2.[16] If we use a range
of 1 to 6 in per capita product between the two groups of countries—
a moderate one after allowing for purchasing power adjustments—
the income elasticity of savings (i.e. the ratio of the proportional
difference in savings to the proportional difference in income, both
taken to geometric means as bases) is about 1.48. A differential in per
capita income equal to a fifth of the larger, or 22.4 percent of the
geometric mean, would then mean a differential in savings of 33.2
percent of the geometric mean, or a differential in the savings *proportion* between 100 and 66.8/77.6, or roughly 14 percent. If the savings
proportion determines the capital formation proportion, and if the
latter, given a fixed incremental capital-output ratio, sets the rate
of growth of total product, a decline of about one-seventh in the savings proportion means an equal drop in the rate of growth of total
product—all of this subject to the qualifications that further discussion
of the relations between capital formation proportions and rates of
growth of product suggests.

Whether or not the effects just indicated—both for the transitional trend caused by a shift to a higher rate of increase of population and for the persistent consequences of a continuing lower than

might have been per unit product on savings, and hence on growth rates—are major, they are based on calculations which assume a direct and close relation between the age distribution and active participation in economic production. Yet there may be little basis for assuming such a close connection, particularly in comparing LD and MD countries, since many differences in economic and social structure, only some of which are connected with differences in birth and natural increase rates, may affect the age-specific economic activity participation rates. In fact, we find (in the source cited in footnote 16) that for 36 LD countries (each with per capita income less than $200 in 1958) the proportion of economically active to total population in recent years averaged 40.7 percent, compared with 44.7 percent in the 20 MD countries (with income over $575 in 1958). The difference is in the expected direction, but it is only a third as wide as the one implied in the calculations above (where, with allowance for the time adult women spend in bearing and rearing children, the implicit percentages of economically active population were 38.5 for the LD and 50.9 for the MD countries). Clearly, the higher proportion of the population economically active in the LD countries—higher than one would expect on the basis of the age distribution—is due to engagement of a larger percentage of the young males (particularly those below the age of 20) and of the old group (much less important statistically). In the LD countries entry into the labor force is at an earlier age and not delayed by as long a period of education as in the MD countries.[17] On the basis of the proportions of the economically active (and the lower consumption requirements of the young and old), the dependency ratios become 1.87 for the LD and 1.74 for the MD countries, and income per consuming unit (on the assumption of the same return per member of the labor force) becomes 53.4 for LD and 57.4 for MD countries, a difference of about 7 percent of the higher figure. Such differentials are of little consequence for the rate of growth of per unit product in a transition period or for the more persisting effects of a slightly lower per unit income.

Thus in any comparison of the LD and the MD groups, the major effect of the high rate of population increase, via the age structure, is on the rates of participation in the labor force, particularly by the younger males. The factors to which the higher birth rates may be a response, viz. those that reduce the value of investment in the younger generation in the way of education, etc., also make for greater participation in economic activity at earlier ages. To the extent that this failure to invest in human capital influences growth in per capita product, it belongs to the second category of effects, those via pressure on capital formation. In dealing with age structure proper, we can infer that, because of different labor force participation rates, the direct economic effects are minor; and that when the participation rates begin to change, and thus lead to higher dependency ratios, the changes will presumably be in response to changes in views on investment in quality of the younger generation, and will also mean changes in the birth rates and rates of natural increase.

(b) High rates of population increase must affect capital requirements if we assume limited substitution of labor for capital, and a minimum level of capital for turning out product. If we assume that the incremental capital-output (c/o) ratio, i.e. the ratio of additions to capital to additions to product, is 3 to 1, and that population grows 3 percent per year, the *maintenance* of per capita product would require additions to capital, i.e. net capital formation, equivalent to 3 percent × 3, or 9 percent of total product. If the net capital formation capacity of an economy were, say, 15 percent of total product, this would leave only 6 percent of total product for capital formation to provide *additions* to product—which would permit total product to grow an additional 2 percent, and per capita product 1.9 percent per year (i.e. 105/103 − 1.00). But if population were growing only 1 percent per year, net capital formation needed to maintain per capita product would be only 3 percent of total product, leaving 12 percent to provide additions to total product of 4 percent, and per capita product would also grow about 4 percent per year. If the net capital formation proportion actually realized were to drop to 10 percent, the residue for increasing per capita product would practically vanish if the rate of population growth was 3 percent, but would still be substantial if it was 1 percent.

In any evaluation of the effect on capital requirements of high rates of population increase, two aspects are important: (1) the degree of fixity in the capital requirements; and (2) the level of the c/o ratio. The more fixed the requirement and the higher the c/o ratio, the greater the pressure of high rates of population increase on capital formation, and hence the greater the constraint on the growth of per capita product. While fixity and level are interrelated, it is best to consider them separately.[18]

(1) Although it appears to be a technological measure, the c/o ratio is largely a social magnitude that is variable over time and differs substantially among countries. Even in the production of a *single* commodity by a standardized method, capital can be utilized with different degrees of intensity (ranging from less than 8 to 24 hours a day); and can be expensive (new, or solid and durable) or inexpensive (secondhand, or less solid and less durable). For several products, all relevant to the same need (e.g. various means of transportation, or

types of shelter) the capital employed may involve significantly different c/o ratios. For an open economy, i.e. one that can supplement domestic production by imports (in return for exports), the choice is extended to that between domestic output and foreign provenance—for the same range of needs for final products; and the c/o ratios can be modified by reliance on a different structure and volume of exports and imports.

It is, therefore, hardly surprising that the observed incremental c/o ratios change markedly over time—usually rising in the course of economic growth as pressure to economize on capital declines; and, in cross-section comparisons, are usually lower in the less developed than in the more developed countries.[19] Of particular interest in the present connection is the evidence for the post-World War II period, for which we have fairly comprehensive estimates at least for the non-Communist world. Gross domestic product (in 1958 prices) for the less developed non-Communist countries (Latin America, Asia excluding Japan, and Africa excluding South Africa) grew from 1950-52 to 1962-64 at the rate of 4.58 percent per year; the comparable rate for the developed non-Communist countries (Europe, North America, Australia and New Zealand, Japan, and South Africa) was 4.02 percent per year.[20] We also know that in the 1950's net capital formation proportions (*domestic*, related to net domestic product, not national as used above) averaged about 10.1 percent in the LD countries and 15.4 percent in the MD countries (the former being countries with per capita GDP below $200 in 1958; the latter with per capitas above $575). The gross domestic capital formation proportions (related to gross domestic product) were 15.9 and 22.2 percent respectively. Since net and gross domestic product have approximately the same rate of growth, the incremental net c/o ratios were 2.2 for the LD countries, and 3.8 for the MD countries—a difference of more than 40 percent of the larger figure (the gross c/o ratios were 3.5 and 5.5 respectively).

This seeming lack of fixity in incremental c/o ratios does not mean that the c/o ratio can be extended downward to some virtually insignificant level close to zero. A sizable chunk of capital, not replaceable by labor, is required if a given group of products, even broadly defined, is to be produced. This irreducible capital, which forms the hard core of the c/o ratio, is presumably found at low levels; and in this sense fixity and level are interrelated. But how low is the low, and how much can the c/o ratio be modified? This question is not easily answered—for it requires knowledge of the effect of the economic and social institutions on the efficiency with which capital can be used in order to optimize economic growth. At this point not only the economic, but also several social factors become important, for they can influence the efficiency of capital use, and fairly significantly on a nationwide scale. All one can say here is that the c/o ratio becomes fixed only at low levels; and that it has a wide range which is affected by social and political factors that far transcend the economic—so that the economic effects via capital requirements become dependent on the social and political system—a conclusion which will only be reinforced by consideration of the questions bearing on the *level* of the capital formation requirements.

(2) Given fixity of the incremental c/o ratio, its level is clearly important in evaluating the economic effects of a high rate of population increase because it reveals the magnitudes of the adjustments required to *compensate* for the greater capital requirements. Thus, if the relevant c/o ratio is 3 to 1, and we compare the effects of two rates of population increase, 1 and 3 percent per year, the difference in capital formation is between 3 and 9 percent of net product respectively; and the additional 6 percent of national product, if these are to be shifted from consumption to capital formation, are only a slightly larger fraction of government and household consumption, which together are well over 80 percent of national product. We can argue that with this c/o ratio, the shift of resources to provide the additional capital formation required seems moderate. But if the c/o ratio is 15 to 1, capital requirements for the same two rates of population increase are 45 and 15 percent of national product, necessitating a shift of over a third of consumption into capital formation. Such a large shift is formidable, and would require major changes in the institutions that govern the allocation of resources.

In order to ascertain the level of the incremental c/o ratio—which must be done before the effects of a high rate of population increase in the LD countries can be evaluated—we must identify the capital required to increase product per unit of labor (in the MD countries) and then accept or adjust the resultant level in application to the LD countries. In attempting this task, we face two distinct, but interrelated, difficulties.

The first, having to do with observation and measurement of the c/o ratio in the past, forces us to define capital. So far we limited ourselves to the narrow, conventional definition, i.e. material investment in construction, equipment, and additions to inventories, and based the ratios on this definition. But the use, in the analysis of economic growth, of capital inputs so defined together with labor inputs (even when the latter are adjusted for differences in compensation and thus implicitly in quality), leaves a large unexplained residual—a rise in output per unit of input—which must be due to other factors.

It is because of this finding that economists have turned to education as a possibly important capital factor. And once capital is defined as any input that raises the productivity of "pure" labor (i.e. labor unaffected by an investment in productivity-raising inputs like education, special health provisions, etc.), its scope is widened to include many uses of product now covered under consumption—ranging from better food, shelter, education, and all such "productive" elements of personal consumption to public outlays, not only on education, etc., but also on other services that increase social, and through it, economic efficiency. With this wider concept of capital, the line of distinction between economic and non-economic shifts, at least as far as analysis is concerned. For in order to measure the relevant capital inputs, we must distinguish within all uses of economic product between "pure" consumption and "pure" capital formation components; and we can do this only through analysis of the content of the activity involved in its bearing upon labor productivity. Even if the specific activity or process requires only a minor input of economic sources, it may have a large effect on productivity. And the analysis clearly points to the next stage, viz. a recognition that economic productivity may be vitally affected by social institutions and processes that in themselves require no or few inputs of *economic* resources. Yet the changes in these institutions and processes required to assure adequate economic productivity may be neither easy nor free, even though the costs are not economic.

The second difficulty is that even if we could identify and measure capital, in terms limited to economic inputs, but corresponding to the broader definition just suggested, the observed measures would relate almost necessarily to the MD countries—not only because the data are available for them, but also because increases in the product of the LD countries are likely to follow the paths already established for the MD countries. But one may argue that, whatever the definition of capital and whatever the levels of the derived incremental c/o ratios, these levels would have to be changed when applied to the LD countries, since, ceteris paribus, these countries can choose more economically among a wider variety of capital uses than their predecessors could in the past. The difficulty, however, is in approximating the magnitude of this downward adjustment, in identifying the minimum requirement in the way of social institutions and other non-economic conditions of economic productivity that were satisfied in the past, and deciding how they can be modified in application to the LD countries.

These rather general comments should serve to indicate the difficulties we face in suggesting the relevant levels of the c/o ratios

—and indeed, in considering the whole question of the effects of a higher rate of population increase in the LD countries on capital requirements. If we limit capital to the narrow, conventional definition, the observed incremental c/o ratios will be fairly low, about 3 to 1 for the net ratios and about 5 to 1 for the gross ratios; and with a further significant reduction in these ratios (which we cannot specify) when applied to the LD countries, the economic effects of the higher rate of population growth are quantitatively minor; and do not necessitate a difficult shift in the allocation of resources even in the LD countries. But this answer is due to the narrow definition of capital, and to the disregard of the other conditions of the efficient use of material capital, that may or may not require substantial economic inputs. And this means that in policy uses one cannot assume that satisfaction of the capital requirements in response to higher rates of population increase and for capital narrowly defined would be sufficient to permit a rise (or even maintenance) of per capita product, despite the high rate of population increase.

The other alternative is to consider the broader definition of capital, which is more realistic but far more demanding. Capital would then include some major uses of product now included under consumption, and consequently the incremental capital-output ratio would be substantially higher. The costs of education alone (including foregone income, which reflects the lower labor force participation ratios among the young and thus reintroduces the age-structure effects of the higher rate of population increase) might double both the capital total and the incremental c/o ratio.[21] And the shift of other "capital-like" elements now classified as consumption (e.g. special health services) would raise the c/o ratio even further. But in drawing the line of distinction between consumption and capital formation, and ascertaining the indispensable elements in the latter, we face the problem of "fixity" in an aggravated form; and we would also face the question of the downward adjustment to be made in applying even the hard c/o ratios observed for the past to the LD countries. Do these countries need the resource-consuming educational, etc., provisions of the MD countries to assure fairly efficient use of material capital to increase economic product? In our present state of ignorance, the relevant incremental c/o ratio, based on this wider concept of capital, cannot be measured with any assurance. It would surely be higher than the ratio under the narrower and more conventional definition of capital, but the orders of magnitude cannot be suggested, although I would guess that the level would not be prohibitively high.

As already indicated, this approach suggests that the purely economic resource requirements of a high rate of population growth, reflected in the c/o ratio which relates *economic* inputs to economic product, would be only moderately high. But, more important, it would stress that the variability of even the broader c/o ratios is due to conditioning of economic efficiency by social institutions and by points of view guiding individuals and societies, aspects of social life that have only minor economic *input* implications and are not likely to be reflected in c/o ratios so long as the numerators of these ratios, even with the widest definition of capital, are *economic* inputs. The belief of East Indians in the sacredness of life, which means a large waste of crops (because of destruction by pests), may significantly affect the c/o ratio in Indian agriculture, and any shift in the ratio in response to a high rate of population growth may necessitate a change in beliefs, which in turn may require only a minor input of economic resources but a large input of other resources in order to modify long-implanted beliefs or to change traditional and respected institutions. The major significance of high birth rates and of a high rate of population increase for growth in per capita product may lie, not in the direct economic effects, which may be moderate even with a wider definition of capital, but in the fact that they reflect a system of views and a set of social institutions unfavorable to modern economic growth.

Concluding Comments

One main theme of this paper is that economic causes do not adequately explain the high levels of fertility in the LD countries, and therefore a more relevant complex of observable and measurable factors than the conventional measures of economic levels or conventional aspects of economic structure (such as per capita income or the share of agriculture) must be sought. A parallel theme is that the economic effects of the high rates of population increase in the LD countries, i.e. greater capital requirements, seem relatively moderate, and emphasis on them oversimplifies the problem. This is because the conventionally measured economic effects overlook other "capital" items required and, in fact, used in the past. This other capital may represent substantial economic inputs, and, if included, would raise the incremental c/o ratio and thus magnify the economic effects of a high rate of population growth by increasing the numerator. On the other hand, it may mean non-economic inputs (e.g. such aspects of the political structure as loyalty and stability) that have a marked effect on economic productivity; and if neglected, may mean a higher c/o ratio because of the effect on the denominator.

If we disregard these non-economic elements, we might find that even with the wider definition of capital, the economic effects of a high rate of population growth would not constitute a major obstacle to an increase in per capita product. And this parallels the conclusion, assumed in the course of discussion, of the technological and economic feasibility of providing the growing population with natural resources. But in both cases the conclusions assume social feasibility, i.e. the capacity of societies to change their institutions and beliefs in order to make more effective use of natural resources or of the economic capital involved in the techno-economic feasibilities. It may well be that social feasibility is more important than the simpler relation of numbers to resources, natural or reproducible; and that if the prospect of changes in social institutions and views is favorable, the LD countries can cope with both the economic effects and the ultimate trend of the present demographic patterns.

Two obvious inferences relating to policy should perhaps be explicitly stated. First, growth policy in LD countries must be geared to a much broader set of determinants and concepts than is, or can be, provided by current economic analysis; which means also that, for lack of such an established framework, conventional economic analysis should be more critically scrutinized and less readily accepted. Second, too much reliance should not be placed on the favorable economic consequences of a lower rate of population increase, in contrast to the unfavorable results of a higher rate of increase. Obviously, this is not to deny that population control would make a large contribution—relieving current social tensions, offsetting failures to exploit the given technological and economic potentials, and forestalling major acute problems in the longer run (longer than the one considered here). But it does suggest a conservative view of the possible benefits of a lower rate of population growth, if the determinants of economic growth other than the simple relations of numbers to economic resources are not transformed to induce greater exploitation of the technological and economic potentials available to the LD countries.

Notes

1. The calculation is based on United Nations, *Demographic Yearbook, 1965* (New York, 1966) Table 1, p. 103. The 1960-64 birth rates shown there were weighted by the arithmetic means of the 1960 and 1964 populations. The LD group is the sum of Africa; Asia except Japan; Latin America, except temperate South America; and Oceania, other than Australia and New Zealand. The MD group is the sum of Western, Northern, and Eastern Europe, the U.S.S.R., Japan, North America, and Australia and New Zealand. Southern Europe and temperate South America are excluded.

2. For 1937 see United Nations, *World Population Trends, 1920-1947* (New York, December 1949), Table 2, p. 10; for 1947 see United Nations, *The Determinants and Consequences of Population Trends,* Population Studies No. 17 (New York, 1953), Table 51, p. 71. For the 1950's see tables in earlier issues of the *Demographic Yearbook* similar to that cited in footnote 1.

3. See United Nations, *Population Bulletin No. 7—1963* (New York, 1965), which is devoted to fertility trends, summarizes a huge volume of data, and contains much analysis relevant to the central theme of this paper.

4. See Simon Kuznets, *Modern Economic Growth* (New Haven: Yale University Press, 1966), Table 8.2, pp. 438-39. The accompanying discussion covers the demographic patterns in the less developed countries; but the grouping used in the table is too broad to reveal the full range of differences among countries.

5. See *Population Bulletin No. 7,* chap. ix, pp. 134-51, which emphasizes this bunching and presents some analytical suggestions as to its implication.

6. In *Population Bulletin No. 7* the correlations for *all* countries between gross reproduction rates and such economic variables as per capita income, the share of non-agriculture in labor force, energy consumption per capita, are all high, negative, and statistically significant (see Table 9.8, p. 148).

7. The death rates were calculated in the manner indicated for birth rates in footnote 1.

In a highly suggestive paper, "Morality Level and Desired Family Size" (presented at the 1966 meeting of the American Association for the Advancement of Science), David M. Heer and Dean O. Smith, of the Harvard University School of Public Health, present a simulation analysis showing gross reproduction rates (GRR) and intrinsic rates of natural increase based on the assumption that the parents, while having a perfect method of birth control, want "to be highly certain that at least one son will survive to the father's 65th birthday." On the assumption of a 95 percent probability of attaining the aim, this simulation analysis for several United Nations mortality models of varying expectation of life at birth shows a steady decline in the GRR as expectation of life rises, but an inverted U shape in the intrinsic rate of natural increase, the latter being low at both very high and very low levels of mortality. The GRR at life expectancy (both sexes) of 35 years is 3.6 and the intrinsic rate of increase is 2.72 percent per year; at life expectancy of 50 years, the GRR declines to 2.4 but the intrinsic rate of increase is still 2.53 percent; at life expectancy of 71.7, the GRR is 1.27 and the rate of increase is 0.9 percent. Although the analysis is subject to several modifications, some of which are presented in the paper, it does demonstrate the effect of changing mortality on birth rates and rates of natural increase when the surviving size of family is being planned. The actual cross-section of countries by rates of natural increase and mortality (for 1946-63) shows the inverted U shape.

8. The limited statistical effects of the economic variables, once other variables are included in the regression equations, are suggested in a paper by Irma Adelman, "An Econometric Analysis of Population Growth,"

American Economic Review, LIII, No. 3 (June 1963), 314-39. A simple regression shows a negative and statistically significant association between age specific (by age of mother) birth rates and per capita income. But a multiple regression equation that includes the share of the labor force employed outside of agriculture, an index of education, and an index of population density, shows that the partial regression coefficient of the age specific birth rates on per capita income is statistically insignificant for all but the two lowest age classes (15-19 and 20-24) and its sign is *positive* (see Table 1, p. 321). On the other hand, the partial regression coefficient for the index of education is consistently negative, large, and statistically significant. But what economic and social variables are represented by the index of education, a combination of a measure of literacy and one of newspaper circulation?

The opaqueness of many of the statistical variables is one persisting limitation of the multivariate statistical analysis so suggestively pursued in the Adelman paper. What is the meaning of the net regression coefficient of the per capita income variable when the effects of an unknown conglomerate represented by an index of education (or of population density) on both the dependent and the other independent variables have presumably been eliminated? Because of this limitation, the analysis and its findings are only barely informative. The unknown interplay of forces reflected in most measurable variables renders such analysis difficult. It would be eased by multiplying the number of variables, which is impractical; or by refining the formulations, which requires the scrutiny of all the statistical measures under widely different social and economic conditions.

9. Per capita GDP is calculated from United Nations, *Yearbook of National Accounts Statistics, 1965,* Tables 9A and 9B, supplemented by data for the Communist countries in my *Postwar Economic Growth* (Cambridge: Harvard University Press, 1964), Table 1, pp. 29-31. The crude birth rates were calculated as indicated in footnote 1.

10. See O. Andrew Collver, *Birth Rates in Latin America,* Institute for International Studies, University of California, Berkeley, 1965.

11. The product figures, from ECLA, are given in Alexander Ganz, "Problems and Uses of National Wealth Estimates in Latin America," in Raymond Goldsmith and Christopher Saunders, eds., *Income and Wealth, Series VIII* (London, 1959) Table XXVIII, p. 260. The death rates and infant mortality are from the Collver monograph.

12. "According to this hypothesis, in a developing country where fertility is initially high, improving economic and social conditions are likely to have little if any effect on fertility until a certain economic and social level is reached; but once that level is achieved, fertility is likely to enter a decided decline and to continue downward until it is again stabilized on a much lower plane" (*Population Bulletin No. 7,* p. 143).

13. If net reproduction rates below 1.5 are taken as moderate, and gross reproduction rates over 2 as high, Table 30 of the *Demographic Yearbook, 1965* shows such a combination for at least six African countries (Central African Republic, Chad, both Congos, Gabon, Upper Volta).

14. For a more detailed discussion of these questions see Simon Kuznets, "Economic Capacity and Population Growth," in Richard N. Farmer, John D. Long, and George Stolnitz, eds., *World Population-The View Ahead,* Indiana University, Bloomington, 1968, pp. 51-97.

15. These and other data in this paragraph are from Kuznets, *Modern Economic Growth*, Table 8.2, pp. 438-40.

In "Population and Economic Growth," *Proceedings of the American Philosophical Society*, 111, No. 3, (June 1967) 170-93, I used a somewhat different set of age classes, assigning the ages 15 through 64 (rather than 15 through 59) to the adult working ages. The results differ little from those shown here.

16. See Simon Kuznets, *Modern Economic Growth*, Table 8.1, pp. 402-8.

17. On this and other demographic aspects of labor force see Jan L. Sadie, "Demographic Aspects of Labour Supply and Employment," Background Paper WPC/WP/84 for Session A.5 of the 1965 U.N. World Population Conference at Belgrade.

18. For a more detailed discussion see Kuznets, "Population and Economic Growth," referred to in footnote 15.

19. For details of these findings see Papers v and vi in the series entitled "Quantitative Aspects of the Economic Growth of Nations," *Economic Development and Cultural Change*, Vol. viii, No. 4, Part ii (July 1960) and Vol. ix, No. 4, Part ii (July 1961).

20. These rates are based on the indexes in the United Nations, *Yearbook of National Accounts Statistics, 1965*, Table 8B, pp. 488-92, with the indexes for the less developed countries brought through 1964 on the basis of data for individual countries in O.E.C.D. Development Center, *National Accounts for Less Developed Countries*, Paris, February 1967 (preliminary). The capital formation proportions are from Kuznets, *Modern Economic Growth*, Table 8.1.

21. See in this connection the illustrative calculation in Kuznets, *Modern Economic Growth*, Table 5.2, p. 231 and the accompanying text.

POPULATION, FOOD AND THE ENERGY TRANSITION

Harrison Brown
California Institute of Technology

Introduction

IT MIGHT WELL TURN OUT that humanity will not be able to extricate itself from its present precarious situation. Increasing population pressures, rising rates of population growth and decreasing per capita availability of food in the poorer regions of the world, a widening economic gap between the rich countries and the poor, a restlessness in the poorer countries stimulated in part by the spreading realization that from a technological point of view they too could lead lives free of deprivation—all of these factors breed political chaos, violence, and unreasoning actions which threaten nations and people. Even a casual survey of current trends indicates that people in the poorer countries will probably be even hungrier a decade from now than they are today, that improvement in economic conditions will take place so slowly that the average individual will not notice much change for the better during his lifetime, that internal political chaos in these areas will increase rapidly, that political differences among the richer nations, when coupled with the tribulations of the poorer ones, can lead to major wars and eventually to the downfall of industrial civilization.

At the same time it is becoming increasingly evident that modern science and technology have given man unprecedented power. We are clearly able from a technological point of view to feed adequately a population considerably larger than that of today, to control its growth, to educate, clothe, and house it. Indeed, we can create a world in which all people, if they wish, can lead free and abundant lives.

In this discussion we will assume that man attempts to make use of these powers and that there will be no major world catastrophe. Within this framework we will attempt to assess world needs for food, energy, and other resources with respect to population and levels of economic and social development. We will then inquire into prospects for increasing the *rate* of improvement of the lot of the average individual. How rapidly can food production be increased? How rapidly can economic improvement be brought about? What are the basic rate-limiting factors in economic development?

"Needs"

The total "needs" of a society for food and other resources can be expressed by the product of population and per capita "needs." Clearly, as the population increases the total demand will increase. Were the population of India, within the framework of today's culture, to increase by 10 percent, the requirements for food would also increase by about 10 percent. Similarly, an increase of population in the United States would have associated with it an equivalent increase in demand for food and other resources.

Granting the general linearity of total requirements in terms of population, the tremendous variation of per capita needs among societies places wide limits upon estimates of future demand. For example, the per capita daily food energy production in India is approximately 2200 calories, while that in the United States is about 10,800 calories. The Indians consume virtually all of their cultivated photosynthates directly. In the United States we consume directly only about 20 percent of our cultivated produce. The balance we feed to animals and obtain, in return, foodstuffs high in protein such as meat, milk, and eggs. In order to provide 940 calories per day of such food to the average person, we feed animals 8600 calories per day per person. As an extreme, were a society to obtain all of its calories from animals, the primary photosynthate would have to total nearly 30,000 calories per day per person. Thus, in terms of basic needs for primary photosynthates, per capita requirements can vary by a factor of 15, from about 2000 to nearly 30,000 calories per day per person.

With respect to material resources, per capita needs can vary over even greater ranges than they do for food. We know that societies which are primarily agricultural can be self-sufficient, reasonably well fed and healthy (provided there is enough food) with virtually no production of iron, steel, and other metals, no electricity, no appreciable consumption of fossil fuels. Yet once the society embarks upon the pathway that leads toward industrialization and the production of a multiplicity of consumer goods, a new ecological system emerges within which items such as telephones, motor vehicles, airplanes, and newsprint become necessities, where formerly they had been luxuries. The United States, which has traveled along this path further than any other nation, has now reached the point where there is nearly one motor vehicle and one telephone in use for every two persons. Altogether well over 10 tons of steel are functioning for every person in the nation. Some 1300 pounds of new steel are produced each year per person, in part to replace the old and in part to add to the capital. In order to power the system some 6000 kilowatt hours of electricity are generated each year per person, and total energy consumption per capita is equivalent to that which would be obtained by burning 11 tons of coal each year.

By contrast, the per capita consumption of material resources in India is tiny. For example, consumption of electricity per head is 100 times less than in the United States and annual per capita steel production is nearly 50 times less.

It is clear, then, that before we can realistically estimate future needs for food, energy, and other resources, we must specify the kinds of cultures we are talking about. Indeed, cultural evolution ultimately is likely to place far more severe demands upon the earth's resources than is population growth. This does not mean, however, that population growth is not associated with grave dangers.

The Energy Transition

To shift to agriculture was the first great human cultural transition following the appearance of tool-using man. The cultivation of the soil made it possible for more than 500 persons to be supported on land which in earlier food-gathering days provided subsistence for but one person. Further, a farmer working in the fields could grow somewhat more food than was needed to support his immediate family. This small surplus made possible the emergence of cities and provided the basis for the flourishing of the great ancient civilizations. From a technological point of view the transition reached its height at the peak of Roman civilization. The Roman engineers went about as far as they could go in the absence of easily available engines powered by other than human beings or animals.

In the soils of the world which are easiest to cultivate the "natural" daily yield of edible photosynthate appears on the average to be about 9000 kilogram calories per hectare. By "natural" we mean the yield which can be maintained without applying chemical fertilizers and pesticides and without benefits of irrigation other than that obtainable from nearby streams. The total area of such land in the world appears to be about 1400 million hectares (including some 200 million hectares of tropical laterites and northern podzols which have not yet been placed under cultivation). Had the agricultural transition continued unperturbed by new technological developments, the population of human beings would probably have grown eventually to a level of about 5000 million persons assuming a daily per capita subsistence availability of primary photosynthate of 2500 calories. This would be 50 percent greater than the population of human beings in the world today.

The ultimate level of population, as well as the worldwide rate of growth, was dramatically changed by the invention and evolution of new ways of concentrating and controlling energy. Starting with the Newcomer engine in 1705 and the near-simultaneous development by Darby of a process for converting coal to coke, a sequence of events took place which has had profound effect upon man's ability to produce food. The new technology made possible the production and distribution of fertilizers and pesticides; the scientific approach made possible the breeding of new varieties of plants. The combination of these developments increased potential average crop yields from about 9000 to more than 30,000 kilogram calories per hectare per year—greater than three times the "natural" level. Under optimal conditions annual yield of edible material corresponding to 150,000 calories per hectare per day are now obtainable (i.e., sugar cultivation in the north temperate regions under cloudless skies).

This second transition, which we will call the energy transition, also has extended in several ways the potential area of cultivatable land. First, the availability of large concentrations of power added a new dimension to our ability to manage water. By mid-twentieth century 11 percent of the world's cultivated acres were supplied with water by conventional irrigation schemes. In recent years the area of irrigated land has been increasing rapidly, particularly in Asia, Africa, and Latin America. The proportion of cultivated land irrigated by conventional means might eventually be expected to rise to about 20 percent. The proportion cannot become appreciably greater than this for there simply is not enough water available in our rivers. In spite of the small proportion of cultivated land under irrigation, however, the total effect of irrigation upon world crop production has been substantial.

Further, the energy transition accelerated the rate of development of new cropland. Forests could be converted to farms more rapidly than previously. Improved transportation made remote areas more easily accessible for settlement.

Altogether, the first phase of the energy transition has increased the "carrying capacity" of the earth for human beings at subsistence levels by a factor of about 4. Some 20,000 million persons could in principle be supported assuming a daily per capita availability of primary photosynthate of 2500 calories. This is some six-fold higher than the present population. Assuming that future per capita requirements for primary photosynthate are those prevailing in the United States today, some 4600 million persons could in principle be supported at U.S. levels of food intake.

The first phase of the energy transition also dramatically altered the ways in which people live. The new machines spread to the farms and rapidly replaced work animals and human beings. Whereas only some 10 percent of the population could live in cities following the agricultural transition, in the more technologically advanced countries we find that most people now live in cities. In such areas the working farm population is destined eventually to represent but a very small fraction of the total labor force.

It is in the highly urbanized technologically advanced nations of the world that per capita demands for raw materials and energy have reached such large proportions. And thus far, there is little indication of a lessening in the rate of growth of per capita needs. Our per capita quantities of steel and other metals in use in the United States are continuing to climb. Our per capita consumption of energy increased by 13.4 percent between 1960 and 1965 alone, corresponding to an annual growth rate of 2.7 percent per year. It is quite possible that by the year 2000 our per capita consumption of energy in the United States will exceed the equivalent of that obtained by burning fifteen tons of coal per person per year.

The Present Food Problem
Thus the first phase of the energy transition worked for the benefit of the people in the technologically more advanced countries. On the whole, they are now adequately fed, housed, and clothed. Their life expectancies appear to be the highest since man appeared on earth.

But in large regions of the world populations came into contact with the energy transition in one-sided ways. Irrigation systems were built and extended. Railroad systems and highways were built. Techniques of public health spread. In part for these reasons and in part for others, which are by no means clearly understood, life expectancy increased and with it rates of population growth. But farming technology did not change very much.

As new lands were put under cultivation in these regions the population continued to grow at such a pace that average levels of food intake remained at subsistence levels. Yet in most such areas the process of industrialization, which is essential if the chemicals and machinery required to produce more food are to be manufactured, has taken place at a rate much too slow to bring about real improvement.

In short, we know that by the uniform application of known technology world food production could be increased several-fold. In fact, however, yields per acre in the developing areas have increased only 8 percent in 10 years, less than 1 percent per annum. New lands have been brought into production only very slowly. The net result has been an actual decrease in per capita food availability in many regions of the world.

Such slow increases in productivity have certainly not been intentional. The development plans of virtually every developing nation have allocated 10 to 30 percent of development funds to agriculture and have anticipated increases of productivity ranging from 5 to 8 percent per year. The subsequent performance has almost always fallen discouragingly far short of the goals. The reasons for the failures have been manifold. The Food and Agriculture Organization of the United Nations has said about the Indian program that there have been "inadequate economic incentives to peasants, inadequate management programs, inadequate extension, inadequate supply of trained personnel at all levels."

Of all of the factors, education and training are perhaps the most critical. They have been key inputs in the rapid rise of productivity in the United States, Japan, and other developed countries. Japan, in order to support its intensive agriculture, produces 7000 college-level agriculturists per year. In all of Latin America, by comparison, only 1100 trained agriculturists are produced annually. In Japan there is one trained farm advisor for every 600 farms. In Colombia the ratio is more like one per 10,000.

People cannot be educated and trained overnight. As the Rockefeller Foundation has demonstrated in Mexico, decades are required to train the people who will have visible impact on agricultural productivity. Yet, we are confronted with the likelihood that the food situation in the developing countries will continue to get worse, at least into the 1980's, no matter what happens with respect to programs of population limitation.

It seems clear that alleviation of these difficulties requires massive action in the developing countries along numerous fronts. The first step is to recognize that the problem of agricultural development cannot be isolated from other problems of economic and social development, that the power plant, the truck, the steel mill, the highway, the pharmaceutical house, and the school are as essential ingredients for increasing agricultural productivity as are irrigation projects and fertilizers. Yet clearly, water, fertilizer, seeds, and pesticides are essential. In short, it would appear that what is needed is sustained general economic and social development at a rate which is considerably greater than the poorer nations of the world are experiencing today.

At the same time it seems obvious that the developing countries themselves cannot do the job alone. They need a great deal of help in the form of technical and capital assistance, help which is given at a rate which greatly transcends today's assistance programs. Indeed it seems doubtful that the major breakthrough can be made, leading to generally improved economic well-being, unless there is a flow of capital assistance from the richer countries to the poorer ones of some $200 billion during the next 20 years. Unless the richer nations are prepared to face up to this necessity the food problem simply will not be solved. Instead, we can look forward to a continuously widening economic gap between the rich countries and the poor and a steadily increasing pressure of population on the available land.

Under these circumstances by the year 2000 we might expect a world population of some 7000 million human beings of which some 20 percent would be classified as "very rich" and some 50 percent would be classified as "destitute."

Needs for World Development

Let us assume for the purpose of discussion that a vigorous program of economic and social development, of a magnitude which is commensurate with the need, is initiated cooperatively between the developed and underdeveloped countries. Presumably such programs would include vigorous birth control programs, the reduction of child and infant mortality, the development of educational systems, industrialization and planned urbanization, extension of cultivated land areas, development of highway and railroad networks, development of water resources, production of improved seed, fertilizers and pesticides, the development of research programs for learning how to do these things. Would the earth's resources permit us to accomplish our objective?

We can appreciate the magnitude of the task when we realize that were all of the persons living in the year 2000 suddenly to be brought up to the level of living enjoyed by the people of the United States today, we would need to extract from the earth over 50 billion tons of iron, one billion tons of copper, an equal amount of lead, over 600 million tons of zinc and nearly 100 million tons of tin, in addition to huge quantities of other substances. These quantities are several hundred times the present world annual rates of production. Their extraction would virtually deplete the earth of all high-grade mineral resources and would necessitate our living off the leanest of the earth substances—the waters of the sea and ordinary rock.

Although depletion of the earth's buried high-grade resources should be a matter of serious concern to us all, and undoubtedly would give rise to serious international competitions, it is by no means an immediate threat, nor is it an insurmountable problem. Given the necessary technology, which can certainly be developed, the earth has ample resources to enable all persons to lead abundant lives, even were the population to grow eventually to a considerably higher level than that now anticipated in the year 2000. Once the world, as a whole, achieves a level of production adequate to feed, clothe, and house the human population comfortably, the problem of continuing production is not great. By far the most difficult problem is that of getting from here to there.

The thought of the entire world living at current American levels of consumption might seem farfetched to many persons. I believe, however, that if development on a world scale is at all successful, something like that will happen, much as it is happening in Japan and in the U.S.S.R. today. Let us remember that Japan already produces more than one-half again as much steel each year as does the United Kingdom (which at one time was the world's largest producer of steel) and that sometime during the early 1970's the Soviet Union may well be producing more steel than will the United States. It is by no means inconceivable that China and India may one day outstrip us all.

The Energy Transition—Phase II

Today in the industrialized part of the world we are passing through a quiet revolution which seems destined to have profound effect upon the future of industrial civilization and which can eventually have considerable effect upon the course of economic development in the poorer countries. In brief, the cost of nuclear-generated power is dropping rapidly and in many areas appears to be less expensive than power generated from coal. The indications are that from now on in the United States more nuclear electrical generating capacity will be installed each year than generating capacity utilizing conventional fuels.

Studies of nuclear power costs suggest that they will continue to decline for some time. They also suggest that it might be possible to design cities in arid coastal regions of certain developing countries which are in effect agro-industrial complexes, completely nuclear powered, with water for agriculture being obtained from the oceans, and with the agriculture itself being highly mechanized.

Should such a development prove to be feasible it might turn out to be a "shortcut" for increasing agricultural production, for decreasing the numbers of required trained agricultural technicians and for integrating the industrial and agricultural sectors. Such a development would open up vast areas of India, Pakistan, the Middle East and North Africa, Brazil, Chile, and Peru for human habitation on a self-supporting basis. Indeed, we can easily imagine this new development doubling again the "carrying capacity" of the world.

Were this to happen, the total "carrying capacity" of the earth would then be eight-fold greater than that obtainable before the energy transition. This is small when compared with the factor of 500 provided by the agricultural transition. But it seems large when we consider that in principle it would make possible the support of a population of 40,000 million persons living at subsistence levels, or a population of 9000 million persons living at present U.S. levels of consumption.

POPULATION AND SOCIETY: AN ESSAY ON GROWTH

Amos H. Hawley

University of North Carolina

INTEREST IN THE RELATIONSHIP between population size and the organization of man's collective affairs is of ancient vintage. In all periods of history human groups have exhibited concern with the control of numbers and have attempted to fit the sizes of their groups to their manpower needs. And every society in its mute wisdom has equipped itself with the cultural means for protection against too few and too many people. Among the first to formulate a principle regarding the relationship was Herbert Spencer. Increase of mass, declared Spencer, is the causal force in social as well as in organic evolution. More specifically, increase in size fosters differentiation thereby converting a human aggregate from a state of incoherent homogeneity to one of coherent heterogeneity.[1] Emile Durkheim went further to point out that population increase is perhaps a necessary but not a sufficient condition for the rise of an "organic" type of social organization. There must be an increase in social or "moral" density, i.e., communication, in order for integration on the basis of differentiation to occur.[2] But Durkheim's view was consulted only by an occasional sociologist, while the principle generalized by Spencer became the prevailing dogma. It had been prominent, of course, in the writings of classical economists on competition before the appearance of Spencer's monumental work, and it persisted in their works well into the twentieth century. Competition, itself a function of numbers, was held to be the great distributor and organizer of men. In due course, however, such an explanation was judged to be far too simple and was set aside for more sophisticated conceptions of societal development.

The years following the speculations of Spencer and Durkheim have brought a surprisingly small amount of empirical investigation into the implications of population size for the organization of society. Most of what has been done is found in studies of social evolution by archaelogists and anthropologists. I will have occasion to refer to some of that work in later pages, but much of it suffers from exceeding breadth and lack of detail. Students of contemporary societies, sociologists for the most part, have avoided the larger issue, preferring to draw the problem down to particular institutions.[3] The relevance of the findings from those studies for present purposes hangs upon an assumption of isomorphism between the parts and the whole of a social system which might better be debated elsewhere. Now and then a student of society at large acknowledges the existence of the demographic factor, but after a few introductory remarks the matter is usually forgotten as attention fastens on the details of social organization.[4]

I confess that the more I have thought about the question the more sympathy I have gained for what seems to be a general avoidance of the issue. Tantalizing as the question is, it casts one upon a sea of uncharted perplexities. The main difficulty, in my judgment, lies in the great disparity between the two terms of the relationship. While population is a relatively specific variable, society, social system or social organization, however we characterize it, is a highly involuted one. There is a great deal of consensus about how to conceptualize and measure the one, but very little agreement on how to treat the other. In fact, our knowledge, or perhaps I should say our conceptual apparatus, has not yet prepared us for the formulation of society as a single variable, if indeed that is possible. What we have, instead, is a set of variables of undetermined number and of unassessed weights and qualities.

Having said as much, it seems more than a little presumptuous to proceed with an examination of the relationship between population change and societal change. Still, the question has enough importance to warrant an exploration, if only in a preliminary fashion. In the nature of the case my procedure will have to be speculative, though it will be possible to supplement the argument here and there with empirical gleanings from available sources. But first I must describe how I intend to view society and population.

Society, or better still, a social system, may be simply described as an arrangement of relationships among a set of mutually complementary parts. This, of course, glosses over a mass of complexity. If we confine attention to its formal aspects alone, there are not less than three broad categories of components in a social system. The first is the division of labor comprising all of the functions routinely performed by individuals and institutionalized groups the fruits of which are exchanged through either formal or informal means. Such is the meaning of economy in the broadest sense of the word. Second, there is what in popular usage is meant by the term social, namely, a number of associations based on common interests which are active by and large in the leisure periods of the weekly round. A third class of elements is interwoven among the preceding two. It embraces all of the canalizing practices and rules that link economic and social parts in a whole—ranging from kinship obligations and incest taboos through standard weights, measures, and coinage to bureaucratic protocol and legal strictures. In some instances this threefold classification may be criticized as an arbitrary cataloging of components that are scarcely distinguishable. In others it may be just as fairly regarded as a vast oversimplification. In all kinds of societies the three classes of elements interpenetrate and complement one another so extensively that there is no clear distinction among them. Although late in man's history the economic and the social sectors have seemed to draw apart as a result of the progress of specialization, even now the separation exists largely in abstraction. Perhaps nowhere else does this become so clear as in the study of population.

The familiar notion of population holds it to be an aggregate of human beings. This immediately raises the question: What is the aggregative principle? How are the class limits defined? In practice we find that the term population is normally used in connection with a territorial boundary of some description. One might suppose that the purpose served by a boundary is to delineate an aggregate possessing unit character. Boundaries, however, may differ widely in their degrees of approximation to unit character in the aggregates they enclose. The "population of Africa" is certainly not comparable to the "population of the United States": the former obtains its unity from a definition, the other from its internal organization. The latter represents unity of the highest order; that is, the members of the aggregate are organized in an inclusive system of relationships such that each member is a participant in a joint enterprise and his welfare depends upon the effectiveness with which the whole operates. The system might be small and simple, as in the case of a semi-independent settlement engaged in a self-sufficient mode of life, or it might be large and complex, as in a modern industrial state. Although the degree of integration may be less than complete, as it is more often than not, and the limits may be vague and unstable, still it is only a population possessing a more or less coherent organization that constitutes an identifiable unit and it is only of such an entity that questions about relationships between properties and characteristics can profitably be asked. It is in this sense that I prefer to use the term population.

In dealing with organized aggregates it is conventional to treat numbers an an independent and organization as a dependent variable.[5] Upon careful consideration that proves to be a naive, though sometimes an expedient, procedure. There is or seems to be a prepossessing concreteness about population, while the social system appears to be irretrievably ephemeral. That these are optical illusions is soon brought home to the observer when he sets out to manipulate one or the other, whether intellectually or practically. To get at the substance of population in its purest form it is necessary to strip away from a community of mankind its institutional clothing, its accumulation of knowledge and opinion and its technological hardware—all that is subsumed under culture, thereby exposing it as merely an assemblage of biological creatures. Population, in short, is an abstraction and a rather rarefied one at that. The term pertains simply to the quantitative aspect of aggregated human beings. Needless to say, in that form the concept is highly useful, if employed with appropriate reservations.

On the other hand, the seemingly unsubstantial character of the organization of man's collective life rests upon a most casual acquaintance with the facts. With closer attention to detail, organization is discovered to be a tough fabric, woven not of warp and woof, but of diverse and ramified strands. Far from being a mere figment of man's conceptual powers, a social system has a longevity that overreaches the life spans of the individuals caught up in it and a resilience that enables it to withstand catastrophic onslaughts. Yet, considered separately from population, social system is also an abstraction. It has no visibility apart from the routine activities of the members of a population.

The relation between population and social system, then, is manifestly an intimate one.[6] Population is delimited by the farthest reach of a network of inter-connections. Social system occurs only in an aggregate whose members staff its roles and engage in the interchanges that form its relationships. The two are by way of being different aspects of the same thing; each presupposes the other and therefore is involved in the definition of the other. Does it follow that neither population nor the organization of a social system, assuming that we can operationalize the two satisfactorily, can be altered without a corresponding change in the other? I will postpone an attempt to deal with this question pending further discussion. What is needed at the moment is a conception of how cumulative change occurs.

From what has been said it appears that social system change or growth must be at least a dual, possibly a multi-faceted, phenomenon. A paradigm would seem to involve a minimum of four interrelated and concurrent processes. There must be an accumulation of culture, non-material as well as material, an increase of population sufficient to take up and put to use the increasing repertory of knowledge and techniques, a broadening territory from which to nourish the growing population and from which also to secure the widening variety of materials that enter into the diversifying culture, and a development of a division of labor together with institutional mechanisms that maintain coherence in the expanding system.[7] The several processes unfold from a focal point, usually at a route intersection where the probabilities of cultural exchanges are greatest. But growth does not necessarily follow from the mere exchange of experiences; it ensues only from innovations that increase productivity or facilitate movement and communication. With gains of these kinds the sustenance base is enlarged, more people can be supported, and a more elaborate organization can be staffed. Population increase stems in part from attenuations of the death rate resulting from a stabilization and increase of the food supply and from the establishment of peace and order in the area. Growth from that source is supplemented by the incorporation of peripheral settlements into the expanding system. It may be supplemented further by net migration, for the new technology may require skills not present in the indigenous population. As a spreading territorial division of labor pushes out from the focal point there develops at that location a more refined functional division of labor addressed to the administration of the growing system, to the processing and distribution of products and to exploiting the opportunities for interest satisfactions created by the concentration of settlement. In other words, population change and social system change are bound together in the same general process. Both, moreover, are provoked by the same cause, cultural infusion and accumulation. Neither has the power to cause itself and neither, therefore, can initiate change in the other.[8] Nothing less than a comprehensive view of change can provide an adequate understanding of growth.

If we accept comparative materials from simple societies as describing an evolutionary continuum, we have at least presumptive, though partial, evidence of how growth progresses. The correlation of population size with type and productivity of economy is abundantly documented.[9] A hunting and gathering economy can support bands of little more than 50 people. A mixed hunting and agricultural economy raises the size of a residence unit to 250 or more persons. Settled agriculture is capable of supporting much larger organized populations. As crafts and trade are added to agriculture the organization is extended beyond a single settlement unit to embrace many such units. The population may number in the tens of thousands. Where trade and industry become predominant there is no known upper limit to population size. Furthermore, over and above its association with numbers, Nimkoff and Middleton have observed that type of family is also contingent on type of economy.[10] Similarly the number of roles in a society[11] and the extent of stratification[12] have been related to measures of population size and of productivity. So confident of that association is Robert Adams that he has employed evidences of stratification as indicators of prehistoric urbanization.[13] And Swanson has demonstrated that the incidence of monotheism varies with the number of levels or strata in societies.[14]

Of these studies one of the more suggestive is that of Naroll. His analysis of data pertaining to 30 different societies led him to the conclusion that with increase in the size of the largest settlement unit in a society the number of crafts is raised to the fourth power and the number of non-lineage associations or "teams" increase as $(\frac{T}{2})^6$. This allometric relationship doubtlessly derives from a multiplication of differentia in a population on the basis of which the number of combinations in which people may group themselves for the pursuit of special interests can increase more rapidly than population size. Since groups of that kind convene intermittently and for short periods of time, an individual may hold memberships in two, three, or more of them in addition to his time-consuming role in the division of labor.

I have sketched in broad outline a conception of growth that seems to have occurred in man's evolution from nomadic hunting and gathering bands to settled village life to agricultural state societies and finally to industrial urban societies.[15] This is not to say that the progression has been a smooth trend; there have been many stops, relapses, and resumptions along the way in the long-run course. Interruptions arise from various sources. For one thing, until a system is highly developed, cultural accumulation is subject to a large element of chance even for a people favorably located relative to paths of diffusion. Much of what comes to it through existing channels is apt to be trivial or otherwise useless. Cultural gains of critical importance are unpredictable; they may be widely spaced in time or occur in the wrong sequence. In that event the long-run trend might be expected to move through a series of Malthusian cycles, i.e., periods of growth ending in somewhat precarious equilibrium states.[16] At each step a system is only a little more able to resist catastrophic epidemics or invasions by hostile neighbors. Not infrequently, too, expansion has been curtailed by the encroaching boundaries of expanding systems in adjacent territories. For one reason or another expansion in the past has flourished in a region for a time, then has faltered and subsided, only to spring up again in another quarter. The scale attainable in these renewals of growth gradually increased as episodic technical advances were slowly assembled and pieced together.[17]

Now and then what seem to be exceptions to the process of growth occur. A striking instance of that nature has taken place in Java. As the Dutch, in the eighteenth century and afterward, developed their policy of large-scale cash crop exploitation on the basis of the traditional domestic unit of production, they inadvertently initiated population increase, mainly through transportation improvements which reduced the frequency of famine. Population increase has continued down to the present, despite the diversion of large amounts of land to non-subsistence uses and the exclusion of Indonesians from direct participation in the Dutch controlled economy. Population growth has been sustained by what Geertz[18] terms "cultural involution." By that he means that there has been, on the one hand, a progressive intensification of subsistence crop cultivation through steadily rising applications of labor and, on the other hand, a fashioning of an extremely intricate communal land tenure system by means of minute elaborations and improvisations in the tissue of rights and duties. Having observed the same phenomenon, Keyfitz reports a trend among the Javanese toward technological retrogression.[19] The plow, he says, is set aside for the spade, harvesting proceeds stalk by stalk while the sickle lies idle, and the backs of men have been substituted for the bullock cart in transportation, all in order to spread the work and thus the legitimate claims to the food supply over an ever larger number of people.[20]

It is more than likely, of course, that the Javanese could not have developed their communal land tenure system as they did without various borrowings from Dutch culture or from one another through the freer communications the Dutch created. It is by no means clear that population pressure was the effective operating force. Left to itself a self-sufficient agrarian community has very limited capacity for absorbing population increments. As a rule, a high and fluctuating mortality rate serves as the regulative instrument. Where that fails, as it has repeatedly in man's past, members of the community resort to migration and colonization. Even so, it is common to find peasant peoples chronically overpopulated, especially where there are sharp seasonal variations. The necessity of having on hand enough manpower to meet the peak word loads of planting and harvesting leaves them with too many people or wide-spread underemployment during the remainder of the year. In contrast, where there is a subservient labor supply, as in Europe from the Middle Ages onward, landed families practiced single inheritance as a way of keeping the domestic enterprise intact. Consequently in each generation there was an outpouring of dispossessed sons and daughters who were forced to live by their wits in the interstices of a rigidly compartmentalized feudal order.[21] That unattached population became the agents of the changes that were to revive the economic and social life of Europe after the eleventh century.[22]

But even though the relationship between population and the social system is close, discontinuities do occur, particularly at the beginnings and at the endings of growth periods. Social systems are seldom completely integrated. Hence change may begin in one or another sector while elsewhere traditional forms persist. In fact, change in population and in organization, though subject to a common cause, proceeds through different mechanisms. In the one, change is basically a biological process;[23] in the other, it is a matter of communication. The two can and often do get out of phase with one another therefore. Variations in population size begin with an alteration of the birth-death ratio from which shifts in age composition immediately follow.[24] The effects of the latter eventually spread over two or more generations, though the circumstance from which the initial change ensued might have long since disappeared. As opposed to the movements of biological events, organization growth feeds on information inputs in the form of new ways of acting. The consequences of innovations entering a system are usually cumulative and are always irreversible.

Their qualitative peculiarities also make for differences in their susceptibilities to change. Population, perhaps because it is a fairly simple phenomenon, is highly unstable. Mortality, for example, is notoriously responsive to variations in life conditions. Therefore in a very short space of time a gap can be opened between birth and death rates resulting in an increase or a decrease of population size. For this reason size variations and shifts in the rates of vital events are sensitive indicators of significant modifications having occurred in the circumstances surrounding a social system.[25] Unlike population, organization is a set of interlocking reciprocities variously weighted with contingencies of many sorts. To overcome the inertia inherent in a matrix of linkages of that kind requires more than just an impress on the system. The impact must be either appropriately timed or strong enough to launch sequences of adjustments reaching through all of the connected parts. The lapsed time between the beginning and the conclusion of organization change differs with the type of change impending, the extent of the integration of the system, whether the process is given guidance and still other conditions.

Once started, organization change may gather a momentum that tends to carry it beyond the rate of population change.

Thus short-run demographic dislocations have been a recurrent feature of human history. At different times they have appeared as too few or as too many people for the changing organization. It may well have been the case, as Boak has argued, that the decline of the Roman Empire, after 300 A.D., was hastened by population decrease brought about by frequent epidemics and military losses. He cites intensified efforts to bind workers to estates, to prohibit migration, and to encourage reproduction.[26] There is the possibility, of course, that one decline was a symptom of the other. In the end, toward the close of the eighth century, when the Roman administrative system had collapsed and the once flourishing towns were in shambles, European population reverted to its primitive density and mode of life. This is but a dramatic instance of what has occurred in many other times and places.[27]

Subsequently, through most of the late Middle Ages, as the resurgent cities were striving to enlarge their domains over surrounding lands, population deficits were felt in many parts of Europe. Frequent wars and high death rates in the unsanitary towns hampered the growth of trade and industry. Towns and kingdoms were in active competition for army recruits, settlers, and laborers.[28] In Prussia towns offered sanctuary to escaped serfs, granting them citizenship, if they succeeded in remaining there for a year and a day. Now and then natural catastrophes aggravated an already difficult situation. In the fourteenth and fifteenth centuries the Black Death carried away one-fourth to one-half of the inhabitants of Europe. Organized life was everywhere disrupted and trade declined. The characters of ruling families, of monasteries, and of other institutions were permanently altered by the ravages of the disease.[29] Buer reports the losses of agricultural techniques which were rediscovered several generations later.[30] Almost a century passed before population regained its pre-plague level. Near the end of the period the expansion of overseas empires placed further strains on limited manpower resources. Portugal found it necessary to prohibit further emigration from its small population to its colonial holdings.[31] Other nations emptied their prisons into the outward streams of migration and all turned to slavery as a solution to their colonial population needs.

After mid-eighteenth century, however, the state of affairs was reversed in northern Europe. There was then a surfeit of population. As the agricultural revolution improved the abundance and stability of the food supply, the death rate went into a protracted decline.[32] The rate of population increase became steadily larger until the birth rate entered upon its decline in the latter part of the nineteenth century. In the meantime the reorganization of agriculture was displacing rural population from traditional employment. Together the two factors produced a surplus of people faster than the industrializing economies could absorb it. Western history would certainly have been different had it not been possible to export the transitional surplus to areas of population deficits.[33] Not until the new economies achieved some maturity and the rate of population increase had subsided was a balance between numbers and organization approximated once again.

In many respects the changes occurring in developing nations today parallel those that took place in Europe 150 or more years ago. To the extent that that is true, current modernization trends permit a closer look at what is involved in the expansion and reorganization of social systems than historical accounts often afford. A major difference lies in the rates of change in the two instances; while in the West the change occupied more than a century, in the new nations the transition is being telescoped into a few decades. That difference generates other differences, some of which will be touched upon in passing.

In both cases the onset of change began in weakly integrated nations; nationhood was often more nominal than real. Consequently sharp discontinuities occurred. That is nowhere better demonstrated than in population growth in the developing nations. Within the brief span of 25 years their death rates have been reduced by 50 percent or more—from 38 or 40 per 1000 population to less than 20 per 1000, while birth rates linger at their old levels of 40 or more per 1000. Population growth rates have soared, therefore, above 2 percent per annum and to as high as 3.5 percent. The abrupt upsurge of population, probably unique in man's experience, is far in advance of complementary changes elsewhere in the respective societies. Levels of living have remained relatively constant, for example, unlike the European experience in which living levels and population growth advanced in rough association with one another. That there should be acute stresses and strains felt throughout the societies affected is to be expected, the more so because they are forced to solve their demographic problems within their own boundaries. There are, however, many other disjunctions encountered in such circumstances. I refer to disparities such as an emerging technical economy under an administrative system dominated by nepotistic practices and tribal loyalties, of mechanized industry and a handicraft agriculture, of a too rapid agglomeration in cities of a people habituated to a village way of life, of enormous intellectual stimulation circumscribed by authoritarian restraints, of diverse and often unreconcilable foreign influences, technical as well as ideological. Obviously in so confusing a welter of uneven movement there can be no easy assignment of effects to population change or to any other one factor at work. One can only try to pick up the thread of population influence here and there and follow it until it is lost once more.

The effects of population growth are easiest to trace from the shifts in age composition that are produced. Each year the number of youngsters who survive to the next year of age exceeds the number who preceded them in that age group. The cumulative result of increasing survival rates, while fertility remains constant at a high level, is a slowly though steadily rising proportion of youth in the population. As is well known, new opportunities and incentives find their readiest reception among young people; they are neither burdened with established habits and memories of precedents nor yet enmeshed in the entanglements of community life.[34] Thus where the numbers of these immanent heirs to the social system are disproportionately large the society is in a favorable position for a quick transition to a different organization.

Furthermore, mortality decline yields greater returns from the investment in new generations. A drop in the death rate from 40 to 20 per 1000 means (in a stationary population) an increase of life expectancy at birth of from 25 to 50 years. Now, if the labor force age begins at 15 years and extends beyond 50 years, the number of productive years realized per birth on the average is more than tripled by the 50 percent decline in the death rate. Or, put another way, a given number of productive years of life is obtained from one period of dependent childhood rather than from three. The society with the higher life expectancy is justified, therefore, in spending larger sums for training its youth. On the other hand, increased longevity brings a greater overlapping of generations and consequently a sharpened contest between generations over the distribution of opportunities for employment and other positions of responsibility.

But the capacity of a developing nation to make the fullest use of abundant and highly adaptable new generations is problematical. According to Rostow a number of preconditions must be met before a society is prepared for rapid and coordinated development.[35] He speaks of the need for the displacement of the old land-based elite by a new class of leaders who are prepared to assemble and allocate surplus income to investments in industrial equipment. That, in turn, calls for a set of new institutions which, though specifically instrumental in facilitating commerce, savings, and investments, also have wide implications for the whole of social life. One is reminded in this connection of Pirenne's account for the struggle between the emergent burgher class and the feudal aristocracy for control of the medieval European city. Ultimately the victorious burghers gained a complement of municipal institutions including a tribunal, a court, a new penal code, and a commercial law.[36] These provided new degrees of freedom on the strength of which expansion surged forward. There is also a precondition in the form of what economists call "social overhead," such as roads and communications, schools and various other citizen service facilities, all of which call for substantial capital outlays. In Western development the capital needed for that purpose was initially provided by joint stock companies and other private sources as governments were slow to assume responsibility for essential services. In contemporary developing nations, however, time does not allow for the slow accumulation of social overhead; large-scale capital funding efforts on the part of central governments must begin early in the process. Yet the simultaneous need for social and industrial capital poses a serious dilemma. Funds needed to prepare the oncoming generations for effective participation in a modernizing society detract from funds that should be invested in ways that will increase per capita income.[37] Pending a resolution of that impasse population controls are clearly imperative, if not by means of a declining birth rate, then through a rising death rate.

Meanwhile the swelling cohorts of youth mature to labor force age, some with, but most without, training for a different type of life. The little family farm, despite the flexibility inherent in its subsistence mode of operation, becomes saturated with labor power and mouths to feed. Traditional leadership in the village—the priest, the headman, the conjurer of the spirit world—having no solution to this and other problems that have arisen, is brought to the brink of discreditation. A deepening poverty, as Banfield observed in southern Italy, threatens village community organization with dissolution.[38] So the excess youth, males primarily, drift away to the metropolis, leaving behind the young women to chafe in marital deprivation.[39]

In the city the migrants gather in village or tribal enclaves, for ignorance of the city and its ways makes the help of a friend indispensible. In the peasant experience, moreover, the work unit is founded on a social unit rather than being something apart.[40] If the migrant finds a job, it is on the lowest rungs of the occupational ladder, usually in the already overcrowded service industries. Or he might find employment in an unmechanized industry, such as construction, where his willingness to accept low wages adds a further deterrent to capital investment in the industry.[41] In the after hours his recreation is uncontrolled by customary sanctions; the paternalism of employer or labor boss is a poor surrogate for family controls. Prostitution, gambling, and idling will occupy his leisure hours. At the termination of the job the newcomer discovers, if he were to look, that the city offers little in the way of welfare services. He drifts back to his village carrying ideas and behavior patterns that challenge folk prescriptions and temper the welcome extended to him.[42] Three or four sojourns in the city may pass before he settles into continuous residence there, though he may never completely sever his rural ties.[43] In the second and later generations of city life the grip of lineage loyalties is weakened as new forms of association take their place.[44]

For its part the city is overwhelmed with the countryside's super-numerary beneficiaries of a falling death rate. It draws to itself most of the educated and promising youth as well as hordes of unprepared, impoverished, yet hopeful, seekers after a foothold in the urban economy. Enriched by the one, the city's undeveloped municipal services—police, fire, health, education, welfare—are severely over-burdened by the other.[45] Where city administration is an adjunct of the national government, as seems to be the rule in new nations, it has no taxing powers and small latitude for the exercise of governmental initiative. Nor has civic consciousness advanced to the point where voluntary groups arise to press for needed social improvements. The middle class is too small and too inexperienced to be articulate in such matters.[46] By and large welfare is left to the family which may or may not extend its protection over a small number of "clients." A strongly family-centered society is characterized by indifference toward the non-kinsman and the body politic. "For in all societies in all ages," said Alfred Zimmern, "the law of the larger unit tends to be held in less esteem than that of the smaller, and progress consists in making the spirit of the smaller, with its appropriate ideas and customs, trans-mute and inspire the larger."[47]

The city is a school. It inculcates habits of mind and behavior that can be learned nowhere else. There the person learns adaptability to the challenge and flux of new experience. He gains a cosmopolitan outlook, the more quickly as he comes to appreciate the need for and the uses of literacy. As he becomes aware of the similarity of his problems with those of others, he is awakened to the bearing that the welfare of the whole has on the well-being of the individual. The widening of his horizon leads him to cultivate the techniques of participation in the complex and highly structured society. This includes not only knowledge of how to extract his satisfactions from among a great variety of specialized services, but also how to employ the principles of organization to serve unmet needs. The formation of voluntary groups—political parties, pressure groups, avocational associations—gives his voice a chance to be heard above the din of urban activity. Harder to learn is the disciplined application of that newfound power in an orderly exercise of influence.

Nevertheless it is unlikely that these lessons can be turned to use without a rise in per capita income or, more particularly, of per capita disposable income. In an urbanized society social enfranchisement rests largely on the degree of one's participation in the monetary nexus. When there are funds left to the worker after the costs of food and shelter are paid he can purchase fuller access to communications and educational opportunity, he can cultivate avocations, contribute to the support of associations of interest to him and even add to the economy's capital account through his small savings. Members of his family may delay or shorten their membership in the labor force, devoting themselves to activities that further expand the service and avocational sectors of organization. Thus the growth of organizational ramification seems to depend less directly on the increase of numbers than on the availability of means for participating in the collective life. In other words, once organization passes a certain level of development, e.g., at which the sustenance problem is solved, proliferations and elaborations may follow at an accelerating rate, outstripping the rate of population growth, as suggested in Naroll's findings.

Unfortunately there are no dependable data available on trends in the number of participant organizational units in advanced societies, to say nothing of societies undergoing development. Such information as we have is obtained from recent cross-sectional observations, based on sample surveys in Western nations, of the frequency and incidence of memberships in formal, voluntary associations. Those studies indicate that approximately 40 percent of adult population belong to no formal associations of any kind. Most of the people who make up that proportion fall at or near the lower ends of the income and educational scales. The higher the income and the educational levels of respondents, the greater is the frequency of memberships per person. If memberships in associations that have no apparent civic significance are excluded, the correlation becomes considerably closer.[48] To construe findings of this character as representing a pattern of change is hazardous, to say the least, though the temptation to do so is not easy to resist.[49]

Once major transitional dislocations are overcome it is to be expected that population and the social system will return to a pattern of close covariation. Then, however, there is the question mentioned earlier of how much change can occur in one without a commensurate change in the other. But we know nothing about the tolerances for independent variability and even less about the conditions that determine the tolerances. Nevertheless, it is apparent that in most populations there are reserves of numbers or of unused time that can be drawn upon to meet emergency needs of organization change. Conversely, every society seems to have means for diverting the energies of excess numbers to unproductive roles. The number of persons who can be so accommodated without changes in the system is probably held within narrow limits. Nor does it seem plausible that the interplay of variations within their restricted ranges can exert a mutual causation; the effect rather should be a balancing of necessary conditions, as with weights on a balance scale. "Growth," said Boulding in his paraphrasing of D'Arcy Thompson, "creates form, but form limits growth."[50]

Still, mature societies are subject to cyclical variations. Economic and political events intrude from time to time to disturb a status quo. A temporary decline in the birth rate, for example, such as results from a separation of the sexes in wartime, is followed by a rise after the restoration of peace and then by another recession after marital relationships are resumed and the backlog of unmarried youth is exhausted. A series of such variations sends waves of dents and bulges through the age structure of a population. Eighteen to 25 years after each deviation from the secular trend the birth cohorts reach marriageable ages. Because of their numbers they will then have relatively few or relatively many births, though age-specific rates might have remained unchanged, and another series of reverberations echoes through the age structure. The institutions that are addressed to the needs of different age groups find themselves alternately over-equipped and under-equipped as the distorted cohorts age into and out of their functional purviews. It is conceivable that the adjustments made to the changing sizes of clienteles leave no permanent marks on the institutions concerned. But again the fluctuations may present opportunities for modifications that have been held in abeyance for lack of sufficient justification.

In general, empirical work on the relationship between population and society is frustrated in varying degrees by the necessity of accepting the nation as the unit of study, for most relevant data are reported only by nations. National boundaries usually exaggerate the scope of the fully organized unit in developing areas, whereas they under-represent the effective unit in advanced nations. In the former case the nation is usually in process of becoming a unit in more than a nominal sense and is still far short of that attainment. A close-knit organization is emerging in the form of an internally expanding urban system that is progressively encompassing a larger proportion of the state's territory, but the margins of the enlarging system are still frayed with partially assimilated villages and districts interspersed with pockets of undisturbed traditionalism. On the other hand, in developed nations political boundaries seldom contain either all of the population that supports the internal organization or all of the organizational elements in which the national population is involved. The completeness of fit in these respects doubtlessly improves with increase in the size of the nation, though it is never perfect. Small developed nations may and do have social systems as elaborate and as advanced as those of large nations. They do so by virtue of extensive international relations, sociocultural as well as economic and political. Interrelations of that order are in effect a means of pooling the resources, manpower, knowledge, and experience of two or more political jurisdictions.[51] The process of development seems to cause obsolescence in national boundaries for an increasing number of purposes.

A further difficulty has its root in conceptualization. I refer to the practice of thinking of population solely in terms of numbers. The alternative, however, leads one into a circular argument. As A. B. Wolfe commented in his critique of optimum theory, whatever significance population might have results not from numbers alone but also from how the members are distributed among activities, how fully their energies are applied, how equitably they share in the products of their efforts and so on.[52] But these are organizational rather than demographic facts. The two variables become confounded when a refinement of numbers is attempted.

There is no purpose to be served by belaboring the point of this discussion any further. Population, as I have tried to show, is endogenous to a social system. Of necessity the relationship between the two must be a systematic one, doubtlessly allometric in form. What is true in principle or in the long run may have its exceptions in the short run. Demographic dislocations do occur. If a social system is unable to overcome such dislocation through cultural infusions of one sort or another, its redundant numbers must be cast out either in migration or in a rise of the death rate. There is no evidence thus far that population can function in social change other than as a necessary condition. But this should not be construed as a deprecation of the importance of population or of the study of population. There is much that needs to be known about how the process of covariation of population with the structure of a social system operates under varying conditions. Here, as in so many other instances, there is a striking disparity. While the study of population as a special field is highly systematized and equipped with powerful tools of analysis, the study of social systems lags in an immature state. Progress of the

kind I consider essential calls for the exercise of a great deal more
constructive imagination about what constitutes a social system and
about how to operationalize its dimensions than has yet been demonstrated.

Notes

1. Herbert Spencer, *The Principles of Sociology* (New York: Apple-
ton-Century-Crofts, 1921), I, 471.
2. Emile Durkheim, *The Division of Labor in Society*, trans. George
Simpson (New York: The Macmillan Co., 1933), pp. 256-63.
3. Philip J. Allen, "Growth of Strata in Early Organization Development," *American Journal of Sociology*, xxviii (1962), 34-46; T. R. Anderson and T. R. Warkov, "Organizational Size and Functional Complexity,"
American Sociological Review, xxvi (1961), 23-28; Roger G. Barker,
"Ecology and Motivation," in Marshall R. Jones (ed.), *Nebraska Symposium on Motivation, 1960* (Lincoln, Nebraska: University of Nebraska
Press, 1960), 1-44; Mason Haire, "Biological Models and Empirical His-
tories of the Growth of Organizations," in Mason Haire (ed.), *Modern
Organization Theory* (New York: John Wiley and Sons, 1959), chap. x;
Amos H. Hawley, Walter Boland, and Margaret Boland, "Population Size
and Administration in Institutions of Higher Education," *American Socio-
logical Review*, xxx (1965), 252-55; N. S. Ross, "Management and the
Size of the Firm," *Review of Economic Statistics*, xix (1952-53), 148;
F. W. Terrien and D. L. Mills, "The Effect of Changing Size upon the
Internal Structure of Organizations," *American Sociological Review*, xx
(1955), 11-13.
4. Cf. Talcott Parsons, "Population and Social Structure," in Douglas
G. Haring (ed.), *Japan's Prospect* (Cambridge: Harvard University Press,
1946), pp. 87-114. In another work Parsons, commenting on Durkheim's
attention to population pressure, describes it ambiguously as a "biologizing
of social theory." [*The Structure of Social Action* (Glencoe, Illinois: The
Free Press, 1944), p. 323]. See also Marion Levy, *The Structure of Society*
(Princeton: Princeton University Press, 1952), p. 151.
5. W. F. Ogburn was a distinguished spokesman for this conception
of the variable. See his "On the Social Aspects of Population Changes," *The
British Journal of Sociology*, iv (1953), 25-30. In his *Social Change* (Englewood Cliffs, N. J.: Prenctice-Hall, 1963) Wilbert Moore expresses the
same view (p. 18), but in another essay ("Sociology and Demography,"
in P. M. Hauser and O. D. Duncan, eds., *The Study of Population*, Chicago: University of Chicago Press, 1959, p. 835), he declares that population is not an exogenous variable.
6. This was appreciated by Thomas Malthus. His limiting assumption
of a "fixed state of the arts" is of central importance in his argument. (*An
Essay on Population*, London: Everyman's Library, I, 9.)
7. Burt Aginsky argues that the amount of culture possessed by a
society is contingent on population, area, and mobility including communi-

cation. ("The Evolution of American Indian Culture: A Method and Theory," *Thirty-Second International Congress of Americanists* (1956), pp. 79-87.)

The concept of expansion is much more fully developed by R. D. McKenzie "Industrial Expansion and the Interrelations of Peoples," in E. B. Reuter (ed.), *Race and Culture Contacts* (New York: McGraw-Hill, 1933), pp. 19-33; and O. D. Duncan, "Social Organization and the Eco-System," in R. E. L. Faris (ed.), *Handbook of Modern Sociology* (Chicago: Rand-McNally, 1964), pp. 36-82.

8. The inability of a population to generate its own characteristics and trends is ably argued by E. T. Hiller, "A Culture Theory of Population Trends," *The Journal of Political Economy*, xxxviii (1930), 523-50. Although they are referring only to low-income economies, E. M. Hoover and Ansley J. Coale discard the possibility that population growth can produce economic growth, in *Population Growth and Economic Development* (Princeton: Princeton University Press, 1958), 21-25. Again, Norman B. Ryder comments that population replacement is not a cause of social change in "The Cohort as a Concept in the Study of Social Change," *American Sociological Review*, xxx (1965), 844.

On the other hand, that the causes of change in a social system are necessarily external in origin, though logically indisputable, is nevertheless often questioned. It is assumed, however, by students in many different fields, such as Arnold Toynbee, *The Industrial Revolution* (Boston: The Beacon Press, 1956), pp. 59-60; W. W. Rostow, *The Stages of Economic Growth* (Cambridge: The University Press, 1960), p. 6; Julian H. Steward, *Theory of Culture Change* (Urbana, Illinois: University of Illinois Press, 1955), p. 40; and Walter Gold;chmidt, *Man's Way* (New York: Holt, Rinehart and Winston, 1959), p. 108.

9. V. Gordon Childe, *Man Makes Himself* (London: Watts and Co., 1936) and *Social Evolution* (New York: Schuman, 1951); Edward Deevey, "The Human Population," *Scientific American* (Sept., 1960), 3-9; O. D. Duncan, *op. cit.*; C. D. Forde, "The Anthropological Approach in Social Science," in M. Fried (ed.), *Readings in Anthropology* (New York: Thomas Crowell, 1959), ii, 59-78; and Julian Steward, *op. cit.*

10. M. F. Nimkoff and Russell Middleton, "Types of Family and Types of Economy," *American Journal of Sociology*, lxvi (1960), 215-25.

11. M. Edmonson, *Status Terminology and the Social Structure of North American Indians* (Seattle: University of Washington Press, 1958); and Raoul Naroll, "A Preliminary Index of Social Development," *American Anthropologist*, lviii (1965), 687-715.

12. Marshall Sahlins, *Social Stratification in Polynesia* (Seattle: University of Washington Press, 1958).

13. Robert McAdams, *The Evolution of Urban Society* (Chicago: The Aldine Press, 1965).

14. G. E. Swanson, *Birth of the Gods* (Ann Arbor: The University of Michigan Press, 1965).

15. Walter Goldschmidt, *op. cit.*

16 See K. W. Taylor, "Some Aspects of Population History," *Canadian Journal of Economics and Political Science*, xvi (1950), 301-13.

17. For an impressive documentation of this accumulation through rises and falls of societies, see William H. McNeill, *The Rise of the West:*

A History of the Human Community (Chicago: University of Chicago Press, 1963).

18. Clifford Geertz, *Agricultural Involution: The Process of Ecological Change in Indonesia* (Berkeley: University of California Press, 1963), pp. 80-82, 90-103.

19. Nathan Keyfitz, "The Growth of Village Populations and Economic Development in South Asia," *Population Review* (Madras), i (1957), 39-43.

20. A parallel to the "closed corporate community," or system of shared poverty, of Java has been noted in Central America by Eric Wolfe, "Closed Corporate Peasant Communities in Mesoamerican and Central Java," *Southwestern Journal of Anthropology*, xiii (1957), 1-18.

21. For a vivid description of how the rural family system applied selective inheritance see Ladislas Reymont, *The Peasants* (New York: A. A. Knopf, 1924-25), iv; and Conrad Arensburg, *The Irish Countryman* (New York: The Macmillan Co., 1937), chap. iii.

22. Cf. H. Pirenne, *Economic and Social History of Medieval Europe* (New York: Harcourt, Brace and World, 1937), pp. 66-67.

23. Substantial changes, of course, do result from non-biological sources, i.e., migration and accretions on the periphery of an expanding system. Such changes are controlled by the same mechanisms that affect organization changes.

24. For a competent discussion of the effects of birth and death rate changes on age composition see Ansley J. Coale, "The Effects of Changes in Mortality and Fertility on Age Composition," *The Milbank Memorial Fund Quarterly*, xxxiv (1956), 79-114, and "How the Age Distribution of a Population Is Determined," *Cold Springs Harbor Symposium on Quantitative Biology*, xxii (1957), 83-89.

25. On this matter I seem to be in disagreement with Josiah C. Russell, who describes population as "a slow, ponderous force," the effects of changes in which may not become apparent until a century or more has passed. ("Demographic Pattern in History," *Population Studies*, iv, 1948, 403.) But Russell is dealing with the long sweep of history in an epoch in which the diffusion of influences over broad areas could only move slowly by permeating from insular locality to insular locality. My concern is with events within a system, not as among systems.

26. A. E. R. Boak, *Manpower Shortage and the Fall of the Roman Empire* (Ann Arbor: The University of Michigan Press, 1955).

27. E.g., A. R. Radcliffe-Brown, *The Andaman Islanders* (Cambridge: The University Press, 1933), 19; and Charles Wagley, "The Effects of Depopulation upon Social Organization as Illustrated by the Tapirape Indians," *Transactions of the New York Academy of Science*, Series 2 and 3 (1940), pp. 12 ff.

It is of interest in this connection that high mortality among the people of Truk makes impossible a consistent observance of the patrilocal residence rule. Very often the father has succumbed before a son can bring a wife to the father's village. (Ward E. Goodenough, "Residence Rules," *Southwestern Journal of Anthropology*, xii, 1956, 22-37.)

28. Herbert Moller, *Population Movements in Modern European History* (New York: Macmillan, 1964), pp. 19-42.

29. "The Black Death," *Encyclopedia Britannica*. Vol. iii (1963).

30. M. C. Buer, *Health, Wealth and Population in the Early Days of the Industrial Revolution* (London: George Routledge, 1926), pp. 67-68.

31. Donald Pierson, *The Negroes in Brazil* (Chicago: University of Chicago Press, 1942), pp. 112-13.

32. The decline began about 100 years before important improvements in medical and sanitary knowledge appeared. A careful examination of the state of knowledge at the time is presented in T. McKeown and R. G. Brown, "Medical Evidence Relating to English Population Change in the Eighteenth Century," *Population Studies*, ix (1955), 119-41.

33. J. Isaacs, *Economics of Migration* (London: Trubner and Co., 1947), pp. 21-22.

34. The significance of cohort succession in the social system for the acceptance of social change is ably treated by Norman B. Ryder, *op. cit.*

35. W. W. Rostow, *op. cit.*, p. 7.

36. Henri Pirenne, *Medieval Cities* (Princeton: Princeton University Press, 1925), pp. 168-212.

37. Ansley J. Coale, "Population and Economic Development," in P. M. Hauser (ed.), *The Population Dilemma* (Englewood Cliffs, N. J.: Prentice-Hall, 1965), chap. iv.

38. Edward Banfield, *The Moral Basis of a Backward Society* (Glencoe, Illinois: The Free Press, 1958).

39. See Geoffrey and Monica Wilson, *The Analysis of Social Change: Based on Observations in Central Africa* (Cambridge: The University Press, 1954).

40. Manning Nash, *Primitive and Peasant Economic Systems* (San Francisco: Chandler Publishing Co., 1966), pp. 23-24.

41. According to Walter Philips, the resistance to technological change in low capital/labor ratio industries often stems from the workers themselves and more directly from the labor entrepreneurs. ("Technological Levels and Labor Resistance to Change in the Course of Industrialization," *Economic Development and Cultural Change*, xi, 1963, 257-66.) An interesting account of the problems encountered in adapting a peasant labor force to the standard procedures of a modern factory system is given by Kuo-Heng Shih, *China Enters the Machine Age* (Cambridge: Harvard University Press, 1944).

E. H. Phelps-Brown and Sheila V. Hopkins describe the wage-depressing effects of rural migrations to sixteenth century European cities in "Wage Rates and Prices: Evidence for Population Pressure in the Sixteenth Century," *Economica, New Series*, xxiv (1953), 289-306.

42. For resumés of investigations of urbanization processes in Africa and in Latin America, see UNESCO, *Social Implications of Industrialization and Urbanization in Africa South of the Sahara* (Paris: United Nations, 1956), and UNESCO, *Urbanization in Latin America* (New York: International Documents Service, 1961).

43. William B. Schwab, "Oshogbo—An Urban Community," in Hilda Kuper (ed.), *Urbanization and Migration in West Africa* (Berkeley: University of California Press, 1965), pp. 85-109.

44. Richard D. Lambert, "The Impact of Urban Society on Village Life," in Roy Turner (ed.), *India's Urban Future* (Berkeley: University of California Press, 1962), chap. vi.

45. The cities of developing areas are not unique in this respect. The appearance of modern municipal services in western cities occurred a half-century or more after the needs for them had become critical. E.g., see Blake McKelvey, *The Urbanization of America, 1860-1915* (New Brunswick: Rutgers University Press, 1963).

46. It is strange, indeed, that in the profuse literature on social stratification almost nothing is said about the contributions social classes make to the development of society. One might suppose, along with Henri Pirenne (*op. cit.*), W. W. Rostow (*op. cit.*) and Harvey Leibenstein (*Economic Backwardness and Economic Growth*, (New York: John Wiley and Sons, 1957), pp. 39-41, that the middle class in particular is an aggressive factor in the emancipation from traditional restraints and in the creation of instrumentalities for enlarging participation in social life.

47. Alfred Zimmern, *The Greek Commonwealth* (Modern Library, 1931), p. 95.

48. Charles R. Wright and Herbert Hyman, "Voluntary Association Memberships of American Adults: Evidence from National Sample Surveys," *American Sociological Review*, xxiii (1958), 284-94; Thomas Bottomore, "Social Stratification in Voluntary Organizations," in David Glass (ed.), *Social Mobility in Britain* (Glencoe, Illinois: The Free Press, 1954), p. 354; Gunnar Hecksher, "Pluralist Democracy: The Swedish Experience," *Social Research*, xv (1948), 417-61; and O. R. Gallagher, "Voluntary Associations in France," *Social Forces*, xxxvi (1957), 154-56.

49. Of interest here is the direct covariation of the frequency of voluntary association memberships with size of city in the United States (see Wright and Hyman, *ibid.*). O. D. Duncan, who has given a great deal of attention to size of city correlates, has also observed that indicators of social organization vary directly and fairly monotonically with size of city. "Optimum Sizes of Cities," in Paul K. Hatt and Albert J. Reiss, Jr., (eds.), *Cities and Society* (Glencoe, Illinois, The Free Press, 1957), pp. 759-72. W. F. Ogburn and O. D. Duncan ("City Size as a Sociological Variable," in E. W. Burgess and D. J. Bogue, eds., *Contributions to Urban Sociology*, Chicago: University of Chicago Press, 1964, p. 142) have noted, too, that the frequency of innovations increases with size of place.

50. Kenneth Boulding, "Toward a General Theory of Growth," *Canadian Journal of Economics and Political Science*, xix (1953), 337.

51. An excellent illustration of this fact is provided by Irene Taeuber, in "Population Increase and Manpower Utilization in Imperialist Japan," *Milbank Memorial Fund Quarterly*, xxviii (1950), 273-93.

52. A. B. Wolfe, "The Theory of Optimum Population," *Annals of the American Academy of Political and Social Science*, (November, 1936), pp. 243-49. See also E. F. Penrose, *Population Theories and Their Application* (Stanford University, California: Food Research Institute, 1934), pp. 47-94.

III. BIOLOGIC ASPECTS OF FERTILITY CONTROL

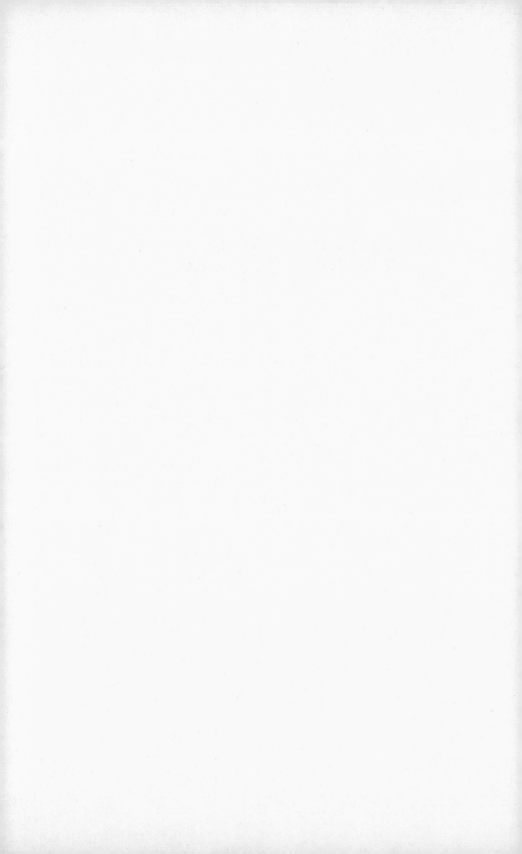

THE EFFECT OF BIRTH LIMITATION
ON GENETIC COMPOSITION
OF POPULATIONS

Jean Sutter
Institut National D'Études Démographiques

Where birth control practices have been well documented, the study of its effect on the genetic structure of populations permits a thorough examination of its development and of its mechanism.

Fertility Decline

France has the most reliable data on the first implementation of birth control and its accompanying phenomena. Historically, the first manifestation of this phenomenon in occidental civilization is found there. The historical surveys made by French demographers were sufficiently advanced, moreover, to prove now that the repercussion of birth control at the demographic level was unusually early and, among some social classes, could be measured as far back as the middle of the seventeenth century.

It is also now fully established that by the end of the seventeenth century birth control had taken root among the upper classes of society, particularly the nobility. L. Henry and C. Lévy (*16*) revealed that contraception was practiced as early as that, particularly among the dukes and peers of the realm. In their study they examined, for the period 1665-1799, 59 families that included at least one duke and peer of the realm. Although marriages in that social class were considerably earlier than for the country as a whole, there was a very pronounced decline in fertility from the middle of the seventeenth century. In the case of complete families (that is, those where the wife married before 20 and the marriage lasted until she was between 45 and 50) the number of children was 6.15 for marriages between 1650 and 1699; 2.79 for the period 1700-1749; and 2.00 for the period 1750-99.

The average age of the wife when the youngest child was born—a marked indication of birth control—was 31.2 for 1650-99; 26.7 for 1700-1749; 25.1 for 1750-99. Family limitation has been general among married couples of the upper classes since at least the beginning of the eighteenth century if not much earlier.

In studies dealing with evidence of contraception in France, all writings, civil, medical, and religious, have been thoroughly investigated (3). These studies show how the concept of birth control spread in eighteenth-century French society.

Numerical confirmation of the state of mind voiced, often only hinted at, in the publications of the day is afforded by very accurate historical demographic studies undertaken for the last 15 years under the auspices of the I.N.E.D. The study of Crulai, a village in Normandy with 1000 inhabitants (12), is the prototype of these studies of rural or semi-urban populations from the seventeenth to the nineteenth centuries. From 1675 to 1760 the crude birth rate was 36 per 1000 of population. From this time there is a slow decrease until the Revolution, apparently as a result of a drop in the proportional number of marriages. After the Revolution the decrease is very rapid. Towards 1810 the birth rate was approximately 20 per 1000 whereas according to age and marital status and the previous fertility rate, it should have been 31 per 1000. Towards 1870 the rate must have been in the neighborhood of 13 per 1000.

A similar state of affairs is revealed by J. Ganiage (11) in his study of 3 villages of Beauvaises. The following table, for example, shows the fertility of women in the eighteenth century, divided into age groups according to the year of marriage.

Women Married	Age Group					
	20-24	25-29	30-34	35-39	40-44	45-49
Before 1780	527	515	448	368	144	21
After 1780	519	431	359	222	109	6

If the line of demarcation between groups is moved back to 1780, the fall in fertility is immediately clear on comparing the fertility rate per 1000 women of the same age, according to whether they were married before or after 1780. The difference for the second period is 16 percent lower for the group aged 25-29; 20 percent lower for the group aged 30-34; and 39 percent lower for the group aged 35-39.

Before 1780 there was an average of 6.7 births per family (complete family); after 1780 it was only 5.3. Ganiage believes that the practice of contraception became evident between 1785 and 1790, after 60 years of demographic development.

Ganiage gives the mother's age at the birth of the youngest child for the two periods. These figures, too, are highly suggestive.

Age group	under 30	30-44	35-39	40-44	45-49	50 and over	Total
Before 1780	1	3	26	37	8	—	75
Percent	1.3	4.2	34.6	49.3	10.6	—	
After 1780	2	3	11	11	1	1	29
Percent	6.9	10.3	38.0	38.0	3.4	3.4	

The same phenomena are revealed in the monographs published on other villages in other parts of France: at Sotteville-lès-Rouen (13); in Quercy (33); and in a village in the north of France from 1665 to 1851 (9). Birth control had such an effect on fertility that its repercussions on French registered fertility statistics was noted unusually early.

Figure 1 represents the evolution of the crude reproduction rate for the whole of France since 1770 (3). The decline continued until 1935. Starting as far back as 1750, it was very rapid in the last 10 years of the eighteenth century. Between 1851 and 1871 there was a slight slackening, but after 1881 the decrease continued at an accelerating rate until 1938. It was in 1881 that fertility began to decline in the other European countries.

We quote Bourgeois-Pichat (3) to show the efficacy of family limitation in France: "If the fertility rate of the 18th century had been maintained up to 1880, France would have had 88 million inhabitants at that date instead of only 38." The demographic result of such a considerable drop in fertility is a fall in the proportion of "the young" and a rise in that of "the old." One might consider these data sufficient for an attempt to demonstrate the effect of contraception on the genetic structure of the population.

Considered from the above viewpoint, the problem of the relationship between family limitation and its results on the genetics of population appears a simple one. By this process there occurred considerable differences in fertility according to whether or not the family groups practiced contraception, that is, whether they were Malthusian or non-Malthusian. Comparison between the genetic contributions of non-Malthusian and Malthusian families could be reduced to a matter of simple arithmetic, but, in fact, such oversimplification is too limiting, and any discussion of the problem based on such data would be a serious mistake. If, ultimately, such data does have to be

used to establish hypotheses on the disturbances induced at the
genetic level by the differential fertility phenomenon, then it becomes
necessary to examine the actual functioning of Malthusianism accompanied by other phenomena—demographic, socioeconomic or cultural—all working towards completing, restraining, or accelerating
the peculiar effect of birth control. Furthermore, with the fall in fertility there was a decline in mortality, causing what Landry (18) has
described as "demographic revolution."

Reduction in Mortality, Demographic Revolution (Cycle)
The decline in fertility through contraception has produced marked
differences in fertility, further accentuated by an accompanying decline in mortality. Hence the phenomenon in France described by
Landry as far back as 1934, which afterwards became widespread and
has since been thoroughly investigated by Bourgeois-Pichat (3). This
is how he puts it:

"The demographic evolution of the last two centuries
amongst nations with a European civilization has become classic.
Let us briefly review its successive phases. On an average there
was a rough equilibrium between a very high degree of fertility
and a very high degree of mortality—such was the basic characteristic of these populations before their 'demographic revolution'
got under way. In the initial phase there was a decline in mortality without any corresponding modification in fertility. Births
steadily exceeded deaths and population increased rapidly. The
decline in fertility that then occurred in its turn, marks the setting
in of the second phase. At first, however, this decline had no apparent effect on births, which continued increasing owing to the
favorable-age structure formed during the course of the preceding phase, as well as because of the continued decrease in
mortality. Finally, as the downward trend in fertility became
more pronounced the excess of births over deaths decreased progressively and in some instances there was even an excess of
deaths. This is the final phase of the phenomenon. Had the trend
continued, a regular decrease in population would have been observed. In actual fact no country has as yet reached this phase in
evolution. With the renewed rise in births in France during the
last years there are grounds for a less pessimistic view. A new
equilibrium between births and deaths appears possible, on a
very different basis, moreover, than that obtaining for the natural
equilibrium of the past.

"Only the last phase can be accurately investigated. It occurred recently, in fact, at a time for which detailed statistics are
available. There is still a fair amount of information about the

second phase which starts with a decline in fertility. For countries other than France the date of this decline is, in fact, set towards 1880, when reliable vital statistics began to be available. But we cannot fix an accurate date for the second phase in France. The first French statistical information permitting an accurate measurement of fertility dates from 1891, and it has been possible to make estimates up to about 1800. Now, all these data show that in France the downward trend in fertility had started before the end of the 18th century.

"Only a few statistical data for the Scandinavian countries show the outset of the first phase. The beginning of this phase, with its initial decline in mortality, can be approximately assigned to about 1750 for these countries.

"To sum up: supposing the above outline to be a qualitatively adequate description of the demographic history of European populations, it remains difficult, at least for the first phase, to give exact details not only about the evolution of those populations, but also, on a quantitative level, about the extent of the variations in mortality and fertility. This is particularly difficult in the case of France whose 'demographic revolution'—considerably earlier than that of other countries—started at a time when statistical data were both infrequent and incomplete. Notwithstanding their paucity by no means all of the data have been utilized."

Bourgeois-Pichat (3) was, however, able to calculate the mortality rates for France since 1771, according to different age groups (Figures 2 and 3). A marked decline in mortality is seen during the whole of the last part of the eighteenth century.

In the 3 age groups, 1-4, 5-14, and 15-24 the evolution of the rate of mortality since 1800 has been very similar, i.e., a gradual reduction until 1890, followed by acceleration with the discovery of preventive treatment for infections.

Before 1800, when the mortality at ages 5-14 remained almost constant, there was a substantial decline in the group aged 1-4, as a result of the disappearance of smallpox.

Infantile mortality for the group aged 0-1 varied very little until the end of the nineteenth century. For groups of over 24 years, the evolution is seen to be the same (Figure 4). Until about 1860 there is a slow decline with a slight difference favoring women. After 1860 the reduction in the rates for women becomes more pronounced in comparison with the rates for men, which remained practically constant until 1945 when antibiotics were introduced.

To sum up, since 1770 mortality in France has been declining steadily. It decreased slowly until 1890, except for the age group 1-4 as we have seen. After 1890 the decline accelerated for both sexes and for all age groups.

The Increase of Internal Migrations

The statement that large-scale internal migrations in France were accompanied by the foregoing demographic phenomena is commonplace. There were great migratory movements from the country to the towns throughout the nineteenth century, but the available numerical data for these phenomena are a long way behind those for mortality and fertility. The difficulty of such historical research doubtless explains why they are so scanty. This is why C. H. Pouthas (24), who gives a picture of the population of France during the first half of the nineteenth century, puts it as follows:

> "The conclusions that can be drawn remain incomplete. Without local studies, neither the origin nor the purpose of these migrations can as yet be known, in particular, can the foreign element in the centres of immigration be told from what came from other departments."

While we cannot ignore the migrations, our knowledge of their extent can only be indirect because of the many variables. The increase in the number of large towns and in their population would be one such variable. While only 8 French towns had more than 50,000 inhabitants in 1801, there were, for example, 15 in 1850.

Another way is to compare the census figures for the emigration of natives of one department to other departments of France. For instance, the 1891 census gives a population of 1,324,660 inhabitants for the Nord department. The distribution of the native emigrants from the Nord department to 11 other departments was as follows (5):

Pas-de-Calais	:	51,492	Meuse	:	3,370
Somme	:	5,990	Meurthe-et-Moselle	:	1,744
Aisne	:	19,621	Seine-et-Oise	:	5,360
Oise	:	4,957	Seine-et-Marne	:	1,470
Ardennes	:	2,189	Seine-Inférieure	:	2,699
Total : 146,319.			Paris	:	47,427

This gives an idea of internal migrations.

The development of Paris affords further conclusive evidence of these migrations. L. Chevalier (5) has contributed valuable data on this. According to the census taken in 1891, for example, 1,659,390 inhabitants of Paris were born in other departments. Of these, 697,-

204, or 42.02 percent, were natives of 18 departments for which the figures are as follows:

Seine-et-Oise	:	89,666	Oise	:	35,469
Seine-et-Marne	:	55,777	Somme	:	32,139
Nord	:	47,427	Pas-de-Calais	:	30,399
Yonne	:	45,811	Haute-Saône	:	29,344
Seine-Inférieure	:	39,696	Côte-d'Or	:	28,450
Nièvre	:	39,263	Creuse	:	28,123
Meurthe-et-Moselle	:	38,888	Sarthe	:	28,065
Aisne	:	38,393	Cantal	:	27,934
Loiret	:	35,624	Aveyron	:	26,736

This gives ample proof of the powerful attraction Paris exerted over the departments as a whole.

The Increase in Endogamy
The fall in fertility, the decline in mortality, and the migration expansions occurred at the same time. After a more or less long latent period there appeared in their wake a striking demographic phenomenon: a considerable increase in the number of consanguineous marriages among the populations concerned. The genetic importance of this phenomenon can be immediately appreciated.

To understand this phenomenon we have to recall the concept of "isolates" put forward by the Swede, Walhund (35). This concept originated in the need to determine population subdivisions within a large population such as that of most modern nations; subdivisions within which it would be possible to make an accurate count of the genetic frequencies in an actual generation and of their evolution in subsequent generations, according to the mode of transmission.

To this end it was necessary to subdivide very large populations into "isolates." In its applications Mendelian population genetics assumes the existence of panmixia in the populations studied. In other words, the basic assumption is that the populations are closed and that the fertility is the same for all their couples. Confronted with the impossibility of measuring over-large populations, Walhund decided on fragmentation. Since marriage plays an important part in hereditary transmissions, Walhund defined the "isolate" as the population inside which each individual has the possibility of marrying.

Dahlberg (7), also a Swede, extended this concept to the human level.

The concept of "isolate" can be easily understood by picturing the life of the inhabitants in the village of Europe before the industrial era. Communication difficulties discouraged barter. Populations from one village were often positively hostile to another. The prospects of marriage were as limited as they can still be today among primitive tribes or within geographically isolated communities. This situation would appear to have imposed strict endogamy on these populations.

Investigations in this field have gradually shown that an isolate could have several origins. An isolate within which it is possible for strict panmixia to exist may be the result of physical isolation and can be qualified as geographic. Such, for example, is an isolated village whose inhabitants can marry only amongst themselves and where the proportion of marriages between cousins is necessarily high.

Not all isolates, however, are geographical. Many religious isolates are known. In some departments of France, for example, Protestants and Catholics often still live side by side, rarely intermarrying and creating imaginary isolates which are nevertheless solid in structure. The existence of professional isolates can also be easily demonstrated. There are families of artists, musicians, doctors, and soldiers in every country. In France there still persists several Polish, Russian, Armenian, and Greek isolates of fairly long standing.

There are also isolates created by a combination of all the causes cited above. The Indian population of Parsi is a striking example of this: immigration, religion, general abilities, and the principle of caste have at one and the same time contributed to create and perpetuate it.

Measurement of the Size of the Isolate
The fact that the size of the isolate can be measured emphasizes the advantages of the concept. In a field where after all it would be vain to look for too great accuracy, this metric element, whatever its degree of approximation, is not negligible. There is, in fact, too often a tendency to speculate on purely imaginary data.

Credit goes to Dahlberg for showing as far back as 1929 that the size of the isolate or, in other words, the number of marriageable individuals can be calculated from the frequency of marriages between first cousins. From these figures he estimated that the average isolate for Sweden consisted of 400 individuals for the period preceding the industrial era. These calculations are based on the following reasoning: there is a relationship between the size of a population, on the one hand, and both the frequency and the distribution of the different degrees of kinship on the other. When the selection of a partner becomes limited because of the small number of marriageable individuals, a high proportion of interbreeding among close kindred is to be expected. Hence the concept of measuring the size of the isolate from marriages between first cousins.

From this angle the evolution of our civilization can be supposed to have increased the possibilities of marriage. The isolate of the past would, because of that, literally have broken up with the coming of the industrial era and there would have been an appreciable decrease in consanguineous marriages.

Dahlberg was the first to express the measure of the breaking-up phenomenon of isolate in terms of the decrease in consanguineous marriages between first cousins. This is how he put it in 1948 (8):

"When out to get an idea of the size of the isolate, it should first and foremost be remembered that this naturally varies to a high degree. The one extreme is the large town with its never-resting human masses. The other extreme is country of wild, deserted nature, e.g. in Northern Europe, with small isolated villages. As well as this, the size of the isolates is at present undergoing violent changes, on account of the development of communications, emigration to towns, etc. Going on available figures, we can probably assume that in older times the marriages between cousins stood at about 1 percent, which corresponds to an isolate of 400 individuals. Nowadays, marriages between cousins seem to approach 0.25 percent, which corresponds to an isolate of 1600 individuals. This would mean that, on an average, a person, contracting a marriage has the possibility of choosing 800 persons nowadays, and from only 200 previously."

It was believed for a long time that consanguinity was very widespread among the populations of Europe before modern times. In 1955 we questioned this in a study on the evolution of the number of consanguineous marriages in a French department: the Loir-et-Cher, between 1812 and 1954 (32). The study involved consanguineous marriages requiring dispensation from the Roman Catholic Church for the following degrees of consanguinity: third degree, (3 D, uncle-niece aunt-nephew) fourth degree (4 D, first cousins), fifth degree (5 D, first cousins once removed), sixth degree (6 D, second cousins with the addition of double cousins as, for example, offspring of the brothers of one family who had married the sisters of another family).

The rate of evolution (Figure 5) is as follows: the constant frequency of consanguineous marriages is between 2 and 3 percent with a higher percentage for only two years. From 1835 to 1870 a regular increase in consanguinity is seen. Between 1870 and 1900 it invariably remains above 3.5 percent, frequently rising to between 5 and 6 percent. After 1900 the percentage of consanguineous marriages decreased slowly until in 1930 it dropped to below 1 percent. The marked rise after World War I should be noted. The increase in consanguinity within the Loir-et-Cher department during the nineteenth century is accordingly very distinct.

We have since, in a study still to be published, investigated the evolution of consanguinity in 272 parishes of the Finistère department over the 103 years from 1859 to 1962. The rate of the phenomenon is comparable for all the parishes. The number of consanguineous marriages increased considerably after 1858. It reached a maximum value around 1900 and then declined for the most part below the initial value after World War II. In Tables 1 and 2, we have grouped the representative random data for 27 parishes of Finistère selected from among the 272 parishes.

Table 1 shows that while there were no consanguineous marriages for 14 out of the 27 parishes during the quinquennial period 1858-63, the percentage for the remaining 13 ranged from 0.8 to 6.4. The other columns give the percentage of consanguineous marriages for these quinquennial periods when these values were highest for each parish. The percentage of the period of consanguineous marriages ranged between 2.8 (for Ploujean) and 50.0 (for Saint-Divy). After 1858-63 it was not long before endogamy reached its peak during the following quinquennial periods: 1874-78, 4 times; 1879-83, 2; 1884-88, 1; 1889-93, 2; 1894-98, 1; 1899-03, 5; 1904-08, 3; 1909-13, 7; 1914-18, 2.

It is between 1900 and 1914 that endogamy is seen to reach its maximum most frequently: 15 times out of 27.

Table 2 gives the percentages in the last period 1958-62 according to the values of the peak.

The extension of endogamy in France during the nineteenth century was also found in other countries. In Italy, L. L. Cavalli-Sforza *et al.* (*4*) and A. Moroni (*21*) showed that in several dioceses the frequency of consanguinity estimated by the special permissions of the Roman Catholic Church followed an evolution similar to the one previously described (Figure 6). In Sweden, Alström (*1*), dealing with marriages of first cousins only, showed that their number increased between 1750 and 1850. In this case, however, the juridical evolution of the special permissions was such that the results should be read cautiously.

Increase in Consanguineous Marriages: Its Mechanism

The demographic phenomenon of an increase in the number of consanguineous marriages is a continuation of the demographic cycle of birth control, decline in mortality, and internal migrations whether working simultaneously or not. Let us examine how they work.

(a) *Birth control*: On the assumption that 20 couples limit their family to 2 children by practicing birth control for one generation, while 80 have 4 children in the first generation, we get 40 children on the one side and 320 on the other. If each child follows in the Malthusian or the non-Malthusian tradition for the next 2 generations, by the fourth generation we get 160 descendants of the original 20 and 5120 of the other group, the original 80.

On the other hand, by assuming that the descendants of the Malthusian 20 remain Malthusian and that every generation 20 percent of the descendants of the original 80 couples become Malthusian, by the fourth generation we get 800 descendants of Malthusian couples as opposed to 3548 of non-Malthusian. This gives an idea of the rapidity with which the demographic situation develops. Such a process clearly brings about marked difference in the fertility of the population.

As we pointed out in 1951 (*31*) the frequency of consanguineous marriages, whatever the degree of consanguinity, depends on the average size of the family. In this way an individual belonging to a group with an average number of 2 children per family has, on an average, 2 uncles or aunts, 4 first cousins, 8 first cousins once removed, and 16 second cousins. In the case of 7 children per family the figures are respectively: 18, 84, 261, and 1176. Doubtless not all of those connected by marriage can be considered marriageable: incompatibilities of sex and age occur. As the average size of the family increases there is a proportionate increase in the age distributions of connections by marriage, and a certain number of them have, consequently, to be ruled out. Thus, from among the 1176 second cousins of an individual belonging to a group where the average number of children per family is 7, half must be discounted as being of the same sex. From among the other half, a further number have to be discounted because the differences in age are too great to permit marriage (Table 3) (*28*).

The calculations show that where the average number of children per family is over 3, age differences produce incompatibilities. In Figure 7, the continuous lines indicate the average number of connections by marriage of every degree for an individual belonging to populations where the average size of the family varies. The pecked lines indicate the average number of connections by marriage of an age compatible with marriage. The very assumption of panmixia makes it easy to understand that the differences in fertility caused exclusively by the advent of birth control should, within two to three generations, be able to produce an increase in the number of consanguineous marriages. By this process every individual belonging to a non-Malthusian family was able to have many cousins descended from the same common ancestors, whereas for the issue of Malthusian families the relative loss of cousins was very marked.

Only the effect on the size of the family has been discussed here.

(b) *The decline in mortality:* Let us see what can happen if there is a decline in mortality only. If mortality declines without a corresponding fall in fertility, there is a rather large increase in the number of children reaching a marriageable age. On the one hand population increases numerically and, on the other, there is an increase in the number of cousins for each marriageable individual. This, for example, is what must have occurred among the French-Canadian peasants (17). At the time of the 1921 census women of 40 had an average of 10 living children. With such norms the population increases very rapidly: it doubles every 16½ years, and the isolates of preceding generations have to split up into several new ones. Starting from this model, J. Hajnal (14) is inclined to believe that the increase in consanguineous marriages noted during the course of the demographic cycle can be attributed exclusively to the drop in mortality. This remains to be proven on the practical level.

(c) *Emigration:* It is with this factor and its effects that we are least familiar. On the assumption that emigration is homogeneous and that 1 or 2 members of each family are known to leave their isolate, families of 2 or 3 will, for example, lose all their virtual cousins within 3 generations. For larger families the loss will be insignificant from the point of view of consanguinity and the number of virtual cousins. A significant and effective differential will then be established.

We now have to consider other factors. We have just seen that the differential phenomena are essential for explaining the points that interest us. The decline in fertility is not global: there are differences in the extent of birth control practiced by families. The result of this differential fertility is known for certain regions of France such as Vendée: the Protestant districts which practice contraception have been literally swamped by the Catholic ones which do not.

The degree to which contraceptive practices prove efficacious in a population where they have become general depends on several factors:

(a) Biological factors. There are, for example, naturally hyperprolific couples, while others are sub-prolific.

(b) Socioeconomic factors. It is well known that the effectiveness of the different contraceptive methods varies according to the socioeconomic level.

(c) Lastly, cultural factors also play an important part: level of education, religious beliefs and whether practicing or not, etc.

What is true for fertility is equally true for mortality. It is unnecessary to dwell upon the differences that can still be observed today, in accordance with all the above factors, for example, in mortality in general and, above all, in infantile mortality.

We can thus surmise that endogamy received a powerful stimulus from these three factors acting singly and independently. With no decline in mortality and efficient contraception it is understandable that an increase in the number of marriages between cousins should have occurred where panmixia existed.

It is likewise conceivable that without contraception the decline in mortality (as in Hajnal's model) should have given a powerful stimulus to endogamy within three generations, by increasing the average size of the family, Similarly, it can be imagined that large-scale and heterogeneous rural emigration per family, unaccompanied by birth control or a drop in mortality, should have produced the same result by creating differences in the size of families at the time of the age of marriage.

It must be emphasized that statistically the three phenomena exert pressure in the same direction, according to the following pattern: At a period when a certain proportion of couples are practicing birth control and others are not there is an accompanying decline in mortality which accelerates the results of control. At a time when 20 percent of families, the Malthusians, have only 2 or 3 children of marriageable age, the others, because the expectation of life has risen, have 5, 6, 7, or even more.

It is evident that these factors have operated simultaneously in France. If Hajnal's hypothesis as represented in the model is correct, we should have witnessed a considerable increase in the French population of country villages, whereas in fact the process has been reversed.

The increase in consanguineous marriages in France occurred at the time of a sharp drop in natality, when France, if we limit ourselves to the population of French origin, became depopulated. The apparent lack of change of the natality in the stationary population is due to the very large number of immigrants.

In many villages the population decreased as endogamy increased. A third element, migration, must, moreover, have played a considerable part. Extensive rural emigration took place simultaneously with the demographic revolution.

A department such as Finistère must have lost close to 200,000 inhabitants between 1850 and the 1914-18 War. The three phenomena—decline in fertility, decline in mortality, and migration—had operated simultaneously.

It is clear that in the future the historical study of demographic facts will justify what we are now putting forward. It is probable, if not certain, that the above factors operated simultaneously to create the endogamous drive of the nineteenth century. In some parts one factor must certainly have had the ascendancy over the other two at a given moment. We believe that it was contraception that had the most influence in some departments. For example, its effect was certainly greater in the depopulated areas of Aquitaine than in Brittany or the Central Massif. The effect of the decline in mortality must also have been more pronounced in Loir-et-Cher. Emigration had become so widespread in the rural departments that its effects are more difficult to localize. It must, however, have operated simultaneously with demographic growth in the department of Finistère, for instance.

In any event, it must be admitted that the process by which endogamy appeared in various parts of France must have been affected by mechanisms that differed according to region while operating in the same direction. This is probably why the rate at which the isolates broke up differed from one department to another and from one region to the next. Different mechanisms operating separately or together are the reason why the endogamous drive has not been homogeneous and simultaneous everywhere. We have seen that in the 27 communes of Finistère maximum growth was not reached at the same period, no doubt, because the mechanism may have varied from village to village.

It is this difference in the mechanism, and the different combinations of the three factors, that must be responsible for the chronological difference in the appearance of endogamy on the one hand, and, on the other hand, in its preservation and in the breaking-up of isolates. As early as 1948 (29) we pointed out that the breakup of isolates varied perceptibly from one department to another in France. In 1955, when we compared the evolution of isolates in Loir-et-Cher with those of Finistère, our calculations showed a difference of 30 years in their endogamic evolution, paralleling the decline in fertility and mortality.

Consequences of Genetics

General Aspect of the Problem

From the foregoing, one can conclude that a precise estimate of the effects of birth control on the genetic structures of populations is not possible today. Birth control is not, indeed, a single manifestation: it has, among other factors, interactions with mortality decline and migrations. It is, however, possible to estimate the exact effects of a contemporary phenomenon from the genetic standpoint; namely, an increase in consanguinity, followed by its gradual disappearance: We can get a general idea of the demographic evolution already described, by noting that generations are replaced unequally and that their numerical increase depends on only a small proportion of women. Consequently, their genetic importance becomes progressively greater with succeeding generations.

P. Vincent (34) published an interesting study on the role of large families considered from this angle. He investigated, from the fertility point of view, the history of 500,000 women born in France during 1881, a demographic generation as it were. From the 1931 census the history of these women showed the following: 140,000 had died before reaching marriageable age (turned 15); 60,000 aged 15-49 had died spinsters; and 270,000 had married.

Table 4 shows the fertility of the married women. Their distribution is according to the number of children born.

It can be seen that families with 0, 1, or 2 children, who constitute over one half of the total (61.1 percent, contribute only a quarter of the descendants of the generation (25.6 percent). Families of at least 7 children, who form considerably less than a tenth of the total number of families (6.3 percent), on the contrary, produce a comparable number of children (20.9 percent). Families of 10 or more children alone, although infinitesimal in number (1.6 percent) contribute almost as many children as families with an only child (7.2 percent as against 8.5 percent). Families with at least four children (24.2 percent) alone account for over half the descendants of the generation (53.1 percent), whereas more than half of the families (61.1 percent) have only 2 children at the most.

The above figures emphasize the importance of the part played by large families, but P. Vincent has emphasized this even more tangibly in the question he asks himself about the generation under consideration: In what proportion would its descendants have been reduced had the largest families abstained from procreating their children of higher order, and what would have been the resulting rate of replacement for that generation? In other words, he posed the following question: By what percentage would natality have been reduced, had such families as had produced more than 7 children limited the number of their children to 7 and not had either their eighth or those following? The answer is given in the two right-hand columns of the preceding table (Vincent has allowed 0.78 as net rate of basic effective reproduction for the 1881 generation).

We see that if there had been no families of 8 or more children in the 1881 generation, natality would have decreased by 4.1 percent.

It would have been reduced by 10.2 percent if there had been no families of 6 or more children. With 3 children per family natality would have been reduced by a quarter (25.2 percent). These figures are very instructive as to differential fertility. They demonstrate the importance of its role in the renewing of human populations, and, from a genetic viewpoint, its fatal repercussions on the composition of populations.

The transformation speed of the human genetic structures, under this influence confirms Pearson's (23) calculations from the Danish Vital Statistics. At first, 25 percent of the parents give 50 percent of the children. In the second generation, if the fertility of the descendants is the same 75 percent will be born of the former 25 percent, 90 percent in the third generation, and 96.4 percent in the fourth.

The opinion held by demographers today is that it was due to the above phenomena that only 10-12 percent of the French of 1789 were represented in the 1880 generation. Several geneticists—even outside of the use of the mathematical models which are the basis of theoretical genetics—have relied entirely on the results of demographic phenomena in their endeavors to demonstrate the genetic incidence of this state of affairs. Thus, Osborn (22) made the following comments:

(a) The transformation of demographic facts provokes a waning in the selective effect of death. When the expectation of life fluctuated between 25 and 40 years, half the number of children died before they had attained half their reproductive age. In the United States, at the time of the foundation of the republic (1793) only 36 percent of those born alive survived until the age of 35. Today, with an expectation of life exceeding 68 for men and 70 for women, 95 percent of the children born alive reach their reproductive period. Death rates are falling very rapidly. Differential mortality, which certainly played a very important part in selection, has practically disappeared. The only remaining mechanism of selection is the mortality during first week of life. Osborn states:

> "We are obliged to admit that when death rates are low, the influence of death functions, above all, is in eliminating genes responsible for premature deficiencies; and that death has little or no effect on the distribution of genes on which intelligence or personality depend."

(b) A probable weakening in the selective effect of births has certainly appeared as well. In the United States, women born between 1905 and 1909 had three children by ages 45-50; those born between 1875 and 1879 had 4.33 by the same age. Simultaneously, there occurred a considerable differential fertility which had passed through several phases of development. At first, fertility was lower among the upper social classes. An equalizing in family sizes was next observed. Now the process is reversed, the upper classes have more children. There is, finally, less and less selection through natality.

Cook (6) published relevant statements on the same topic.

Increase in Consanguineous Marriages and Its Effects

If the foregoing observations are clearly important to a global appreciation of the genetic transformations arising in the population through the demographic events described, the study of the effects of consanguineous marriages is even more conclusive.

We have seen how consanguinity increased among the 27 Finistère parishes representative of the 272 parishes (Tables 1 and 2). The main effect of consanguinity is as follows: it brings about a tendency towards homozygosity. The closer the ties of consanguinity and the lower the frequency of the gene, the stronger this tendency will be. For example, if the frequency of a gene, p, is 1/100 (which roughly corresponds to the frequency of the gene leading to albinism) the odds are 10,000 to 1 against the appearance of an albino among the descendants of a couple whose ties of consanguinity are negligible. In the case of a couple who are first cousins, however, the odds are 1380 to 1, or seven times greater.

If the frequency of the gene is 1/100, the chances of producing a homozygote are 195 times greater in a marriage of the third degree, between uncle-niece or aunt-nephew, than when the parents are not related by marriage. If the frequency is 1/10, however, the chances in favor of a homozygote carrier are only 2.35 times greater.

If the parents of an individual, x, are not related by marriage, the probability of his receiving a certain gene in a chromosome is independent of the probability of his receiving another gene in the homologous chromosome, since there is no relationship between the chromosome inheritance of his two parents. This no longer holds true if the two parents of the individual x are related by marriage. In this case the probability that two homologous loci of the individual x will be identical (homozygosity), that is to say, obtained from an ancestor common to both his parents, and is expressed by his coefficient of consanguinity. The value of these coefficients is $\frac{1}{8}$ for uncle-niece or aunt-nephew couples (or for the children born of them), 1/16 for couples who are first cousins, 1/32 for couples who are first cousins once removed, and 1/64 for couples who are second cousins.

The mean coefficient of consanguinity for a population, Wright's F or Bernstein's a, represents the probability that 2 homologous loci of an individual taken at random in a population will be identical.

The mean value of this probability can thus be evaluated a priori for any individual or a couple; on the other hand, involve an a posteriori evaluation with the genealogy as starting point.

Table 5 gives the values for the mean coefficients of consanguinity F or $a.10^5$ for each of the 27 parishes of the Finistère sample for the 3 periods (a) 1859-63, (b) the period of maximum endogamy, and (c) 1958-62. Elsewhere Table 5 shows 2 values corresponding to F or $a.10^5$: K_1 the rate of the increase in homozygotes due to consanguinity where the gene frequency is 1/500; and K_2 the rate of increase where the gene frequency is 1/5,000.

It can be seen that during the first period of the coefficient F, among the 13 parishes out of the 27 to have one, varied between 13 and 231, with a value of 63 for the 13 parishes. During the period of maximum endogamy all the parishes showed a coefficient. The latter varied between 49 and 1989 with an overall value of 264. During the most recent period, 1958-62, only 8 out of the parishes had a coefficient. The value of F ranged between 20 and 80 and its overall value has only 11.

The rates of increase K_1 and K_2 represent the numbers by which the frequency of homozygotes increases through the action of consanguinity in a population where panmixia obtains. The value of K_1 ranges between 1 and 2.1 for the first period, with an overall value of 1.3. It is between 1.2 and 11 for the second, with an overall value of 2.3. During the third period K_1 varies between 1.1 and 1.4, with an overall value of 1.05. For the value of K_2, corresponding to a frequency of 1/5,000, the following facts can be observed. During the first period its value ranged between 2 and 12, with an overall value of 6. During the second period it was between 3 and 100, for an overall value of 14. During the third, it ranged between 2 and 5, and its overall value was 1.5.

The consequences produced by such a considerable increase of homozygotes in the population through the action of this endogamic drive can be only briefly indicated here if the coefficients of consanguinity and the mode of transmitting a character are both known. It is then possible to calculate the probability of an individual's belonging to a genotype as well as the distribution of various genotypes in the population.

As shown by J. B. S. Haldane (15), the consequences of consanguinity are intensified when several characters are considered. Assume that the two characters are monohybrid and autosomal and that the frequency of the recessive gene of the one is 0.01 and that of the recessive gene of the other is 0.003. Then, the chances that a couple who are first cousins will transmit both characters simultaneously are

156.5 times greater than for a couple who can be considered as non-consanguineous. If we consider the proportion of marriages of the third to the sixth degree noted among the Catholic marriages in France from 1926 to 1945, we find, assuming the family relationship to have been negligible for the marriages beyond those degrees, that 72 percent of those carrying both characters are offspring of unions of the third to the sixth degree only. Thus, less than 2 percent of those marriages account for over half of the descendants carrying the two characters.

Owing to 20 years of remarkable advancement in population genetics we can understand the effect of the phenomena previously described upon the qualitative aspect of populations from 1850 to 1940. An appreciation of the phenomena created by endogamy is possible only in the light of practical observations of the consequences produced by consanguineous marriages. In the fields of mortality and recessive malformations, the increase of homozygosis has led to an increase in undeniably high frequencies. Under conditions described earlier on, recessive mutations, latent perhaps for centuries, have become manifest.

Clearly, many instances of mortality have resulted from such a considerable increase of homozygotes. Lethals or semi-lethals have also manifested themselves, with or without consequent premature mortality. As we have shown (27), mortality increases with the degree of consanguinity. Infant endogenous mortality is particularly high among the descendants of consanguineous marriages. This is true not only for the mortality of the younger ages but also the mortality in general (Tables 6 and 7).

Table 7 also shows that the distribution of mortality according to age is proportionately the same for consanguineous and non-consanguineous families. But since mortality is always higher among consanguineous families their expectation of life is consequently appreciably lower. This satisfactorily explains the fact that the endogamous drive of the nineteenth century checked the drop in mortality associated with such advances as higher standards of sanitation, and thus slowed down the rise in the expectation of life in the zones of greatest endogamy as compared with zones where there was less inbreeding.

From the standpoint of pathology, consanguineous marriages give rise to many abnormalities, especially by way of recessive homozygosity. It is difficult to determine specifically the malformations that have appeared and the statistics extant are few. Nevertheless, we now possess some very valuable data from work carried on in Sweden since 1931, following up the remarkable researches made by

Sjögren (26) on juvenile amaurotic idiocy. It would appear that under the existing frequency conditions diseases of the nervous system and tuberculosis are those which increase most as a result of endogamy. Doctors in the nineteenth century had for a long time observed the prevalence of tuberculosis manifestations among the descendants of consanguineous marriages. This fact has been pointed out by a good many investigators including Puffer (25) among others. We ourselves called attention to this in 1951 (30) and again in 1958 when we were investigating the effects of consanguineous marriages on descendants. The closer the degree of consanguinity the greater the increase in tuberculosis among the descendants.

Dronamraju (10) has recently made a study of Andhra Pradesh in India. The percentages of consanguineous marriages among the parents of different diagnosis groups of patients are shown:

Diagnosis of patients	Percentage of consanguinity
Cancer	25.0
Pulmonary T. B.	42.1
Other kinds of T. B.	30.8
Diseases of C. V. S.	23.0
Diseases of C. N. S.	21.0
Respiratory Diseases	36.2
Deficiency Diseases	31.4
Injuries	20.0
Malformations	41.7

None of these percentages, except for pulmonary tuberculosis, is significantly different from the average.

The fact is all the more conclusive, as in this region of India, with its very old tradition of endogamy, many of the deleterious genes must have been eliminated by natural selection in the course of continuous inbreeding for many hundred years.

Under the influence of the endogamic drive, a virtual increase has thus been observed in instances of mortality as well as in pathological conditions. Table 8 (27) makes an analysis of these observations in the endogamous rural zones of France. A comparison is made between consanguineous and non-consanguineous families, the latter acting as a control group. The distributions for the control families and the consanguineous families, just as for the children corresponding to them, show a difference with a probability of over 90 percent. At the level for the families, the greatest differences are noted between the two "normal" and "abnormalities + deaths" categories. In the former the control group is the more numerous, while in the latter, the consanguineous group is very much greater. The "with deaths" categories, without abnormalities, show no statistical differences.

At the level for children the differences between "control" and "consanguineous" are real for the four categories.

Other Manifestations

In the foregoing we have outlined the genetic consequences partly attributable to the manifestation of birth control among families in western populations. Much still remains to be said on this subject by going beyond the data established at present, likewise by working from the determinist or stochastic models generally employed in population genetics. It is, for instance, clear that the appearance of homozygotes in great numbers among populations has appreciably disturbed the genetic homeostasis as understood by Lerner. The question presents itself, briefly, as follows:

By genetic homeostasis should be understood "the tendency of a Mendelian population as a whole to retain its genetic composition arrived at by previous evolutionary history" (20). A great many naturalists have studied the problem, noting that nature seems to prefer the average. Attempts have been made, including the use of models, to explain what the genetic mechanism of this operation was. The part played by heterozygosis in the appearance of this phenomenon has proved important.

Since Weismann, all the great modern biologists, R. A. Fisher, S. Wright, H. J. Muller, Th. Dobzhansky, and J. Huxley have established that bisexual reproduction confers plasticity to populations on a large scale, and facilitates the transformation of genetic composition in response to environmental changes. Its action also constitutes a stabilizing, conservative force in relation to events considered over a short period.

These favorable conditions combine with the presence of heterozygotes. The vital superiority of the former over homozygotes is evident. Heterozygosis favors ontogenic self-regulation (homeostasis of development) because the organism is in this case more apt to remain within the norms of canalised development. It also favors self-regulation of populations (genetic homeostasis) by which average types are preferred to extreme types.

It has been recognized by scientists that the depression due to consanguinity is accompanied by a phenotypic variance, environmental in origin. As the genetic variance decreases, the reduction in vitality renders organisms more sensitive to environmental influences. Homozygotes are less adaptable and become more sensitive to variations.

The phenomenon of polymorphism—that is to say, the incidence of the fact that heterozygotes show certain vital advantages over homozygotes—is a recent discovery of importance to mankind. Because of its generalized character, this phenomenon has further upset such logical conclusions as might have been possible.

Since, for the moment, we can speak only from an imaginative point of view or else engage in science fiction, we have preferred to restrict ourselves to the field best known. Assuming we have made some new contributions, we have elected to limit our interpretation to a strict conformance with reliable scientific findings, without any speculation as to what will be known tomorrow.

It must again be emphasized that the appearance of endogamy, largely due to birth control, has had important social repercussions in the family organization; as stressed by Mr. Aries (personal communication), this phenomenon has given rise to patriarchal families that did not exist in the last century. There is, however, no agreement about the social repercussions of the above phenomena.

It should, moreover, be stressed that genetic facts cannot be isolated from the sociological, economic, and cultural whole in which modern populations evolve. Larsson (19) has been able to isolate thirteen orders of factors operating in the realm of these ideas. We cannot refer to this in greater detail because of lack of space.

General Survey and Conclusion

As early as the end of the eighteenth century, largely, no doubt, to family limitation, a differential fertility became evident in the population of France. Starting from this fact, together with its verified demographic consequences, we have outlined the genetic consequences of these circumstances. Our present degree of information prevents us from separating the specific effects of birth control from those produced by the decline in mortality and by migration, which established themselves in the French population at the same time. The three phenomena have operated in the same direction, producing in the end, differences in the ranks of individuals of reproductive age. This has resulted in a considerable endogamic drive, manifested by the appearance of a great number of consanguineous marriages in the population.

It can be calculated that the mechanism described on the demographic level has been widespread among the populations of western Europe. It can consequently be propounded that the endogamic drive is an element that should now be integrated into the demographic revolution or cycle. From now on a new element can therefore be considered to be an integral part of this revolution. In the light of the genetic consequences of this situation, it must be conceded that the consequences of the demographic revolution pattern extends to a considerable degree at the population level.

By this very fact a great body of qualitative phenomena, that had until now resisted every attempt to be classified as concepts of demographic significance, proves to be an integral part of conventional demography. The introduction of this new element may in the future establish a bridge between crude demographic data and the phenomena of sanitation that have up to now remained obscure. It seems more rational, for instance, to explain the increase in cases of tuberculosis from the end of the nineteenth century up to the introduction of antibotics in western populations, as well as the increase in abnormality and backwardness in the zones where endogamy was most flourishing. Likewise, data on the development of qualitative and sanitary phenomena are recorded in a new and much more realistic spirit. It is also clear that the problems set by this phenomenon have, in the aggregate, had great repercussions on the composition of populations. However, an estimate of these repercussions will, doubtless, always remain impossible. The fact that, through this phenomenon, one half of the children in practically every generation are produced by one quarter of the parents implies rapid genetic transformations whose exact incidence cannot be specified.

Unfortunately we cannot expound upon these phenomena now, for to treat them adequately would require a volume. For instance, since Galton and his "Hereditary Genius" (1869), there exists a whole literature in the realm of psychology which holds that the average intelligence of the population must have declined in the course of generations since intellectuals have fewer children. The question has still not been settled.

We could mention many other fields where analogous ideas have been provoked by the fact that the renewing of generations depends on only an infinitesimal part of families. We cannot, however, define the mechanisms of this as yet, any more than we can know what happens to natural selection in such a situation.

Finally, our opinion is that the endogamic drive should, undoubtedly, be integrated into the demographic cycle. It is a necessity of our epoch to integrate genetic facts into demographic structures. The distinction often made between quantitative and qualitative demography is somewhat of a convention. Elements considered for a long time to be qualitative are gradually entering the quantitative domain. This is essential to the understanding of the biological import of the evolution of modern societies. The fall in fertility, a phenomenon widespread throughout the world in our epoch, implies profound qualitative transformations. The present and future evolution of underdeveloped areas is also giving rise to many demographic observations. We hope that everyone responsible will pay the greatest attention to the genetic phenomena involved in these transformations: this is the price to be paid for the future quality of man.

REFERENCES

1. Alström, C. H., "First Cousin Marriages in Sweden 1750-1844" and "A Study of the Population Movement in Some Swedish Subpopulations from the Genetic-Statistical Viewpoint," *Acta. Genet.*, 8:295-369, 1958.

2. Bergues, Hélène, *et al. La prévention des naissances dans la famille Ses origines dans les temps modernes.* Paris, P.U.F., I.N.E.D., 1 vol. in-8°, p. 400, 1960.

3. Bourgeois-Pichat, J. "Evolution générale de la population française depuis le xvIIIème siècle," *Population*, 6:635-62, 1951.

4. Cavalli-Sforza, L. L., Moroni, A., Zalaffi, C., and Zei, G. "Analisi della consanguineita osserrata in alcune diocesi dell'Emilia," *Atti Ass. Genet. Ital*, 5:305-16, 1960.

5. Chevalier, L. *La formation de la population parisienne au xIxème siècle.* Paris, P.U.F., I.N.E.D., 1 vol. in-8°, p. 312, 1950.

6. Cook, R. C. "Changing Patterns of Selection," *Acta. Genet.*, 6:349-53, 1956-57.

7. Dahlberg, G. "Inbreeding in Man," *Genetics*, 14:421-54, 1929.

8. Dahlberg, G. *Mathematical Methods for Population Genetics.* Karger, Basle; London, New York, Interscience Publ, 1 vol. in-8°, p. 93 and 182, 1948.

9. Deniel, L. and Henry, L. "La population d'un village du Nord de la France. Sainghin-en Mélantois de 1665 à 1851," *Population*, 20:563-602, 1965.

10. Dronamraju, K. R. "Genetic Studies of the Andhra Pradesh Population," in *The Genetics of Migrant and Isolate Populations* (E. Goldschmidt, ed). New York, Williams & Wilkins, vol. 1 in-8° ccII p. 369, 1963.

11. Ganiage, J. *Trois villages de l'Ile-de-France. Etude démographique.* Paris, P.U.F., I.N.E.D., 1 vol. in-8°, p. 148, 1963.

12. Gautier, E. and Henry, L. *La population de Crulai, paroisse normande, étude historique.* Paris, P.U.F., I.N.E.D., 1 vol.-8°, p. 269, 1958.

13. Girard, P. "Apercus de la démographie de Sotteville-lès-Rouen vers la fin du xvIIIème siècle," *Population*, 14:485-508, 1959.

14. Hajnal, J. "Concepts of Random Mating and the Frequency of Consanguineous Marriages: A Discussion on Demography," *Proc. Royal Soc. B.*, 159:125-77, 1963.

15. Haldane, J. B. S. "The Association of Characters as a Result of Inbreeding and Linkage," *Ann. Eugen.*, 15:15-23, 1950-51.

16. Henry, L. and Lévy, C. "Ducs et Pairs sous l'Ancien Régime. Caractèristiques démographiques d'une caste," *Population*, 15:807-30, 1960.

17. Laberge, C. "La consanguinité des Canadiens Français," *Population, 22*:861-96, 1967.

18. Landry, A. *La révolution démographique. Études et essais sur les problèmes de population.* Paris: Recueil Sirey, 1 vol. in-8°, p. 231, 1934.

19. Larsson, T. "The Interaction of Population Changes and Heredity," *Acta. Genet., 6*:333-48, 1956-57.

20. Lerner, I. M. *Genetic Homeostasis.* Edinburgh, London: Oliver & Boyd, 1 vol., p. 134, 1954.

21. Moroni, A. "Evoluzione della frequenza dei matrimoni consanguinei in Italia negli ultima cinquant'anni," *Att. Ass. Genet. It. Pavia, 9*:208-23, 1966.

22. Osborn, F. "Changing Demographic Trend of Interest to Population Genetics," *Acta. Genet., 6*:354-62, 1956-57.

23. Pearson, K. "Reproductive Selection" in *The Chances of Death and other Studies in Evolution.* Vol. 1, pp. 63102. London: Cambridge. Univ. Press, vol. 2, 1897.

24. Pouthas, Ch. H. *La population française pendant la première moitié du xixème siècle.* Paris, P.U.F., I.N.E.D., 1 vol. in-8°, p. 227, 1956.

25. Puffer, R. R. *Familial Susceptibility to Tuberculosis.* Harvard Univ. Press, 1 vol. in-8°, xii, p. 106, 1944.

26. Sjögren, T. "Die juvenile amaurotische Idiotie. Klinische und erblichskeitsmedizinische untersuchungen," *Hereditas, 14*:197, 1931.

27. Sutter, J. "Recherches sur les effets de la consanguinité chez l'homme," *Biol. Med., 47*:563-660, 1958.

28. Sutter, J. and Goux, J. M. "L'aspect démographique des problèmes de l'isolat," *Population, 16*:447-62, 1961.

29. Sutter, J. and Tabah, L. "Fréquence et répartition des mariages consanguins en France," *Population, 3*:607-30, 1948.

30. Sutter, J. and Tabah, L. (a) "Les notions d'isolat et de population minimum," *Population, 6*:481-98, 1951.

31. Sutter, J. and Tabah, L. (b) "Effets des mariages consanguins sur la descendance," *Population, 6*:59-82, 1951.

32. Sutter, J. and Tabah, L. "L'évolution des isolats de deux départements français: Loir-et-Cher et Finistère," *Population, 10*:645-74, 1955.

33. Valmary, P. *Familles paysannes au xviiième siècle en Bas-Quercy. Étude démographiques.* Paris, P.U.F., I.N.E.D., 1 vol. in-8°, p. 192, 1965.

34. Vincent, P. "Le rôle des familles nombreuses dans le renouvellement des générations," *Population, 1*:148-54, 1946.

35. Wahlund, S. "Zusammensetzung von Populationem und Korrelationserscheinungen von Stanpunkt der Vererbungslehre ausbetrachtet," *Hereditas, 11*:65-106, 1928.

Table 1. Frequency of consanguineous marriages in 27 parishes of Finistère (French
Department) for two periods: 1859-63 (2), (3), (4), and of maximum
endogamy (6), (7), (8)

(1) parish, (2) (6) total of marriages, (3) (7) number of consanguineous marriages,
(4) (8) percentage, (5) period of maximum endogamy

(1)	(2)	(3)	(4)	(5)	(6)	(7)	(8)
Bodilis	72	0	0	1889-1893	61	5	8,2
Carhaix	88	4	4,5	1914-1918	83	4	4,8
Collorec	51	2	2,0	1874-1878	48	4	8,3
Edern	99	2	2,0	1874-1878	78	3	3,8
Fouesnant	90	3	3,3	1899-1903	123	6	5,7
Guilers	75	0	0	1909-1913	69	3	4,3
Huelgoat	77	0	0	1904-1908	82	3	3,7
Kernilis	35	0	0	1899-1903	20	1	5,0
Landivisiau	130	1	0,8	1899-1903	117	4	3,4
Lannédern	23	0	0	1909-1913	27	2	7,4
Loc Eguiner Saint-Thégonnec	41	0	0	1909-1913	25	2	8,0
Logonna-Daoulas	78	1	1,3	1879-1883	73	5	6,8
Mellac	75	0	0	1894-1898	78	3	3,8
Penmarc'h	109	7	6,4	1874-1878	123	14	11,4
Plogonnec	118	4	3,4	1904-1908	110	6	5,5
Ploudaniel	127	0	0	1884-1888	110	2	1,8
Plougastel-Daoulas	249	2	0,8	1899-1903	343	28	8,2
Ploujean	114	2	1,8	1899-1903	103	3	2,8
Plouvorn	126	0	0	1879-1883	100	2	2,0
Port-Launay	45	0	0	1909-1913	28	3	10,7
Rédéné	51	0	0	1904-1908	75	6	8,0
Saint-Divy	19	0	0	1914-1918	4	2	50,0
Saint-Pabu	42	1	2,4	1909-1913	50	10	20,0
Saint-Thonan	16	0	0	1889-1893	17	1	5,9
Spézet	120	3	2,5	1909-1913	164	6	3,7
Trégarvan	15	0	0	1909-1913	22	5	22,7
Le Trévoux	51	1	2,0	1874-1878	64	2	3,1
	2136	33	1,54		2197	135	6,22

Table 2. Frequency of consanguineous marriages in 27 parishes of Finistère (French Department) for two periods: Maximum endogamy (2), (3), (4), (5) and 1958-62 (6), (7), (8)

(1) parish, (2) maximum endogamy, (3), (6) total of marriages, (4), (7) number of consanguineous marriages, (5), (8) percentage

(1)	(2)	(3)	(4)	(5)	(6)	(7)	(8)
Bodilis	1889-1893	61	5	8,2	52	0	0
Carhaix	1914-1918	83	4	4,8	118	0	0
Collorec	1874-1878	48	4	8,3	30	0	0
Edern	1874-1878	78	3	3,8	68	0	0
Fouesnant	1899-1903	123	6	5,7	128	2	1,6
Guilers	1909-1913	69	3	4,3	54	0	0
Huelgoat	1904-1908	82	3	3,7	43	1	2,3
Kernilis	1899-1903	20	1	5,0	32	0	0
Landivisiau	1899-1903	117	4	3,4	126	0	0
Lannédern	1909-1913	27	2	7,4	13	0	0
Loc-Eguiner Saint-Thégonnec	1909-1913	25	2	8,0	10	0	0
Logonna-Daoulas	1879-1883	73	5	6,8	38	1	2,6
Mellac	1894-1898	78	3	3,8	60	0	0
Penmarc'h	1874-1878	123	14	11,4	203	0	0
Plogonnec	1904-1908	110	6	5,5	79	1	1,3
Ploudaniel	1884-1888	110	2	1,8	72	0	0
Plougastel-Daoulas	1899-1903	343	28	8,2	163	3	1,8
Ploujean	1899-1903	103	3	2,8	47	0	0
Plouvorn	1879-1883	100	2	2,0	100	2	2,0
Port-Launay	1909-1913	28	3	10,7	23	0	0
Rédéné	1904-1908	75	6	8,0	37	0	0
Saint-Divy	1914-1918	4	2	50,0	28	1	3,6
Saint-Pabu	1909-1913	50	10	20,0	39	2	5,1
Saint-Thonan	1889-1893	17	1	5,9	32	0	0
Spézet	1909-1913	164	6	3,7	101	0	0
Trégarvan	1909-1913	22	5	22,7	11	0	0
Le Trévoux	1874-1878	64	2	3,1	40	0	0
		2197	135	6,2	1747	13	0,74

Table 3. Number of cousins of a given degree (D) with whom a given individual, in an isolate of 1000 members, may marry, panmixia assumed (From J. Sutter & J. M. Goux, 1961)

Family size	Uncle-niece Aunt-nephew 3th D	1st Cousins 4th D	1-1/2 Cousins 5th D	2nd Cousins 6th D
2	1	2	4	8
3	2	6	14	36
4	4	12	32	96
5	5	20	57	200
6	7	30	90	360
7	9	42	130	500

Table 4. Fertility of 270,000 married women born in 1881. Proportion of the families (2) according to live births (1). Proportion of children according to family size (3). Effects of an hypothetical reduction of the maximum number (n) of children per family (4) (5) (From P. Vincent, 1946)

Live births	Proportion of the families (percent)	Proportion of children according to family size (percent)	Hypothesis of reduction to n of the maximum number of children per family	
(1)	(2)	(3)	(4)	(5)
Illegitimate children out of the statistic of families		4.4	Reduction in the number of descendants (percent)	Net reproduction rate
0	16.5	—	—	—
1	22.2	8.5	63.8	0.28
2	22.4	17.1	40.2	0.47
3	14.7	16.9	25.2	0.58
4	9.0	13.8	16.0	0.65
5	5.4	10.4	10.2	0.70
6	3.5	8.0	6.5	0.73
7	2.2	5.9	4.1	0.75
8	1.5	4.5	2.5	0.76
9	1.0	3.3	1.5	0.77
10 and more	1.6	7.2		
Total........	100.0	100.0	—	0.78

Table 5. Coefficient F ou α. 10^5 and rates of increasing of homozygoty K_1 (gene frequency 1/500), K_2 (gene frequency 1/5,000) for 27 parishes of Finistère (French Department) during three periods: 1859-1863 (2), (3), (4), for period of maximum endogamy (5), (6), (7) and 1958-1962 (8), (9), (10)

(1) parish (2) (5) (8) F ou α (3) (6) (9) K_1 (4) (7) (10) K_2

(1)	(2)	(3)	(4)	(5)	(6)	(7)	(8)	(9)	(10)
Bodilis	—	—	—	333	2.7	18	—	—	—
Carhaix	231	2.1	12	301	2.5	16	—	—	—
Collorec	184	1.9	10	228	2.1	12	—	—	—
Edern	79	1.4	5	240	2.2	14	—	—	—
Fouesnant	104	1.5	6	203	2.0	11	61	1.3	4
Guilers	—	—	—	204	2.0	11	—	—	—
Huelgoat	—	—	—	229	2.1	12	36	1.2	3
Kernilis	—	—	—	313	2.5	17	—	—	—
Landivisiau	24	1.1	2	93	1.4	6	—	—	—
Lannédern	—	—	—	231	2.1	12	—	—	—
Loc-Eguiner Saint-Thégonnec	—	—	—	750	4.7	38	—	—	—
Logonna-Daoulas	80	1.4	5	321	2.6	17	41	1.2	3
Mellac	—	—	—	280	2.4	15	—	—	—
Penmarc'h	158	1.8	9	267	2.3	14	—	—	—
Plogonnec	53	1.2	4	99	1.4	6	20	1.1	2
Ploudaniel	—	—	—	85	1.4	5	—	—	—
Plougastel-Daoulas	13	1.0	2	251	2.2	13	29	1.1	2
Ploujean	27	1.1	2	145	1.7	8	—	—	—
Plouvorn	—	—	—	78	1.4	5	42	1.2	3
Port-Launay	—	—	—	725	4.6	37	—	—	—
Rédéné	—	—	—	333	2.6	18	—	—	—
Saint-Divy	—	—	—	781	3.9	40	56	1.2	4
Saint-Pabu	149	1.7	8	1219	7.0	62	80	1.4	5
Saint-Thonan	—	—	—	184	1.9	10	—	—	—
Spézet	78	1.3	5	124	1.6	7	—	—	—
Trégarvan	—	—	—	1989	1.1	100	—	—	—
Le Trévoux	31	1.1	3	49	1.2	3	—	—	—
	63	1.3	4.2	264	2.3	14	14	1.07	1.7

Table 6. Endogenous, exogenous, and perinatal mortality for three categories: control groups, first cousins, second cousins, in three French rural departments: Morbihan (M), Finistère (F), Loir-et-Cher (L.C.). From J. Sutter, 1958 (The rates are for 1000 live births)

	Total control	Total Cons.	Total 1st C.	Total 2nd C.	(Control group) M.	F.	L.C.	Total CSG M.	F.	L.C.	1st C. M.	F.	L.C.	2nd C. M.	F.	L.C.
Stillbirths (c)	21	37	43	33	21	22	20	52	29	26	57	34	29	55	23	21
Endogenous Mortality (a)	13	26	32	16	16	9	15	34	20	19	49	27	21	15	12	17
Infant Mortality (b)	46	75	87	68	54	39	41	83	83	56	99	86	69	65	81	51
Exogenous Mortality (b − a)	33	49	55	52	38	31	26	49	63	37	50	59	48	50	69	34
Perinatal Mortality (c + a)	34	63	75	49	37	30	35	86	49	45	106	61	50	70	35	38

Table 7. Distribution of mortality per age groups in two categories of families— control-group and consanguineous From J. Sutter (1958)

	Control group crude number	percent	Consanguineous crude number	percent
Stillbirths	84	17.0	80	18.6
1 to 30 days	79	16.0	75	17.4
2 to 12 months	106	21.4	91	21.1
1 to 10 years	111	22.4	96	22.3
11 to 30 years	115	23.2	89	20.6
Total	495 deaths		431 deaths	
	$x^2 = 1.29$ (4 d.l.)		$P > 0.90$	

Table 8.

(a) Number and percentages of the totality of the families in each category: Normal, with deaths only, with abnormalities only, with abnormalities + deaths (classified according to the degree of consanguinity). (From J. Sutter, 1958)

	Control Group	4th D	5th D	6th D	Total CSG
Normal	902	139	45	178	362
	(66,32)	(41,1)	(54,2)	(58,0)	(49,9)
With deaths only	309	72	15	74	161
	(22,71)	(21,4)	(18,1)	(23,8)	(22,2)
With abnormalities only	77	43	8	16	67
	(5,76)	(12,8)	(9,6)	(5,2)	(9,2)
With abnormalities + deaths	72	82	15	39	136
	(5,31)	(24,4)	(18,1)	(13,0)	(18,7)
Total	1.360	336	83	307	726

Comparison of two distributions: $x^2 = 13,5$ (3 d.l.) $- P > 0.90$.

(b) Number and percentages of children in the above families

	Control Group	4th D	5th D	6th D	Total CSG
Normal	2.302	335	114	451	900
	(56.2)	(32.1)	(44.0)	(47.3)	(40.0)
With deaths only	1.188	243	46	288	577
	(29.0)	(23.3)	(17.8)	(30.2)	(25.6)
With abnormalities only	273	117	26	51	194
	(6.7)	(11.2)	(10.0)	(5.3)	(8.6)
With abnormalities + deaths	330	349	73	163	585
	(8.1)	(33.4)	(28.2)	(17.2)	(25.8)
Total	4.093	1.044	259	953	2.256

Comparison of two distributions: x^2 100 (3 d.l.) $- P > 0.90$

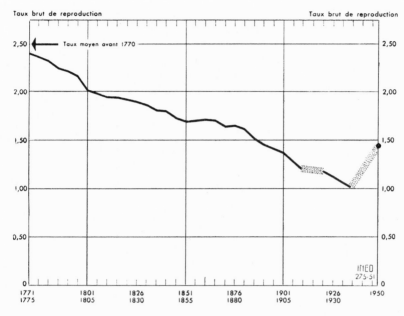

Figure 1. Evolution ot net reproduction rate in France 1770-1950.
(From J. Bourgeois-Pichat, 1951)

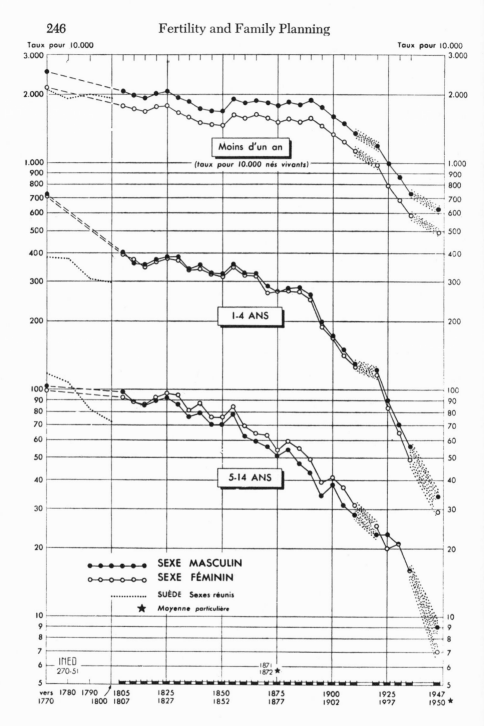

Figure 2. Mortality rate per 10,000 inhabitants, age-group 1-14.
(From J. Bourgeois-Pichat, 1951)

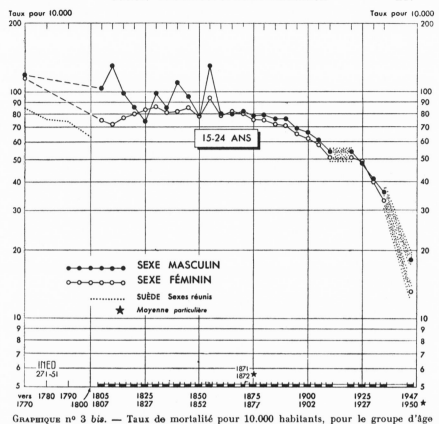

GRAPHIQUE n° 3 *bis.* — Taux de mortalité pour 10.000 habitants, pour le groupe d'âge
15-24 ans.

Figure 3. Mortality rate per 10,000 inhabitants, age-group 15-24.
(From J. Bourgeois-Pichat, 1951)

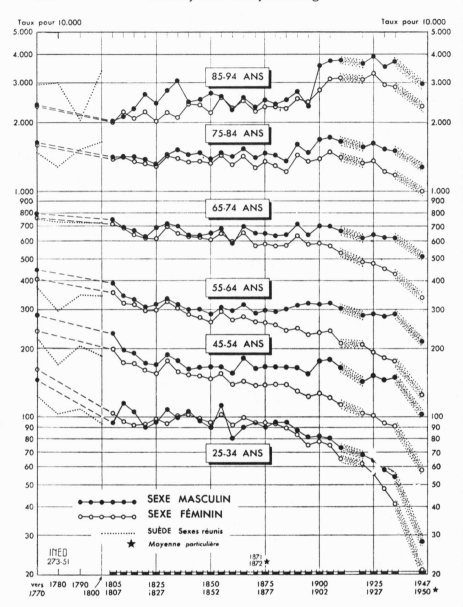

Figure 4. Mortality rate per 10,000 inhabitants. Each age-group.
(From J. Bourgeois-Pichat, 1951)

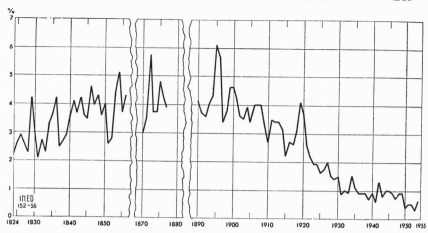

Figure 5. Evolution (percentage) of consanguineous marriages in a French department (Loir & Cher, 1824-1955).
(From J. Sutter et L. Tabah, 1955)

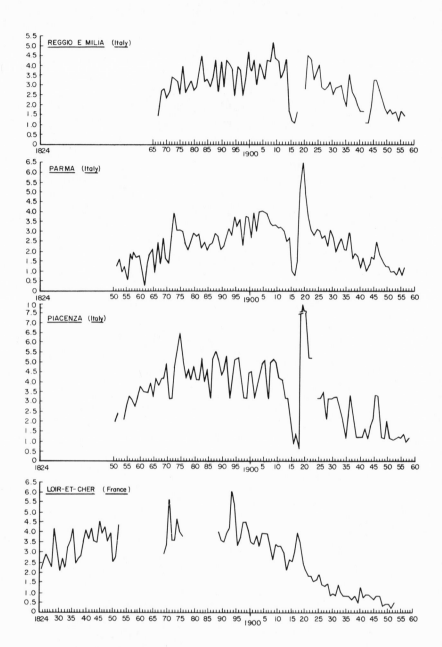

Figure 6. Evolution of consanguineous marriages (percentage) in French and
          Italian dioceses for the last 100 years.
          (From A. Moroni, 1964)

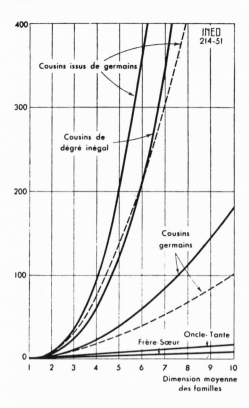

Figure 7. Mean number of relatives for an individual according to the mean family-size of the dwelling population.
(From J. Sutter et L. Tabah, 1951)

BIOCHEMICAL CHANGES AND IMPLICATIONS FOLLOWING LONG-TERM USE OF ORAL CONTRACEPTION

Celso-Ramon Garcia and
Edward E. Wallach

Department of Obstetrics and Gynecology,
School of Medicine;
Hospital of the University of Pennsylvania

Introduction

FOLLOWING REPORTS (57,176) of the effective inhibition of ovulation in regularly ovulating women, through the use of synthetic steroids which mimicked the action of the natural female sex steroids, and the subsequent report of their contraceptive application in fertile human subjects in Puerto Rico and Haiti, the era of endocrine control of fertility was begun. Earlier, Sturgis and Albright (202) had suggested that estrogens might be used for this purpose but only applied them for relatively short intervals. It is indeed surprising that their observation was not seized upon and an attempt made to apply it for longer intervals. It must be kept in mind, however, that progress in this aspect of medical science has been very slow because of the enormous lack of knowledge of the effects of these substances on the various body systems, not to mention the social encumbrances which their use implies. It was not until population pressures became sufficiently convincing that significant efforts were more universally applied.

The earliest oral contraceptive studies, in reality, simply were limited extensions of the more detailed observations which had been carried out on smaller groups of women in Massachusetts, over more confined intervals of time. In recent times, use of many newer available progestogens, with and without estrogens, has provided a wider array of hormonal contraceptive preparations. Further, the ingenious variations in their application through different dosages and regimens tend to complicate the situation, not to mention the confusion attendant upon the introduction of trade names. The list is too lengthy to discuss or even to mention each of these individually. The interested reader can refer to current listings of these agents (*129,36*). It is remarkable that these numerous progestogen-estrogen combinations have many similar basic effects, despite the varied pharmacological action of the individual ingredients (*44,110,47,202,75*). However, one must hasten to point out that the observations of the numerous comparative clinical studies must be interpreted as only being suggestive. There are, as yet, no rigidly-controlled, experimentally suitable studies which eliminate any potential, albeit unintentional, selective or other biases and permit a more precise evaluation of the "true" effects of the various agents. Nevertheless, for practical purposes certain broad conclusions and concepts are possible. That these approaches are very effective in reducing fertility is universally accepted. That the principal mechanism through which this is achieved is ovulation inhibition is also accepted. Still, despite the similarity of the various progestogen-estrogen formulations, one cannot be assured that they can be used interchangeably without altering their effectiveness. Some evidence suggests reduction of contraceptive efficacy through such changes (*130*); other sources refute this concept (*67*). Oral contraceptive practice has become so complex that it is imperative to know not only the basic ingredients of the formulation but also the specific regimen used. A summary outline of the various regimens is given in Table 1.

The progestogen-estrogen combinations have been ascribed many therapeutic applications (Table 2); however, the greatest acclaim for these agents has been associated with their contraceptive efficacy. The lower-dosage forms exemplify the contraceptive use of such compounds. The contraceptive effectiveness reported for these lower dosages of the oral contraceptives is listed in Table 3. The progestogen-estrogen form of contraception is the most effective method of contraception available (Table 4). Little difference, if any, has been demonstrated between the contraceptive efficacy of the combined as compared with the sequential regimens; both are more protective than the continuous low-dosage progestogen regimen. Nonetheless, adequate comparative data are not available.

Crude estimates suggest that over 14 million women throughout the world have used these agents for contraception. In the recent survey of the Fellows of the American College of Obstetricians and Gynecologists, to which 83.7 percent responded, 94.8 percent reported the oral contraceptives as the most frequently prescribed family planning modality and that in the preceding year 1.5 million women had been started on an oral contraceptive method (*165*). Thus, it is understandable that such wide acceptance and usage should foment an interest in learning more about the detailed effects of these substances. With ever-increasing populations, any and all sorts of correlative or associated effects can be expected. Since correlation and causality are not always synonymous, it is imperative that a better understanding of these effects be attained. This is all the more urgent in view of the number of women who are taking these compounds continuously for a number of years, although in most regimens one week lapses between medicated cycles. It is noteworthy that so few proven contraindications have been noted in so large a group of users. Moreover, never have so many healthy women within the reproductive ages been taking any pharmacologic agent for as long a period of time. On the other hand, never have the alternative hazards of pregnancy itself been so vividly assessed. Nevertheless, the fear of the relative unknown has raised much concern. Beclouding the issue is the fact that much of the criticism of these compounds has been raised by those opposed to contraception in any form. Within the limits of propriety, if not sobriety, such criticism or questions are healthy. All new approaches must be reviewed critically. It is gratifying that to date no valid evidence has supported the possible irreversibility of the induced effects. The intended temporary sterility itself has been challenged as a possible irreversible effect (221,39,187). Reminiscent of these criticisms are the implications of a noted gynecologist, in a letter to the editor of the JAMA in 1945 (79), that the use of contraceptive practices available in that day contributed to infertility. At this point, it seems safe to state that fertility potential is neither enhanced nor reduced after discontinuation of oral contraceptive use. Furthermore, in spite of the observed alterations induced by the progestogen-estrogens, there is no scientific evidence which validly demonstrates a significant pathological effect in the normal healthy female.

In summarizing the extensive data of numerous investigators, a composite of the effects of these agents will be presented. The minor individual specific pharmacologic differences cannot be stressed, since no truly reliable comparative studies in the human are available to permit this. Furthermore, it is essential to remember that the changes noted in any individual at a specific time represent the summation of the total dynamic picture as of that moment. For example, variations among individuals can be noted on the same day of parallel cycles. Even in the same individuals, physiologic differences may be noted in a specific phase of one cycle in comparison with the same phase in a cycle many months later. These differences are further compounded by the variations in regimen, ingredients, and dosage. Because of such limitations, the conclusions stated will necessarily be broad generalizations. The biochemical changes during long-term use will be considered in the light of reported observations of the effects of these agents not only on the reproductive tract and the related structures, but also on the general endocrine and metabolic systems. Consideration will be given also to the implications of these alterations.

Effects on the Reproductive Tract and Related Target Areas

Ovarian Effects   Since it is rarely feasible to observe the ovarian changes themselves, it is often necessary to rely on indirect indices of ovulation. It must be stressed that many difficulties are encountered in attempting to draw valid conclusions, since these indices may not give a clear picture of ovarian function. The effects observed may be produced by the agents themselves rather than by alterations in ovarian function. The action of the progestational agents on the thermal regulatory centers, the endometrial histology, and the vaginal desquamation may mask the ovarian-induced effects and in some instances lead to misinterpretation. Urinary pregnanediol excretion, however, is usually low in the absence of ovulation and, since the customary oral contraceptive compounds are not excreted as this metabolite, the presence of pregnanediol in the urine in elevated amounts has been considered as evidence of ovulation. Pregnanediol has been reported to be elevated in the later phase of the cycle on combined therapy in 6.8 percent of norethindrone-mestranol cycles (68) and 2.3 percent of norethindrone acetate-ethinylestradiol (170) cycles tested: It was also elevated in 11 percent of cycles with sequential therapy (13). Accordingly, it has been concluded that ovulation escape does occur. However, during the use of combined formulations, at least, the infrequent occurrence of pregnancy (0.2 per women years of use) is invariably associated with omission of tablets. Moreover, fresh corpora lutea have not been observed at laparotomies performed at times in which their presence might be anticipated, except in one instance (38), where combined therapy is presumed to have been used. Thus, the source of pregnanediol must be considered as possibly arising from either luteinized atretic follicles or from extra-ovarian sources such as the adrenal cortex. While it is possible that ovulation escape may occur, there is little supporting evidence for this phenomenon. The consensus of the investigators is that these ovaries subjected to estrogen-progestogen effect present a gross appearance of relative inactivity (57,179,123,160,161,235,141). There is minimal follicular development, and this is to diameters rarely more than a centimeter. Follicular atresia is believed to follow. Similar follicular activity and atresia have been described during pregnancy, as well as with treatment on the pseudopregnancy regimen. (48). The ovaries of contraceptive users are small and present a "compact" histologic appearance, presumably secondary to the absence of corpora lutea, larger follicles, stromal edema, and other morphologic features normally seen during the untreated cycle. Review of ovarian sections from treated women, although limited in numbers, does not suggest any difference in the relative degree of follicular atresia in comparison to tissues obtained from untreated women of similar age groups (58). Studies from many clinics (57,179,123) (160,161,235) lend support to this view.

The excretion patterns of estrone, estradiol, and estriol, as well as pregnanediol, are usually low in the medicated cycles of oral contraceptive users in comparison with normal cycle data (15). However, variable patterns are observed, during treatment with any single agent, from patient to patient, in addition to variations secondary to differences in medication, dosage, and regimen used (14,113). Although, in the first post-medication cycle these urinary estrogens are excreted in greater quantities than during medicated cycles, these levels are still lower than the mean values for normally menstruating women (15). By the second cycle these values have reached a slightly higher level than found during the normal menstrual cycle. Pregnanediol excretion, however, is within the normal range during the later phases of the first two post-medication cycles (15).

If medication is continued according to regimen, the contraceptive efficacy is not altered, despite prolonged use (169,58,211). However, if medication is not resumed, ovulation most often occurs within a few weeks. To insure optimum contraceptive efficacy, the medication must not be suspended for longer than 7 days at any one time. A shorter interval is recommended for sequential therapy.

On occasion, but infrequently, cyclic follicles have been noted after treatment with these anovulants (124). In patients who were treated with these agents prior to hysterectomies, for whatever reason, different degrees of focal cortical stromal thickening have been observed (124,74,179,156). In contraceptive users, where ovarian sampling was carried out at the time of elective tubal ligation in the absence of pathology of the pelvic structures, this finding has not been observed (160,58).

Upon withdrawing from oral contraceptive practice, the first cycle is usually prolonged and the menses delayed, but in most instances the cycle is less than 8-10 weeks (168) in length. A return to the previous catamenial habit follows. Seventy-eight and six-tenths percent of the patients formerly on combination, and 76.3 percent of those previously on a sequential regimen, showed indirect evidence of the return of ovulation in the first post-treatment cycle, and up to 98 percent by the third post-treatment cycle. No difference was observed in resumption of ovulation between sequential and combination therapy in some 163 randomly-selected women studied (168). Moreover, the promptness of return of ovulation was the same for those who used contraception from 1-4 years as it was for those who had used it for 5-6½ years.

Nonetheless, the patient who has an antecedent history of ovarian irregularities prior to the use of the antiovulants cannot be expected to return to a normal, regular catamenial habit after cessation of oral contraceptive use. Since recall of the past menstrual habit is not very accurate, one cannot know the meaningfulness of observed delays in return of normal catamenia if the patient history is the only evidence of prior normal ovulatory habit (221,39). Our impression is that anovulation following discontinuation of oral contraceptives is usually associated with similar dysfunction prior to institution of these agents. Moreover, anovulation can occur spontaneously at any time in any regular ovulator. Nevertheless, while correlation and causality may not be synonymous, it is well to be alert for the rare patient who may present such a delay. If the amenorrhea persists, it is prudent to rule out intercurrent pathologic causes, whether related or unrelated to the therapy. This is particularly so if the amenorrhea persists for 6 months or more. Therapy with clomiphene citrate, where no significant pathology was noted, has had very salutary results.

Gonadotropin Effects   An accurate assessment of the effects of these agents on gonadotropin excretion is not available. Patient variability in response to medication, dosage, and regimen, together with the technical deficiencies of the assay procedures, complicates the matter (113,217). Daily variations are observed not only from subject to subject but even in the same subject. Thus, dependent on these many variables, there have been reports of no change in total urinary gonadotropins (113), reduction in the mid-cycle peak of total gonadotropins (148), some reduction in FSH (14), abolition of the LH mid-cycle peak (217), or even complete reduction of total gonadotropins (54). No changes in prolactin levels were found in either the first 5 or the last 10 days of treated cycles (188). Increase in human growth hormone levels has also been observed (194). During pregnancy, increases in HCG levels have been attributed to the medication (205). To attempt to generalize and summarize the present situation would be an oversimplification and probably result in inaccuracies; but, for what it may be worth, one can state that high-dosage or continuous administration of the progestogen-estrogen combinations leads to gonadotropin repression approximating undetectable levels (54). With the usual low-dose combined oral contraceptive regimen the mid-cycle LH peak is not detected and FSH may be slightly repressed (14), although not in the early and late phases of the cycle (198). With sequential therapy no detectable alteration of urinary LH has been noted, but some repression of FSH may occur (217,94). No increase in gonadotropin excretion has been reported in the early post-with-drawal cycles, except in situations where the medication was administered for 3- or 4-month intervals. In such cycles, Flowers (51) reports an occasional patient presenting a surge of FSH during the first post-treatment cycle.

It should be mentioned in passing that the ovarian inhibition with oral contraceptives has been overcome by the administration of exog-enous gonadotropins. Earlier reported failures to achieve this were probably a result of inadequate dosage of the exogenous gonadotropin (113,198,37,92). These more recent data point to a central effect of the progestogen-estrogens in inhibiting ovulation, probably through hypothalamic-pituitary inhibition of gonadotropin release. Nonetheless, it must also be kept in mind that certain of these anovulants may reduce the ovarian responsiveness, requiring a greater amount of exogenous gonadotropin.

Vaginal Effects   The appearance of the vaginal epithelium, and particularly the changes shown in the vaginal desquamate, are a summation of the effects of the endogenous as well as the exogenous steroids.

Hertz and Bailar (81), on the basis of normal estrogen secretion rates, conclude that the exogenous estrogen administered exceeds normal endogenous estrogen production. These excretion rates are limited to but three of the total estrogens and do not account for the presumed drug-induced suppression of endogenous estrogen forma-tion as well as the anti-estrogenic effects, particularly with the combined formulation. It should be pointed out, also, that endogenous estrogen production in women on oral contraceptives has not been evaluated. Also, the conclusion of Hertz and Bailar is at variance with many of the physiologic effects noted during long-term therapy. The changes in the vaginal desquamate discloses an increase in the ma-turation of the vaginal epithelium, on occasion with a combined regimen, and more frequently with the sequential regimens. How-ever, with virtually all combined formulations, a low maturation index is reported (89,90). The cytologic ovulation peak is abolished and infrequently, a tendency to vaginitis exists (6,219). It is of some interest that an improvement has been reported by these women when treated with topical estrogen cream or converted to an estrogen-dominant form of therapy such as a sequential schedule.

Cervical Effects During the normal untreated cycle, cervical mucus changes reflect the hormonal status of the particular phase of the cycle. Thus, during the preovulatory, proliferative, or estrogen phase, an increase in the amount, liquefaction, and clearness of the mucus is observed in contrast to the postovulatory, luteal, or progestational phase, when the mucus becomes thick, cellular, and scant. The significance of this biochemical-pharmacological relationship is curious, since the greatest penetration of spermatozoa is assessed about or immediately before ovulation (196). Following ovulation, sperm penetration is generally decreased. These changes persist until the approach of the ensuing ovulation. The thick, scant, cellular mucus, which is relatively hostile to spermatozoal penetration, is a progestational effect which can be mimicked by the combined oral contraceptive therapy or with the administration of the progestogens alone (234,77,131). This is particularly so with those exhibiting a greater anti-estrogenic activity of the progestational component (90). The production of copious, thin, clear mucus with increased spermatozoal penetration is an estrogenic effect which can be induced by exogenous estrogens. It is also seen during the estrogen phase of sequential therapy, where sperm penetration does not appear to be diminished until the progestational portion of the sequence is reached.

Although combined oral contraceptive therapy produces what might be considered a sperm barrier at the level of the cervical mucus, it must be borne in mind that not only is there considerable daily variability, but also one progestogen (Ethinyltestosterone) has been reported to increase spermatozoal penetrability of cervical mucus (16). With the norethindrone-acetate-ethinyl estradiol combination, active motile spermatozoa were noted in the higher regions of the endocervix (28). Zañartu (230) reports that from the 7th to the 18th day 22 percent of the patients observed had from 1 to 5, but less than 15, spermatozoa per high power field of the cervical mucus specimens obtained from women on combined oral contraceptives. Seventy-eight percent of these women, however, had a non-motile spermatozoan present in one or more specimens. A less meticulous worker than Zañartu could easily have failed to locate these enthusiastic but ill-fated gametes.

With continuous "micro" therapy, alterations in sperm penetration are also reported. With chlormadinone acetate used in this manner, spermatozoal penetration was reported absent in only 17 percent of the women observed (178). Further, the mere fact that these gametes are not found in the cervical mucus is insufficient evidence to conclude that they are absent from the endometrial cavity and the fallopian tube as well. In fact, spermatozoa have been localized in the oviducts when their presence could not be confirmed in the cervix (115). Moreover, pregnancies occur with greater frequency among the women using the continuous "micro" progestogen than among those using combined formulations, in spite of the altered sperm penetration of cervical mucus. Such a local "condomatic" effect cannot really be viewed as a potentially significant mechanism in the temporarily induced sterility, since pregnancies can and do occur with such low endocervical sperm densities.

Uterine Effects   With long-term use of the oral contraceptive, the initial softening and questionable increase in size of the uterus is less apparent (148). Leiomyomata, particularly at sustained high dosage, can enlarge, but at the low contraceptive doses this is a rare occurrence (94,134). This is generally seen in the early cycles of contraceptive usage and is felt to be an estrogen effect.

Despite the length of therapy, typical endometrial histological changes are repeated cycle after cycle (150). The particular sequence (153,43,111) which is found depends on the progestogen used and the dosage of the preparation, as well as the regimen (178,119). After the first few cycles of administration, the endometrium becomes thinner with the combined formulation. This is questionably less so at the lower-dosage levels. With sequential regimens, changes in the thickness of the endometrium are less obvious. The sequence of glandular changes with combined therapy is one of moderately prompt progression from a proliferative pattern through a progestational one. The continuing action of the progestogen-estrogen combinations then presents varying degrees of mixed hormonal effect, leading on to secretory exhaustion in the late phases (153). With most of the combined formulations, a marked deciduation of the stroma is exhibited toward the later phase of the cycle (43,111). With sequential therapy, varying degrees of hyperestrinism are seen during the later phase of estrogen action (119). During the later phase of the cycle, under the influence of both progestogen and estrogen, mild progressive progestational glandular, but not stromal, activity is observed (118). Stromal deciduation and exhausted or atrophic glands are absent with sequential therapy (43,119). Here again, particularly with combined therapy, there is a moderately antiestrogenic effect displayed by the progestogen in the later phase of tablet-taking. The glandular atrophy and secretory exhaustion pattern can be overcome by increasing the amount of estrogen ingested (47). Varying degrees of glandular dilation as well as increased stromal vascularity can be observed, with the increases in estrogen content administered along with the progestogen. This would suggest that the combined progestogen-estrogen formulations in the available contraceptive dosage exert an antiestrogenic effect. Further similar suggestive evidence is provided by the slightly more than 1 percent of cycles in which there is a failure of withdrawal bleeding, and in which the endometrium invariably is very scant and atrophic in histologic appearance. Depending upon the dosage of the estrogen and the specific progestogen-estrogen combination, varying incidences of spotting and breakthrough bleeding have been reported (*153,101,126*). With combined formulations, the amount of blood loss at each flow is notably less than previously experienced prior to use of the medication. With sequential regimens, the flow may be slightly heavier than, or similar to, that prior to therapy. Survey of the literature suggests spotting and bleeding to be greatest with the medroxy-progesterone acetate-estrogen combination (*6,65,112*). It has also been suggested that the lynestrenol-estrogen combination has the highest incidence of failure of withdrawal flow. While not clearly understood, it appears that the antiestrogenic effect of the progestogen, as well as the physiologic dose, is closely related to these endometrial effects.

The endometrial histological sequences regress promptly upon cessation of medication. Very scant evidence is suggestive of any carry-over effect, and even this is short-lived (*70*). Pregnancies occur not only in treated cycles, but also in cycles where medication is begun after ovulation, as well as in the very first cycle after cessation of the regimen. The changes produced by these agents do not appear to impede implantation in these instances. The trophoblast seeks out the vascular areas of the endometrium and invades these structures (*19*). Certainly, these vessels are not appreciably altered until late in the tablet-taking cycle (*135*). It is doubtful that even these alterations interfere with the possibility of pregnancy, in the light of the occurrences of pregnancy in the instances outlined above. Moreover, pregnancies have become implanted in the endosalpinx, on the ovary, and on peritoneal surfaces where endometrial structures are absent. Despite endometrial morphologic changes following the postovulatory use of the oral contraceptives, used to regulate the catamenia, pregnancies are not prevented unless abstinence is practiced or ovulation is inhibited.

It has been claimed that a fair regularity of catamenial habit is maintained with continuous low-dosage progestogen. The low dosage is believed to alter the fertility without inhibiting ovulation. According to the report on the experience with the daily use of 500γ of chlormadinone acetate in 1123 women during 13,202 cycles, only 65.5 percent had cycle lengths of between 25 and 35 days (*122*). The cycle lengths following combined and sequential formulations show that at least 95 percent (*169,55,69*) have cycles which fall into this pattern, while approximately 83 percent of vaginal contraceptive users fall within these cycle limits. There is little doubt that the low-dosage continuous progestogen produces greater catamenial variability. Almost 2 percent of the women studied (19 of 1123) while using the "mini" dose had to stop medication because of profuse flow (*122*). Such occurrences of increased flow associated with the contraceptive use of the combined formulations are exceedingly rare (*94*); scanty flow or failure of withdrawal flow is encountered more often. The frequency of hypermenorrhea with the sequential formulations appears to fall between that of the "mini" dose and the combined formulations.

Oviduct Effects   Virtually no data exist which demonstrate the effect of these agents on the human oviduct. Studies on rodents suggest rapid transport of gametes with estrogens (*140*). While progestogens at high doses impede gamete transport, at low, or sub-ovulation inhibiting doses, they produce a prompt ejection of ova into the uterine cavity similar to that of estrogen (*26*). There are, unfortunately, no similar observations in the human which might afford an interpretation of the effects of these agents on oviduct secretions, motility, or gamete transport.

Breasts   Scant data exist on the effect of these agents on mammary glands. While initially there is a mild enlargement (*66,167,182,-214*) and increase in the sensitivity of the breasts (*60*) reported by the patient, these effects at the lower dosages are milder and relatively short-lived. A slight breast enlargement may be noted, especially with the larger doses and particularly when the progestogen and estrogen administration is not cyclic but is sustained over a prolonged interval. However, with combined formulations, the diffuse nodularity of the breasts recorded at the pretreatment examination was less frequently recorded in subsequent examinations while on the oral contraceptives (*149*).

Admittedly, it is not easy to assess the effect of the oral contraceptives on lactation. There is concurrence, however, that at large doses suppression is achieved while perhaps not at the lower doses (*54,186*). If there is a suppressive effect, it is usually not manifest until after 15 or 16 months, and not sooner than 7 months, of breastfeeding in mothers using low-dosage oral contraceptives (*186,80*). No appreciable alteration was noted in milk production, as assessed by the infant weight changes obtained pre- and post-breast feeding, when the low-dosage oral contraceptives were initiated immediately after delivery or after the 10th day, when lactation had been well established (*186*). However, reduction in breast engorgement has been observed when low-dosage contraceptives were initiated 2 hours postpartum in a non-breast-feeding group of patients (*18*).

Only one male breast-fed infant, whose mother was taking oral contraceptives, has been reported to have developed gynecomastia (33). It is unlikely that the gynecomastia is secondary to the oral contraceptive usage by the mother. The quantities of radioactive tracers in breast milk among small groups of lactating women who have been given oral radioactively-labeled progestational steroids have been small (151,206) and are considered of little significance. Only one recent report (107) is at variance with the previous studies. However, these workers failed to assess the biological activity of the steroids in the breast milk such as had been done by the previous workers. Since no such biologic activity as might be inferred from these recent radioactive data has been observed, it is unlikely that there are significantly active hormonal levels in the breast milk obtained from these users of oral contraceptives.

General Metabolic and Endocrine Effects
General Comments   While side effects are associated with the use of any medication, including the ingestion of inert ingredients, considerable apprehension exists regarding the long list of associated effects purportedly occurring secondary to the use of the oral contraceptives. Very early in the contraceptive studies, considerable variations were noted in the incidence of these effects from one center to another, and even in the same center from one group of women to another. This led to a small study in which the blind randomized distribution of either a placebo or an active ingredient was administered to groups of volunteers. For their protection, these women were advised to use a non-chemical method for contraception during the interval that they were to be evaluated for the effects of the tablets being studied. In addition, some groups were forewarned of possible side effects, while others were not similarly admonished. Even with the objective parameter of breakthrough bleeding, an increase in its occurrence was noted in the groups forewarned of possible side effects (154). Similar psychogenic features were observed in Switzerland in a study where a variety of formulations was used under code. The women were noted to present increases in nausea, breakthrough bleeding, and libido loss, with each occasion that medication was changed (173).

The most frequently encountered side effects reported with the use of the progestogen and estrogen combinations are nausea, dizziness, headaches, breakthrough bleeding, mastalgia, weight change, and melanosis. In most instances, although not all, these are secondary effects of the agents. There is, however, a much larger number of infrequently encountered complaints, and in some instances more serious reactions, where an association has never been definitively established. Some reports suggest or imply a meaningful correlation not present in others. These associations must not be excluded even when the infrequency of occurrence casts some doubts. It is the infrequently encountered condition which presents the most difficulty in evaluating the possible cause-and-effect relationship. While scientific data may not support definitive correlation, the clinician should be cautiously alert. Again, one should be reminded that truly reliable comparative studies are not available to make accurate assessment of specific differences between one formulation or regimen and another. Moreover, the personal bias, as well as the well-intended selective process which caution dictates, may of itself confound the issue, making it increasingly difficult or even impossible to prove or disprove cause-and-effect relationships.

Central Nervous System Effects, Including Emotional Effects It has been postulated that these steroids affect the hypothalamus (187). Electroencephalographic findings are variable (220,125). The patterns in the oral contraceptive users are characterized as intermediate when compared with the tracings obtained in the anovulator versus the regular ovulator. Similarly, hypothalamic alterations have been noted in animal studies (50,183). The thermogenic action of these agents has been described as a central nervous system effect. The observation of galactorrhea (76), during prolonged continuous or cyclic use, and on cessation of these agents, suggests the release of lactogenic hormone, probably secondary to a central nervous or hypothalamic influence. In passing, it should be noted that further emphasis of a central effect is supported by the reversal of ovarian inhibition by exogenous administration of gonadotropins.

Changes in mood have been noted during the premenstrual phase of the normal cycle, during pregnancy, the puerperium, and the menopause. Considerable variations of sex steroid levels occur in all of these states. It is felt, however, that emotional depression is associated with the occurrence of falls in urinary estrogen excretion. While depression (76) has been noted during contraceptive usage, psychic improvement has also been reported (224). Of course a lowered level of urinary estrogen is observed with the use of oral contraceptives; however, the correlation of this laboratory observation with the emotional state is yet to be confirmed. Recent reviews cover this aspect thoroughly (63,218).

Increased grooming of males by the female has been observed in the subhuman primate at mid-cycle, and in castrates after estrogen administration (133). This latter effect is reduced by the addition of progesterone to the therapy. Sexual and other behavior has been quite variable in the human when related to the menstrual cycle (232,117). Attempts to quantify cyclic behavioral effects are undoubtedly masked by the preponderance of the cerebral cortical influences, which overshadow any potential or actual endocrine action. It is difficult, if not impossible, to separate the physiologic effects of these contraceptive agents from the psychologic status of the individual. The reported effects of oral contraceptives on libido and coital frequency are so variable that no meaningful alterations have been reported in the large-scale trials (6,155,177,215,229). To date, detailed actuarial, gynecic, psychiatric, and psychologic testing reviews have been unable to demonstrate any significant changes (232,231,10,11). However, double-blind, controlled assessment has not been possible as yet.

Hematologic Changes   Reported hematologic changes are quite varied (23). While no significant changes in hemoglobin levels are noted (155,171), a slight but significant rise in hematocrit has been observed (55,23). Serum iron and serum total iron-binding capacity are also increased in oral contraceptive users. The latter appears to be well above the upper limits of normal. The mean corpuscular hemoglobin concentration is not altered; however, the serum iron was strikingly elevated. Elevations in the erythrocyte sedimentation times have been reported in patients using the combined and sequential formulations (191).

Slight serum calcium and phosphorus decreases have been noted in oral contraceptive users. While there have been some variations of K+, Na+, or Cl− ion levels noted, none of these has deviated from the limits of the accepted norm (21).

Changes in blood serum proteins have been reported as showing a striking rise in alpha-1-globulin, accompanied by a fall in albumin and a rise in beta-globulins (174). By starch gel electrophoretic technique, mobilization of serum proteins produces a discrete protein band localized in the region of the alpha-2-globulins in pregnant women, as well as in oral contraceptive users, in about 92 percent of those observed (35). These protein mobility changes are reversible on cessation of medication. Alterations in protein-bound iodine (85) and cortisol protein binding in plasma are also noted (181). Despite plasma elevations, cortisol secretion rates are not altered (55). The alterations and significance are not clearly understood. To date, a raised serum iron, together with an elevated total iron-binding capacity, has been observed only with hepatitis (108). Such alterations in association with the use of the oral contraceptives are still not clearly understood and warrant further study, particularly with reference to a possible interrelationship.

Carbohydrate Metabolic Effects   The effect of the oral contraceptives on carbohydrate metabolism is not clearly understood. While a diabetogenic effect has been considered as a possibility, the inference is arrived at through circumstantial evidence. Since estrogens and progestogens mimic some of the effects of pregnancy, the diabetogenic action of the latter is ascribed to these hormones. Wynn (227) put forth the hypothesis that since estrogens prolong the biological half-life of cortisol (205), which in turn may potentiate the chemical and diabetic-like state (138), estrogens are therefore diabetogenic. Several workers have demonstrated the glucose intolerance in some women receiving the progestogen-estrogen combinations (22,62,145, 158,159). These effects are even more striking in those women with a diabetic family history (62). It has been pointed out that increases in plasma insulin are also observed in these women demonstrating the glucose intolerance (192). Buchler and Warren (227) did not find differences in the K values, when evaluating the response to intravenous glucose tolerance among treated and non-treated women. However, others have noted abnormally low K values (227,158,159).

Since human growth hormone has been ascribed a diabetogenic activity as well, and it is known that the estrogenic activity of the oral contraceptive causes an elevation in the circulating HGH levels, it is hypothesized that it in turn antagonizes the insulin action. This, it is felt, results in an elevation of the blood glucose level producing a resistance to an insulin-induced hypoglycemia (194).

In appraising the effects of the oral contraceptives on carbohydrate metabolism, a review of the consequences of these agents on the plasma non-esterified fatty acids and blood pyruvate levels, in a test group of women during an intravenous glucose tolerance evaluation, describes significant alterations in their levels, in contrast to the control group (228). This is consistent also with the findings of elevated levels of human growth hormone (193). It is apparent therefore that, although not necessarily consistent nor marked, some alteration in carbohydrate chemistry does occur. From these observed chemical changes, it can be theorized that a diabetogenic action may exist. However, there is insufficient evidence to be conclusive. In women on extended long-term contraceptive usage, and in particular the few who have been on these agents for 10-12 years, as those in Massachusetts, overt diabetes has not been demonstrated. Likewise, there are no reports from any of the centers evaluating the long-term users, as for example in Puerto Rico, Massachusetts, California, and the like, where the norethynodrel-mestranol combination has been used at the 5 or 10 mg dosage level for at least 6 to 10 years. Reversibility of these chemical changes in the parameters measuring or related to carbohydrate metabolism is seen to occur promptly on discontinuing these medications (192,228).

Although increases in insulin requirements may be needed by some diabetic women on oral contraceptives, many are able to take them without altering their insulin needs (*41*).

Effects on Lipid Metabolism   Changes in the lipid profile in women taking the oral contraceptive have been described by Wynn (*228*) as simulating an androgen-like profile. Perhaps this should be described as an antiestrogenic effect of these combinations, since they produce a decrease in urinary estrogen excretion, but an increase in androgens has not been demonstrated. Much speculation has been entertained regarding the significance of these alterations in lipid chemistries, together with the chemical diabetic-like changes of these contraceptive agents, with specific reference to cardiovascular disease. The longitudinal Framingham study (*95*) has found that the antecedent level of serum cholesterol does correlate with the risk of subsequent atherosclerotic cerebral infarction when measured prior to age 50. More recently, serum triglycerides, total and free cholesterol, phospholipids, fatty acids, and skin-fold thickness have been measured relative to the occurrence of cerebral infarction. No correlation existed between the various serum-lipid levels or skin-fold ratio and patients with high or low incidence of occlusive vascular disease. Neither were these two groups different from the control group (*32*). Although the implications are grave, they are not conclusive and, moreover, are not supported by the studies of Jennett and Cross (*91*). More intensive study is desirable.

Thyroid Effects   Thyroid function has been evaluated by means of the BMR, blood cholesterol, triiodothyronine resin uptake, PBI, T4, and radioactive iodine (I_{131}) uptake, as well as by the clinical evaluation of the patient, including evaluation of the Achilles tendon reflex as measured by the photomotogram (*83,222*). With oral contraceptives, the evaluation of the thyroid status is not simple. The basal metabolic rate is not readily used in this country because of the numerous factors which can produce artefacts but, with precautions, it can be used to evaluate the patient on oral contraceptives. Blood cholesterol values, however, are of limited significance, since estrogen may reduce serum lipids. It has long been noted that there were slightly elevated protein-bound iodine values, together with a drop in the triiodothyronine (T_3) resin uptake, resulting from the progestogen-estrogen combinations. However, the radioactive iodine (I_{131}) uptake and the Achilles tendon reflex are not altered by this form of hormonal action (*83,222*). Through indirect means, one may calculate a free thyroxin factor which suggests a normal thyroid state in women taking oral contraceptives (*72*). Normal free thyroxin levels and free T_4 indices have been observed in patients on estrogen therapy. It has been contended that the thyroid function tests reflect alterations in protein-binding secondary to the estrogen content of the compounds. There is no indication from these, nor from the clinical evaluations, that there is any activation of the thyroid state. The shift in the compartmentalization of the thyroxin as produced by the oral contraceptive appears without alteration in the metabolic rate.

Cardiovascular and Related Effects   Venous engorgement has been reported in oral contraceptive users (*71*). It should be pointed out, however, that the parameters of measure are grossly variable and do not afford more than relative conclusions. An increase in forearm blood flow with the progestogen-estrogen contraceptives has also been noted (*127*). On the other hand, a reduction in femoral venous blood flow (*137*) has been reported in animals treated with 2 mg of Enovid intramuscularly daily for 6 weeks. Admittedly, parenterally administered progestogens and progestogen-estrogen combinations have a more profound and prolonged effect than those observed after oral use. Connective tissue changes in rodent arteries suggestive of vessel wall damage have been reported in association with the progestogen-estrogen combinations (*34*). In the discussion of the latter report, each of the discussants seriously questioned the implied conclusions and particularly the inference of the hormonal induction of these changes.

Specific alterations in the endometrial arterioles in women complaining of headaches have been reported only by Grant (*73*). Improvement, aggravation, and no effect on migraine headaches have been noted with the use of progestogen-estrogen combinations (*84, 114*). A more consistent suppressive effect of severe migraine has been suggested with continuous low dosage of progestogen.

Hypertensive development or aggravation has been suggested in rather isolated groups of patients (*102,225*). Certain estrogen-related alterations on the renin-angiotensin-aldosterone system, and their effects on electrolyte and fluid balance, as well as increased sensitivity of vascular smooth muscle, have been theorized as possible mechanisms wherein these women have pressor effects after administration of a progestogen-estrogen preparation. While there may be occasional hypertensive effects, it must also be remembered that the study of angiotensive episodes is so easily influenced by the autonomic system that it is not a simple matter to evaluate the pharmacologic action of an agent on this system. Moreover, there is no evidence of an inciting, continued, or progressive effect reported in any but these rare, isolated subjects. In the Rio Piedras trials, 96.8 percent of 312 control or premedication blood pressure recordings fell within normal range. Only 17 out of 316 Enovid users showed an abnormal elevation at any time in the study. No significant increases were observed on serial follow-up relative to long-term use.

Blood Coagulation and Thrombophlebitis Further confusion referable to hematological changes is encountered in alterations in the blood coagulation factors noted in association with the use of oral contraceptives. A vast number of blood coagulation studies have been carried out in an attempt to assess a possible association of oral contraceptive use and the occurrence of thromboembolic cardiovascular or arterial thrombosis (*8,210,27,163,172,184,195,198,223,233, 175.*) Some blood factor changes suggest a tendency to hypercoagulability; however, increased fibrinolytic activity is also reported. There is no complete agreement in the reports of the observed blood factor alterations secondary to the effects of the oral contraceptives (*4,20, 40,45,87,116,120,146,147,189,208.*) The many alterations in the evaluations of these numerous factors during use of progestogens and estrogens, as well as during pregnancy, have been summarized concisely elsewhere (*42*) and are too lengthy to include in this summation.

In addition to the inconsistency of the reported variations, there is even less concurrence with the significance of these blood coagulation observations, especially with reference to their role in producing thrombophlebitis and embolization.

Caution has been urged lest the thrombotic tendency of the sickle cell hemoglobinopathies be aggravated by the progestogen-estrogen combinations (*78*). In a similar vein, therapeutic usage is suggested for patients with hemophilia (*142*). Increases in factors vii and x in carriers of hemophilia have been observed with oral contraceptive therapy. In the hemophiliacs, oral contraceptive therapy permitted surgery but was also accompanied by gynecomastia and some behavioral changes. Lest it be forgotten, caution should be emphasized regarding the irreversible testicular changes produced by the estrogens in these compounds.

The present concept of the causality of thrombophlebitis is poorly understood. Virchow's triad of 1856 still remains as the foundation of the present concepts (*137*). With some effort, since the data are inconsistent, Virchow's triad could be pictured in action in patients using the progestogen-estrogen combinations. The correlation between the use of these combinations and the occurrence of thrombophlebitis, embolization, and cardiovascular accident has been based on inadequate data. Nonetheless, there are insufficient data to exclude conclusively a possible correlation (*226*). Until recently, all attempts to confirm or exclude an association have failed to support either thesis (*226,2,24*). Recently, however, three separate retrospective epidemiologic studies (*29,164,132*) were reported from the United Kingdom. Morbidity investigations carried out in two, and a mortality study in the third, suggest very similar qualitative conclusions, namely that an association exists between the occurrence of thrombophlebitis, thromboembolic and cardiovascular deaths, and oral contraceptive use. No association of coronary thrombosis deaths was established. From these analyses, it would appear that the risk of venous thrombosis or pulmonary embolism is increased threefold in oral contraceptive users over non-users, but a risk eight times that of the user is faced by the pregnant woman! While the sampling is small, the proportion of women who admitted to taking oral contraceptives paralleled the estimate derived from the total sales of oral contraceptives for the country, giving support to the statistics. It was felt by the reviewing committee that it is unlikely that substantial bias was introduced. The numbers are small and support the earlier reports of an association. Nonetheless, in a retrospective review (91) from a large neurological institute, no relation to cerebral arterial occlusion in young women was supported.

The summation of these three implicating studies suggests that the risk of death may be of the order of 3 per 100,000 users per year, in comparison with the calculated mortality rate for England and Wales of 25 per 100,000 completed pregnancies. Moreover, during the similar time interval, the annual death rate from all causes in women ages 15 to 44 was 97 per 100,000. Thus, if as these studies indicate there is an association between the use of the oral contraceptives and the thromboembolic complications, the risk is indeed small. This is further compounded when one considers that *the risk of becoming pregnant while using contraceptive methods other than the orals is increased many fold.* It is probably not reassuring enough for some that, in reality, the theoretical risk is indeed this small.

Hepatic Effects It has long been known that the 17-alkyl substituted steroids are potential cholestatic agents. Moreover, all of the synthetic sex steroids fall into this category by virtue of their structural configuration. Although the early evaluation of liver function studies failed to detect any deviation from the norm, it is not surprising that alterations are being observed with the use of these agents in occasional women and that these abnormalities are noted with particular reference to hepatic excretory function. The parenteral administration of estriol and estradiol, however, when given to a group of predominantly postmenopausal women, likewise produced a fairly consistent decrease in the hepatic BSP excretion, with 50 percent showing an alkaline phosphatase abnormality (136). It should be pointed out that these naturally occurring estrogens lack a 17-alkyl substitution, indicating that alterations in hepatic function studies are not confined to steroids containing this radical. It was Eisalo (46) who called attention to the fact that when postmenopausal women in Finland were administered an oral contraceptive, elevations in serum transaminase, as well as occasional observations of BSP retention, were observed. Subsequently, isolated sporadic occurrences of jaundice in association with the use of these steroids were reported. Articles appeared with great frequency in a flurry of controversy (1,9,17, 103,109,144,166,190,200,203,212). As the data were accumulated. it soon became apparent that the hepatic alteration which was noted more frequently in the Scandinavian (103) countries, and also in Chile (97), appeared to be related to the greater prevalence of hepatic excretory dysfunction in both of these areas. The genetic implications that appeared likely were subsequently supported by Larsson-Cohn (104). The hepatic alterations return to normal after discontinuation of therapy. Not only has long-term use not shown any deterioration of the laboratory assessment of the sequential liver profile studies (3,56), even among the few with deviations from the norm, but patients with prior evidence of alteration of hepatic function have indeed improved while on these oral contraceptives (59,61). Serial evaluation of the 2-hour BSP retention, SGOT, and SGPT among Scandinavian women has revealed a progressive increase in BSP retention during the first three months of follow-up (105). The BSP retention was maintained thereafter, while the transaminase reached its peak of abnormality within the month and then continued to show a progressive return to normal levels. At the recent IPPF meeting in Santiago, Chile, in April, 1967, Dr. Ricardo Katz (96) reported on 173 subjects who were taking oral contraceptives among 2343 subjects in a study in which gamma-globulin was being evaluated in the prevention of post-transfusion hepatitis. Seven cases, none of whom was on oral gestagens, developed anicteric hepatitis, in contrast to the 27 of 173 women on oral gestagens, who presented laboratory evidence consistent with anicteric hepatitis. There was further histologic confirmation by liver biopsy showing evidence of serious liver damage. Studies with parenterally administered long-acting progestogens and estrogens have failed to support any such alteration in patients observed at the hospital of the University of Pennsylvania (61), who are being studied in serial fashion, with a repeated battery of liver function studies. The situation is still inadequately clarified. Greater alterations appear to be noted during the luteal phase and during the late phase of tablet-taking each cycle (3). As is mentioned above, with reference to the hematologic alterations (174), a fall in serum cholinesterase, albumin, and albumin-globulin ratios, with a rise in serum alpha-1-globulin and beta-globulin, are but a small number of the additional changes associated with the raised serum iron and total iron-binding capacity usually seen only in the presence of hepatitis. The specific significance of these individual laboratory alterations needs much clarification, even though they may not be considered of clinical significance by some. Nonetheless, the occurrence of jaundice or of the symptoms of anicteric jaundice, such as fever, rash, pruritus, arthralgias, and dark urine, contraindicates further use of the oral contraceptives. In instances where a histologic sampling of the liver has been obtained, electron microscopic evidence of some hepatic damage has been reported (106,157). It is of some significance that the use of oral contraceptives by Puerto Rican women, where schistosomiasis is endemic, has not been associated with any instance of jaundice. In the light of this confused situation, while not contraindicated, it may of course be prudent to avoid the use of these agents in women with a prior history of acute hepatic dysfunction. It cannot be over-stressed that these agents are contraindicated in women with a history of recurrent jaundice of pregnancy and in those with chronic defects in hepatic excretory function such as the Rotor or the Dubin-Johnson Syndromes. Women without a past history of jaundice, or without evidence of liver disease, need not be subjected to liver profile studies routinely. Moreover, mild alterations of liver function studies are not an indication for the discontinuance of these drugs, unless otherwise clinically justified. It is of interest that concern exists regarding the repeated use of the BSP test. Despite its diagnostic sensitivity, one cannot recommend this study without some reservations, since it has been associated with reactions serious enough to provoke investigators to terminate, prematurely, the previously planned extensive follow-up study (105).

Integumental Effects   Melanosis, similar to that associated with pregnancy has been ascribed to the use of the oral contraceptives (30,162,177). It appears more noticeably among women with an olive complexion. Since it is seen more notably in the summer months and in southern areas where the intensity of the sun is greatest, exposure to ultraviolet irradiation is implicated. Rice-Wray suggests that there is a nutritional component to melanasia, since it is seen less frequently in patients treated with the Vitamin B complex (170). Objective assessment as with a reflectometer has been unsatisfactory (53). Nonetheless, despite the abatement or relief through early and continued applications of Monobenzone, the condition often leads patients to discontinue medication.

Androgens have the property of producing increases in sebum secretion in the sebaceous glands of the skin, while estrogen administration reverses this effect (201). With the lower doses, the progestogen-estrogen combinations in fact have a predominant estrogen action, even though at elevated levels some of these progestogens would exhibit an androgen-like effect, as judged by sebum production. Of all the progestogens studied, only norethynodrel does not produce such androgenic effects, even at doses of 20 mg/day. Dermatologists have extended these observations, and clinical claims of therapeutic effects in the treatment of acne with low-dosage orals have been reported (49,143,201). On occasion, however infrequent, dermatologic reference should be correlated with possible bilirubinemia. An eczema, neurodermatitis, urticaria, pruritus, or formication may herald an unsuspected anicteric hepatitis. Infrequent and possibly unrelated alopecia of many varieties has been observed during oral contraceptive use (31). While alopecia resembling a male pattern suggests an androgenic effect, such effects have also been seen in association with norethynodrel, a progestogen with intrinsic estrogenicity. These conflicting reports point out the complex problems encountered in attempting to define a cause-and-effect relationship.

Carcinogenic Effects   To date, there is no valid evidence to support a carcinogenic effect of the oral contraceptive, despite much theoretical speculation. While certain objective evidence suggests a suppressive effect by the progestogens and the progestogen-estrogen combinations, this should not be taken to imply that these agents will prevent or forestall the occurrence of these dysplastic changes. Gregory Pincus was impressed with the reduction in the numbers of suspicious or positive smears among oral contraceptive users in comparison with non-oral users. Much as many tried to impress upon him the vagaries of cytologic interpretation, in contrast with the histologic review, he claimed that it was a statistic and should be reported. His implications referable to so vague a parameter were questioned by most. The status of oral contraceptives and cervical neoplasia was by no means considered resolved by Pincus and, because of the important implications of the initial results, further investigations were planned and initiated. These studies, now in progress, utilize a population of women in the reproductive age group randomly assigned intravaginal or oral contraceptives. At present, the data available do not permit the drawing of significant conclusions. Despite the fact that his persistence may still prove to be justified, to date there is insufficient evidence to support or reject his contention. Recent reports point to infrequent polypoid endocervical hyperplasia which, while histologically disturbing, discloses a benign interpretation (207). There is, however, a considerable amount of suggestive and some objective evidence of a suppressive effect on endometrial glandular dysplasias and carcinomas, particularly the metastatic lesions (5,98,99,199). Less emphatic but still impressive are the remissive effects of many of the

progestogens and even combinations on advanced mammary carcinoma (109,185). Much remains to be studied. The existence of a
possible latency effect, pointed to by some, may be important only if
these are significant enough to modify the human life span.

Miscellaneous Little is known about the urological effects of
the oral contraceptives. Ureteral dilatation following their use has
been described (121), and implications are made referable to increased urinary tract infection. Insufficient data are available to comment on supporting or rejecting these claims. Like the urological
system, there are a raft of conditions or states wherein little, if any,
valid information exists. The nutritional status, particularly in de-
pressed areas, is such an example. A similar situation exists with
respect to the supposition of the direct or induced effects of these
agents on the primordial germ cells. While the data are indeed limited, no evidence of increased abortions nor congenital anomalies are
reported (55,69). However, attention is drawn to a suggestive increase
in chromosomal abberations (25) noted in abortus material recently
studied among women who had previously used oral contraceptives
similarly for 11 to 30 months and had stopped for 2 to 4 months. Only
2 types of anomaly were found: triploidy and x-monosomy. While
the study in question is small, it is reassuring, since no trisomic aber-
rations were noted. It is generally accepted that the trisomic specimens of all types equal the overall incidence of triploid and XO
abortuses. Trisomy is the only common type of choromosomal defect
at birth. Again, much exploration in this area is needed.

General Concluding Comments
It is becoming increasingly more difficult to remain abreast of the vast
ever-enlarging literature referring to the enormous numbers of laboratory studies and clinical observations being carried out on the
effects of the old and the development of the newer oral contraceptives. Combined sequential and continued low-dose progestogen regimens are most widely used and sufficiently effective to justify their
recommendation. Parenteral endocrine approaches are exceedingly
effective and may also prove to have even wider applications, if not
acceptance, than presently envisioned. Other oral contraceptive
approaches can not as yet be recommended as safe and effective
methods. No male oral contraceptive is available which can be considered practical and effective. At present, it rests upon women to
sustain the responsibility of effective family planning. It is estimated
that, in the United States, this responsibility is being accepted by the
younger female. Over 40 percent of the women under 30 years of age
have already used the pill (180). Lest it be misinterpreted, let it be

stressed that although there has been a rise in illegitimate births, this rise is parallel with the rise in all births and, moreover, the majority of unmarried mothers are not teen-agers (82). It is not reasonable to assume a direct influence of the oral contraceptives on the situation represented by these facts. However, with judicious application, the problem of an unwanted pregnancy could be overcome. Greater efforts are needed to increase the motivation of not only the patient but also the medical and paramedical personnel to encourage and facilitate responsible parenthood.

The seriousness of the implication of the unwanted pregnancy appears to be far in excess of the potential hazards of the oral contraceptives. Nonetheless, much more effort is needed to define the exact cause-and- effect relationship suggestive for many clinical conditions, and especially for hepatic excretory dysfunction and thromboembolic phenomena. The ability to pre-select those susceptible to the potential hazards needs to be developed. While there are a varied number of hormonal alterations during oral contraceptive use (Table 5), the implications of all of these are as of this date not clear. Despite moderately extensive long-term follow-up and most extensive short-term review, these effects are reversible and appear to present no valid direct evidence of definitive pathological significance. The present oral contraceptives have in addition provided a stimulus to explore the physiology of reproduction.

Greater efforts must be taken to improve the safety screening of newer agents. One avenue of approach is through improvement in the clinical design of the early studies along with more uniform, widespread, and precise evaluation. Such accomplishments will facilitate more accurate retrieval of data in a shorter period of time. Concurrent metabolic studies and greater use of double-blind evaluations are also needed.

The agents available today will undoubtedly give way to better ones, for the ingenuity of man is infinite, and untold technologic resources remain to be tapped by his wisdom.

Table 1. Endocrine Contraceptive Regimens*

I. *Combined Formulations*
   1. Day 5 to 25 (20- or 21-day scheme)
   2. 20 or 21 days on and 7 days off
      (a) Without placebos ⎫ During the 7-day-off period
      (b) With placebos ⎭
   3. Day 5 continuous daily tablet to onset of flow
   4. "Postovulatory" or Catamenial Regulator (day 16 to 25; accompanied by fertile-period abstinence)

Table 1.—Cont.

---

5. Lunar scheme—Start each 21-day schedule with the new moon
6. Intramuscular each month
    Dihydroprogesterone acetophenide 150 mg
    Estradiol enanthate   10 mg
        Given on Day 7, 8, or 9
7. Once-a-month pill (Long-acting pill)
    A progestogen (Chlormadinone, retroprogesterone, 16-17α -dimethyl-6 retroprogesterone, or the 18 homologue of norethisterone), together with a long-acting oral estrogen (3-cyclopentyl ether of ethinyl estradiol) Administered on day 21 of cycle

II. *Sequential*
1. *Classic Sequential*
    (a) Day 5 to 20 or 21—Estrogen alone
    (b) Day 20 or 21 to 25—Combined Estrogen and Progestogen
2. *Modified Sequential*
    (a) Day 5 to 16—Estrogen alone
    (b) Day 16 to 25—Combined Estrogen and Progestogen
3. *Step-up Sequential*
    (a) Day 1 to 5—"Micro" Estrogen dosage
    (b) Day 5 to 16—First Estrogen elevation
    (c) Day 16 to 20—Second Estrogen elevation
    (d) Day 20 to 25—Estrogen and Progestogen
    (e) Day 25 to 30—"Micro" estrogen

III. *Progestogen Alone*
1. "Micro" doses continuous at 0.5 mg daily
2. I.M. Provera 150 mg every 3 months or 400-800 mg every 4 to 6 months

IV. *Estrogens and Non-steroidal Anti-fertility Agents*
1. Cyclic
2. Post-coital

V. *Clomiphene Citrate*
1. To regulate ovulation timing; accompanied by fertile-period abstinence

---

*Not all the above methods have proven effectiveness or safety.
Several of the above regimens have been used only in early clinical trials. Their inclusion is not to be interpreted as a recommendation of effectiveness, safety, and reliability.

Table 2. Clinical Uses of Progestogens

Effective
    Contraception
    Dysmenorrhea
    Benign menstrual irregularities
    Postmenopausal symptoms (with estrogens)
    Suppression of lactation
        (large doses)

Table 2.—Cont.

Possibly Effective
  Pregnancy testing
  Amenorrhea
  Endometriosis
  Acne
  Galactorrhea
  Precocious puberty
  Endometrial hyperplasia and carcinoma

Questionably Effective
  Induction of ovulation
  Therapy of apprehended abortion
  Premature labor
  Premenstrual tension

Table 3. Low-Dosage Oral Contraceptives—Unplanned Pregnancies

| Preparation | Investigator | *Combined Formulations* | | Women Years Use | No. Un- plan. Preg. | Preg. per 100 Women Years |
		No. Pts.	No. Cycles			
Orthonovum	Behrman (*13*)	459	9345	719	0	0
(2 mg)	Goldzieher (*67*)	NA	2953	227	0	0
	Hutcherson (*88*)	306	1825	140	0	0
	Krueger &					
	Sanders (*101*)	79	593	46	0	0
	Matthews (*126*)	107	873	67	0	0
	Mears (*128*)	89	630	49	0	0
	Newland (*139*)	206	2169	167	0	0
	Rice-Wray (*68*)	NA	3464		1	0.3
	Rovinsky (*177*)	235	2234	172	0	0
	Satterthwaite (*182*)	190	2776	214	0	0
	Tyler (*215*)	435	6455	497	0	0
Total			33317	2563*	1	0.04
Enovid	Andrews (*6*)	66	308	24	0	0
(2.5 mg)	Flowers (*52*)	259	3510	270	0	0
	Mears (*128*)	479	4360	335	3	0.9
	Pincus (*152*)	NA	2613	201	3	1.4
	Pullen (*162*)	183	1114	86	2	2.3
	Satterthwaite (*182*)	201	2755	212	1	0.5
	Wiseman (*224*)	NA	1166	90	0	0
Total			15826	1217*	9	0.7
Ovulen	Andrews (*6*)	410	9931	764	0	0
(1 mg)	Holmstrom (*86*)	195	4502	346	2	0.6
	Pincus (*152*)	126	1136	87	0	0
	Satterthwaite (*182*)	164	2071	159	1	0.6
Total			17640	1357*	3	0.2
Norlestrin	Behrman (*13*)	275	5910	455	0	0
(2.5 mg)	Diddle (*38*)	247	1699	131	0	0
	Kloss (*100*)	92	631	48	0	0
	Mears (*128*)	161	615	47	0	0
Total			8855	681*	0	0
GRAND TOTAL			75638	5818*	13	0.2

Table 3.—Cont.

Preparation	Investigator	Combined Formulations				
		No. Pts.	No. Cycles	Women Years Use	No. Un-plan. Preg.	Preg. per 100 Women Years
Sequential Formulations						
C-Quens	Balin & Wan (*12*)	130	545	42	3	7.1
	Goldzieher (*66*)	1191	11730	902	13	1.4
	Goldzieher (*67*)	6070	82085	6314	82†	1.3
	(collab. study)	—	—	—	—	—
	Mears (*128*)	92	435	34	0	0
	Tyler (*213*)	491	7704	593	9	1.5
Total			102499	7885*	107	1.4
Ortho-	Andrews (*6*)	294	2091	161	0	0
Sequential	Behrman (*13*)	254	3116	240	4	1.7
Total			5207	401*	4	1.0
Oracon	Aydar & Greenblatt (*7*)	50	167	13	0	0
	Jungck (*93*)	514	3880	299	3	1.0
	Palva & Onetto (*144*)	150	1179	91	4	4.4
	Young (*229*)	410	6038	465	6	1.3
Total			11264	867*	13	1.5
GRAND TOTAL			118970	9152*	124	1.4
"Mini" Dose Progestogen						
Chlormadinone	Martinez-Manautou (*122*)	1123	13202	1016	40	3.9

*Calculated on the basis of the total or grand total number of cycles of use and 13 cycles = 1 year.
†Calculated on the basis of total cycles and pregnancy rate.

Table 4. Comparative Pregnancy Rates in the Various Contraceptive Methods

Method	Average Pregnancy Rate Per 100 Women Years
Douche (*209*)	37.8
Foam tablets (*209*)	22
Jelly alone (*216*)	20
Withdrawal (*209*)	16
Condom (*209*)	14.9
Safe period (*199*)	14.4
Diaphragm (*216*)	12
Intrauterine device (*199*)	3.9
"Mini" dose orals (*122*)	3.9
Sequential orals*	1.4
Combined orals*	0.2

Table 5. Estrogen-Related Hormone Alterations*

Target Organ	Increased Levels	Para-Endocrine Changes
Pituitary	Growth hormone	Increased extra-cellular glucose
Thyroid	P.B.I.	Thyroxin binding globulin (liver)
Adrenal	Cortisol (PSC)	Trancortin (liver)
	Aldosterone	Renin (kidney)
Pancreas	Plasma insulin	Increased intra-cellular glucose

*Adapted from Gold, E.M. (64)

REFERENCES

1. Adlercreutz, H. and Ikonen, E. "Oral contraceptives and liver damage," *Brit. Med. J.*, ii:1133, 1964.

2. Advisory Committee on Obstetrics and Gynecology, *Food and Drug Administration Report on the Oral Contraceptives*, U. S. Government Printing Office, Washington, D.C., 1966.

3. Allan, J. S., and Tyler, E. T. "Biochemical Findings in Long-Term Oral Contraceptive Usage: I. Liver Function Studies," *Fertil. Steril.*, 18:112, 1967.

4. Amundson, B. A. and Pilgeram, L. O. "Observations on a Relationship Between Steroid Metabolism and the Concentration of Plasma Fibrinogen." *Thromb. Diath. Haemorrh.*, 10:400, 1964.

5. Anderson, D. G. "The Management of Advanced Endometrial Adenocarcinoma with Medroyprogesterone Acetate," *Amer. J. Obstet. & Gynec.*, 92:87, 1965.

6. Andrews, W. C. and Andrews, M. C. "Reduction of Side Effects From Ovulation Suppression By the Use of Newer Progestin Combinations," *Fertil. Steril.*, 15:75, 1964.

7. Aydar, C. K. and Greenblatt, R. "Clinical and Experimental Studies With a New Progestin-Dimethylsterone," *J. Med. Ass. Alabama, 31*:1, 1961.

8. Baines, G. F. "Cerebrovascular Accidents and Oral Contraception," *Brit. Med. J.*, i:189, 1965.

9. Bakke, J. L. "Hepatic Impairment During Intake of Contraceptive Pills—Observations in Post-Menopausal Women," *Brit. Med. J.*, ii:631, 1965.

10. Bakker, C. B. and Dightman, C. R. "Psychological Factors in Fertility Control," *Fertil. Steril.*, 15:559, 1964.

11. Bakker, C. B. and Dightman, C. R. "Side Effects of Oral Contraceptives," *Obstet. Gynec.*, 28:373, 1966.

12. Balin, H. and Wan, L. S. "Chlormadinone, A Potent Synthetic Oral Progestin," *Int. J. Fertil.*, 10:127, 1965.

13. Behrman, S. J. "Choice of an Oral Contraceptive," *Obstet. Gynec. Digest*, 8:37, 1966.

14. Bell, E. T. Herbst, A. L., Krishnamurti, M., Loraine, J., Mears, E., Jackson, M. C. N., and Garcia, C-R "The Effect of the Long Term Administration of Oral Contraceptives on Excretion Values for Follicle-Stimulating Hormone and Luteinizing Hormone," *Acta Endocr.* (Kobenhavn), 54:96, 1967.

15. Bell, E. T. and Loraine, J. "Urinary Steroid and Gonadotropin Excretion in Women Following Long-Term Use of Oral Contraceptives," *Lancet*, ii:442, 1967.

16. Birnberg, C. H., Kurzrock, R. and Weber, H. "Effect of Pregneni-nolene (Ethinyl Testosterone) Upon Human Cervical Secretion," *Amer. J. Surg.*, 57:180, 1942.

17. Boake, W. C., Schade, S. G., Morrisey, J. F., and Schaffner, F. "Intrahepatic Cholestatic Jaundice of Pregnancy Followed by Enovid-Induced Cholestatic Jaundice: Report of a Case," *Ann. Intern. Med.*, 63:302, 1965.

18. Booker, D. E. and Pahl, I. R. "Control of Postpartum Breast Engorgement With Oral Contraceptives," *Amer. J. Obstet. Gynec.*, 98:1099, 1967.

19. Böving, B. "Endocrine Influences on Implantation," in Lloyd, C., ed. *Endocrinology of Reproduction*. New York: Academic Press, 1959, p. 205.

20. Brakman, P. and Astrup, T. "Effects of Female Hormones, Used as Oral Contraceptives, On the Fibrinolytic System in Blood," *Lancet.*, II:10, 1964.

21. Brehm, H. and Kaser, O. "New Facts on Short- and Long-Term Administration of Hormonal Contraceptives" in Dukes, M. N. G., ed., *Social and Medical Aspects of Oral Contraception*. Int. Cong. Series 130, Excerpta Medica Foundation, Amsterdam, 1966, p. 112.

22. Buchler, D. and Warren, J. C. "Effects of Estrogen on Glucose Tolerance," *Amer. J. Obstet. Gynec.*, 95:479, 1966.

23. Burton, J. L. "Effect of Oral Contraceptives on Haemoglobin, Packed-Cell Volume, Serum-Iron, and Total Iron-Binding Capacity in Healthy Women," *Lancet*, II:978, 1967.

24. Cahal, D. A. "Safety of Oral Contraceptives," *Brit. Med. J.*, II:1180, 1965.

25. Carr, D. H. "Chromosomes After Oral Contraceptives," *Lancet.*, II:830, 1967.

26. Chang, M. C. "Effects of Certain Antifertility Agents on the Development of Rabbit Ova," *Fertil. Steril.*, 15:97, 1964.

27. Cohen, M. G. and Sajid, M. H. "Thromboembolic Phenomenon Associated With the Use of Progestational Drugs," *Delaware Med. J.*, 36:81, 1964.

28. Cohen, M. R. and Perez-Pelaez, M. "The Effect of Norethindrone Acetate and Ethinyl Estradiol Clomiphene Citrate and Dydrogesterone on Spinnbarkeit," *Fertil. Steril.*, 16:141, 1965.

29. College of General Practitioners, *J. Coll. Gen. Practit.*, 13:267, 1967.

30. Cook, H. H. Gamble, C. J. and Satterthwaite, A. P. "Oral Contraception By Norethynodrel," *Amer. J. Obstet. Gynec.*, 82:437, 1961.

31. Cormia, F. E. "Alopecia From Oral Contraceptives," *J. A. M. A.*, 201:635, 1967.

32. Cummings, J. N., Grundt, I. K., Holland, J. T. and Marshall, J. "Serum Lipids and Cerebrovascular Disease," *Lancet.*, II:194, 1967.

33. Curtis, E. M. "Oral-Contraceptive Feminization of a Normal Male Infant: Report of a Case," *Obstet. Gynec.*, 23:295, 1964.

34. Danforth, D. N., Manalo-Estrela, P. and Buckingham, J. C. "The Effect of Pregnancy and of Enovid on the Rabbit Vasculature," *Amer. J. Obstet. Gynec.*, 88:952, 1964.

35. De Alvarez, R. R. and Afonso, J. S. "Production of Pregnancy Zone Protein by Contraceptive Steroids," *Penn. Med., 70(7)*:43, 1967.

36. Diczfalusy, E. "Mode of Action of Contraceptive Drugs," *Amer. J. Obstet. Gynec.*, 100:136, 1968.

37. Diczfalusy, E. "Probable Mode of Action of Oral Contraceptives," *Brit. Med. J.*, II:1394, 1965.

38. Diddle, A. W., Watts, G. F., Gardner, W. H. and Williamson, P. J. "Oral Contraceptive Medication: A Prolonged Experience," *Amer. J. Obstet. Gynec., 95*:489, 1966.

39. Dodek, O. I., Jr. and Kotz, H. L. "Syndrome of Anovulation Following the Oral Contraceptives," *Amer. J. Obstet. Gynec.*, 98:1065, 1967.

40. Donayre, J. and Pincus, G. "Effects of Enovid on Blood Clotting Factors," *Metabolism.*, 14:418, 1965.

41. Drill, V. *Oral Contraceptives.* New York: McGraw-Hill Book Co., 1966, p. 144.

42. Drill, V. *Oral Contraceptives.* New York: McGraw-Hill Book Co., 1966, p. 183.

43. Durkin, J. W., Lin, T. J. and Kim, Y. J. "Endometrial Effects Produced by the Oral Administration of Steroids to Control the Reproductive Cycle: The Use of Sequential and Combination Regimens," *Amer. J. Obstet. Gynec., 91*:110, 1965.

44. Edgren, R. A., Jones, R. C. and Peterson, D. L. "A Biological Classification of Progestational Agents," *Fertil. Steril., 18:*238, 1967.

45. Egeberg, O. and Owren, P. A. "Oral Contraception and Blood Coagulability," *Brit. Med. J.*, I:220, 1963.

46. Eisalo, A., Jarvinen, P. A. and Luukainen, T. "Hepatic Impairment During the Intake of Contraceptive Pills: Clinical Trial with Post-Menopausal Women," *Brit. Med. J.*, II:426, 1964.

47. Ferin, J. "Antagonism of Sex Steroids as Determined on the Genital Tract," *Europ. Rev. Endocrin.* Suppl. 2, Part 1:135, 1966.

48. Ferin, J. "Synthetic Progestogens as Ovulation or Conception Inhibitors," in Palmer, R., ed., *La Contraception.* Paris, Masson et Cie, 1964, p. 117.

49. Finnerud, C. W. and McGrae, J. D., Jr. Enovid in Der acnetheratie ein bericht iiber klenisch erfahrunzen. Hautarzt. 15:677, 1964.

50. Flerko, B. "The Central Nervous System and the Secretion and Release of Luteinizing Hormone and Follicle-Stimulating Hormone" in Nalbondov, A. V., ed. *Advances in Neuroendocrinology.* Urbana: University of Illinois Press, 1963, p. 211.

51. Flowers, C. E., Jr. Workshop Clinical Session, IPPF, Santiago, Chile, April, 1967.

52. Flowers, C. E. "Effects of New Low Dosage Form of Norethynodrel-Mestranol: Clinical Evaluation and Endometrial Biopsy Study," *J.A.M.A., 188:*1115, 1964

53. Garcia, C-R and Curet, J. Unpublished data.

54. Garcia, C-R, and Pincus, G. "Ovulation Inhibition by Progestin-Estrogen Combination," *Int. J. Fertil., 9*:95, 1964.

55. Garcia, C-R., Pincus, G., Rocamora, H. and Merrill, A. "Effects of Hormonal Steroids Upon Ovarian and Endometrial Cycles—Long-Term Effects," *Proc. of the 2nd Int. Cong. on Hormonal Steroids, I.C.S.*, No. *132*, Excerpta Medica, New York, 1966, p. 858.

56. Garcia, C-R., Pincus, G., Rocamora, H. and Wallach, E. "Control of Ovulation. Long-term Effects With a Progestin-Estrogen Combination." *Proc. VI Pan American Congress of Endocrinology, I.C.S.,* No. *112,* Excerpta Medica, Mexico City, 1965, p. 138.

57. Garcia, C-R, Pincus, G., and Rock, J. "Effects of 3 19-Noresteroids on Human Ovulation and Menstruation," *Amer. J. Obstet. Gynec.,* 75:82, 1958.

58. Garcia, C-R, Rocamora, H., and Pincus, G. "Long-term Effects of Oral Contraception," *Advances in Planned Parenthood, I.C.S.* No. *138,* Excerpta Medica, New York, 1967, p. 51.

59. Garcia, C-R. and Wallach, E. "Liver Function Studies and Progestogen Contraception," *Fertil. Steril.* In press.

60. Garcia, C-R. and Wallach, E. Unpublished data.

61. Garcia, C-R. and Wallach, E. Unpublished data.

62. Gershberg, J., Javier, Z. and Hulse, M. "Glucose Tolerance in Women Receiving an Ovulatory Suppressant," *Diabetes, 13:*378, 1964.

63. Glick, I. D. "Mood and Behavioral Changes Associated With Use of the Oral Contraceptive Agents," *Psychopharmacologia* (Berlin). *10:*363, 1967.

64. Gold, E. M. "Studies of Adrenal Function During Use of Oral Contraceptives," *Hormone Contraception Studies of Adrenal Function, Professional Series Conference,* Excerpta Medica, Los Angeles, February, 1967.

65. Gold, J. J., Smith, L., Scommegna, T. and Borushek, S. "The Efficacy of Provest in Inhibiting Ovulation," *Int. J. Fertil.,* 8:725, 1963.

66. Goldzieher, J. W., Becerra, C., Gual, C., Livingston, N. B., Maqueo, M. Moses, L. E. and Tietze, C. "New Oral Contraceptive: Sequential Estrogen and Progestin," *Amer. J. Obstet. Gynec., 90:*404, 1964.

67. Goldzieher, J. W. and Maas, J. "Clinical Evaluation of a Sequential Oral Contraceptive." Preprint—vith Pan American Congress of Endocrinology, Mexico City, October, 1965.

68. Goldzieher, J. W., Moses, L. E. and Ellis, L. T. "Study on Norethindrone in Contraception," *J.A.M.A, 180:*359, 1962.

69. Goldzieher, J. W. and Rice-Wray, E. *Oral Contraception: Mechanism and Management.* Springfield: Charles C. Thomas, 1966, p. 55.

70. Goldzieher, J. W., and Rice-Wray, E., Schulz-Contreras, M. and Aranda-Rosell, A. "Fertility Following Termination of Contraception With Norethindrone. Endometrial Morphology and Conception Rate," *Amer. J. Obstet. Gynec.,* 84:1474, 1962.

71. Goodrich, S. M. and Wood, J. E. "Peripheral Venous Distensibility and Velocity of Venous Blood Flow During Pregnancy or During Oral Contraceptive Therapy," *Amer. J. Obstet. Gynec.,* 90:740, 1964.

72. Goolden, A. W. G., Gartside, J. M. and Sanderson, C. "Thyroid Status in Pregnancy and in Women Taking Oral Contraceptives," *Lancet.,* i:12, 1967.

73. Grant, E. C. G. "Relation of Arterioles in the Endometrium to Headache From Oral Contraceptives," *Lancet.,* i:1143, 1965.

74. Graudenze, M. G. and de Almeida, A. B. "Nor-esteróides anticoncepcionais, Estudo experimental baseado na histologia de útero, ovário e embriao," *Rev. Ginec. Obstet., 116:*108, 1965.

75. Greenblatt, R. B. and Mahesh, V. B. Pituitary-Ovarian Relationships," *Metabolism, 14:*320, 1965.

76. Gregg, W. I. "Galactorrhea After Contraceptive Hormones," *New Eng. J Med., 274:*1432, 1966.

77. Guard, H. R. "New Technic for Sperm--Mucus Penetration Tests Using a Hemo-Cytometer," *Fertil. Steril., 11:*392, 1960.

78. Haynes, R. L. and Dunn, J. M. "Oral Contraceptives, Thrombosis and Sickle Cell Hemoglobinopathies," *J.A.M.A., 200:*994, 1967.

79. Hefferman, R. J. "Female Infertility," *J.A.M.A., 128:*613, 1945.

80. Hefnawi, F. E. "Four Years Field Study With Oral Contraception in Egypt" in Dukes, M. N. G., ed. *Social and Medical Aspects and Oral Contraception.* Int. Cong. Series *130,* Excerpta Medica Foundation, Amsterdam, 1966, p. 42.

81. Hertz, R. and Bailar, I. C. "Estrogen-Progestogen Combinations for Contraception," *Proc. of the 2nd Int. Cong. on Hormonal Steroids, I.C.S.* No. *132* Excerpta Medica, New York, 1966, p. 841.

82. Herzog E. "The Chronic Revelation: Births out of Wedlock," *Clin. Pediat.* (Phila.) *5:*130, 1966.

83. Hilgers, T. Crutchfield, C. and Spellacy, W. "Achilles Tendon Reflex to Evaluate Thyroid Function During Pregnancy and in Subjects Taking Oral Contraceptives," *Obstet. Gynec., 30:*83, 1967.

84. Hockaday, J. M., Macmillan A. L. and Whitty, C. W. M. "Vasomotor Reflex Response in Idiopathic and Hormone-Dependent Migraine," *Lancet.,* I:1023, 1967.

85. Hollander, C. S., Garcia, A. M., Sturgis, S. H. and Selenkow, H. A. "Effect of an Ovulatory Suppressant on the Serum Protein-Bound Iodine and the Red Cell Uptake of Radioactive Tri-Iodothyronine," *New Eng. J. Med., 269:*501, 1963.

86. Holmstrom, E. G. "The Long-Term Use of Ovulen for Contraception," *Metabolism, 14:*444, 1965.

87. Hougie, C., Rutherford, R. N., Banks, A. L. and Coburn, W. A. "Effects of a Progestin-Estrogen Oral Contraceptive on Blood Clotting Factors," *Metabolism, 14:*411, 1965.

88. Hutcherson, W. P., Schwartz, H. A. and Smith, L. "Norethindrone with Estrogen as an Oral Contraceptive: A Preliminary Report," *Southern Med. J., 56:*1357, 1963.

89. Jackson, M. C. N. "Oral Contraception in Practice," *J. Reprod. Fertil., 6:*153, 1963.

90. Jackson, M. C. N. "Optimum Dosage for Estrogen—Progestogen Balance to Inhibit Ovulation," *Int. J. Fertil., 9:*75, 1964.

91. Jennett, W. B. and Cross, J. N. "Influence of Pregnancy and Oral Contraception on the Incidence of Strokes in Women of Childbearing Age," *Lancet,* I:1019, 1967.

92. Johanisson, E., Tillinger, K-G, and Diczfalusy, E. "Effect of Oral Contraceptives on the Ovarian Reaction to Human Gonadotropins in Amenorrheic Women," *Fertil. Steril., 16:*292, 1965.

93. Jungck, E. C. "Sequential Estrogen-Progestogen Therapy in Gynecology," *Amer. J. Obstet. Gynec., 94:*165, 1966.

94. Kahn, S., Novick, O. and Diamond, S. "Severe Uterine Bleeding Following the Prolonged Use of Norethynodrel-Mestranol" *Obstet. Gynec., 25:*298, 1965.

95. Kannel, W. B. "Epidemiology of Cerebrovascular Disease: An Epidemiologic Study of Cerebrovascular Disease," in Millikan, C. H., ed. *Cerebral Vascular Diseases.* London, 1966, p. 53.

96. Katz, R. "Anicteric Hepatitis and Oral Contraception," *IPPF Medical Bulletin 1*:4, 1967.

97. Katz, R., Velasco, M. and Reyes, H. "Jaundice During Treatment With Oral Contraceptives," *Gastroenterology, 50*:853, 1966.

98. Kelley, R. M. and Baker, W. H. "Progestational Agents in the Treatment of Carcinoma of the Endometrium," *New Eng. J. Med., 264*:216, 1961.

99. Kennedy, B. J. "A Progestogen for Treatment of Advanced Endometrial Cancer," *J.A.M.A., 184*:758, 1963.

100. Kloss, W. "Erfahrungen mit einem niedrig dosierten Gestagen-Ostrogen-Gemisch zur ovulationshemmung," *Med. Klin. Muncih, 60*:1029, 1965.

101. Krueger, H. G. and Sanders, J. H. "Norethindrone and Mestranol: Experience in Private Practice With a New Low-Dosage Oral Contraceptive," *Ohio Med. J., 60*:548, 1964.

102. Laragh, J. H., Sealey, J. E., Ledingham, J. G. G. "Oral Contraceptives; Renin, Aldosterone and High Blood Pressure," *J.A.M.A., 201*:918, 1967.

103. Larsson-Cohn, U. "Oral Contraception and Liver Function Tests," *Brit. Med. J.,* 1:1414, 1965.

104. Larsson-Cohn, U. "Jaundice and Oral Contraceptives," *Lancet,* 1:679, 1967.

105. Larsson-Cohn, U. "The 2-Hour Sulfo-Bromophthalein Retention Test and the Transaminase Activity During Oral Contraceptive Therapy," *Amer. J. Obstet. Gynec., 98*:188, 1967.

106. Larsson-Cohn, U. and Stenram, U. "Liver Ultrastructure and Function in Icteric and Non Icteric Women Using Oral Contraceptive Agents," *Acta Med. Scand.,* 181, fasc. 3:257, 1967.

107. Laumas, K. R., Malkani, P. K., Bhatnagar, S. and Laumas, V. "Radioactivity in the Breast Milk of Lactating Women after Oral Administration of H-Norethynodrel," *Amer. J. Obstet. Gynec., 98*:411, 1967.

108. Laurell, A. "Plasma Iron and the Transport of Iron in the Organism," *Pharmacol. Rev., 4*:371, 1952.

109. Lewin, I., Spencer, H. and Herrmann, J. "Clinical and Metabolic Effects of 17 -ethinyl Nortestosterone in Mammary Carcinoma," *Proc. Amer. Assn. Cancer Res., 3*:37, 1959.

110. Liggins, G. C. "The Effect of Variation in Estrogen Dosage on the Pregnancy Rate During Sequential Oral Contraception," *Fertil. Steril., 18*:191, 1967.

111. Lin, T. J., Durkin, W. and Kim, Y. J. "The Control of Reproduction and of the Functions of Certain Endocrine Organs as Reflected by Biochemical and Biological Assays," *Curr. Ther. Res., 6*:225, 1964.

112. Livingston, N. B. "Medroxyprogesterone Acetate and Estrogen to Inhibit Fertility," *Int. J. Fertil, 8*:699, 1963.

113. Loraine, J. A., Bell, E. T., Harkness, R. A., Mears, E. and Jackson, M. C. N. "Oral Progestational Agents Effects of Long-Term Administration on Hormone Excretion in Normally Menstruating Women" *Lancet,* II:902, 1963.

114. Lundberg, P. O. "Progestogen and Relief of Migraine," in *Social and Medical Aspects of Oral Contraception,* I.C.S. *94*:167, Excerpta Medica, New York, 1965.

115. Malkani, P. J. and Sujan, S. "Sperm Migration in the Female Reproductive Tract in the Presence of Intrauterine Devices: A Preliminary Report," *Amer. J. Obstet. Gynec.,* *88*:963, 1964.

116. Mammen, E. F., Aoki, N., Oliveira A. C., Barnhart, M. I. and Seegers, W. H. "Provest and Blood Coagulation Tests," *Int. J. Fertil.,* *8*:653, 1963.

117. Mandell, A. J. and Mandell, M. P. "Suicide and the Menstrual Cycle," *J.A.M.A.,* *200*:792, 1967.

118. Maqueo, M., Becerra, C., Munquia, H. and Goldzieher, J. W. "Endometrial Histology and Vaginal Cytology During Oral Contraception with Sequential Estrogen and Progestin," *Amer. J. Obstet. Gynec.,* *90*:395, 1964.

119. Maqueo, M., Perez-Vega, E., Goldzieher, J. W., Martinez-Manautou, J., and Rudel, H. "Comparison of the Endometrial Activity of 3 Synthetic Progestins Used in Fertility Control," *Amer. J. Obstet. Gynec.,* *85*:427, 1963.

120. Margulis, R. R., Ambrus, J. L., Mink, I. B. and Stryker, J. C. "Progestational Agents and Blood Coagulation," *Amer. J. Obstet. Gynec.,* *93*:161, 1965.

121. Marshall, S., Lyon, R. P. and Minkler, D. "Ureteral Dilatation Following Use of Oral Contraceptives," *J.A.M.A.,* *198*:782, 1966.

122. Martinez-Manautou, J. "Low Dose Oral Products," *IPPF Medical Bulletin 1*:1, 1967.

123. Martinez-Manautou, J., Cortez, V., Ginner, J., Aznar, R., Casasola, J., and Rudel, H. "Low Doses of Progestogen as an Approach to Fertility Control," *Fertil. Steril.,* *17*:49, 1966.

124. Matsumoto, S., Ito, T. and Inoue, S. "Studies on the Ovulation-Inhibiting Effect of 19-Norsteroids in Laparotomized Patients," *Geburtsh u Fraenheilk,* *20*:250, 1960.

125. Matsumoto, S., Sato, I., Ito, T. and Matsuoka, A. "Electroencephalographic, Changes During Long Term Treatment with Oral Contraceptives" *Int. J. Fertil.,* *11*:195, 1966.

126. Matthews, J. G., Jr. "Ortho-Novum 2 mg in Conception Control," *J. Amer. Osteopath Assn.,* *63*:920, 1964.

127. McCausland, A. M., Holmes, F. and Trotter, A. Jr. "Venous-Distensibility During the Menstrual Cycle" *Amer. J. Obstet. Gynec.,* *86*:640, 1963.

128. Mears, E. "Clinical Application of Oral Contraceptives," *in* Austin, C. R. and Perry, J. S., eds. *Agents Affecting Fertility.* Little, Brown & Co., Boston, 1965, p. 211.

129. Mears, E. *Handbook on Oral Contraception,* IPPF Oral Advisory Group of the Medical Committee. London: J. and A. Churchill, Ltd., 1966.

130. Mears, E. "Ovulation Inhibitors: Large Scale Clinical Trials," *Int. J. Fertil.,* *9*:1, 1964.

131. Mears, E. and Grant, E. "Anovular" as an Oral Contraceptive," *Brit. Med. J.,* ii:75, 1962.

132. Med. Res. Council, Statis, Res. Unit. "Venous Thrombosis and Pulmonary Embolism Study: Risk of Thromboembolic Disease in Women

Taking Oral Contraceptives: A Preliminary Communication," *Brit. Med. J.*, II:355, 1967.

133. Michael, R. P., Herbert, J. and Wellegalla, J. "Ovarian Hormones and Grooming Behaviour in the Rhesus Monkey (Macaca mulatta) Under Laboratory Conditions," *J. Endocr., 36:*263, 1966.

134. Mixson, W. T. and Hammond, D. O. "Response of Fibromyomas to a Progestin," *Amer. J. Obstet. Gynec., 82:*754, 1961.

135. Morley, F. "Histological Appearance of the Endometrium With Combined Ethynodiol Diacetate Mestranol at Different Dose Levels." Presentation at the International Symposium on Oral Contraception, Folkestone, England, November, 29-30, 1966.

136. Mueller M. N. and Kappas, A. "Estrogen Pharmacology: I. The Influence of Estradiol and Estriol on Hepatic Disposal of Sulfobromphthalein (BSP) in Man," *J. Clin. Invest., 43:*1904, 1964.

137. Neistadt, A., Schwartz, R. W., and Schwartz, S. I. "Norethynodrel With Mestranol and Venous Blood Flow," *J.A.M.A., 198:*784, 1966.

138. Nelson, D. H., Tanney, H., Mestman, G., Gieschen, V. W., and Wilson, L. D. "Potentiation of the Biologic Effect of Administered Cortisol by Estrogen Treatment," *J. Clin. Endocr., 23:*261, 1963.

139. Newland, D. O., Marshall, L. L., Rodger, L. D. Way, F. R. and Webber, R. L. "Effectiveness of a Low Dose Oral Contraceptive Tablet," *Obstet. Gynec., 23:*920, 1964.

140. Noyes, R. W. "The Endocrine Control of the Passage of Spermatozoa and Ova Through the Female Genital Tract," *Fertil. Steril., 10:*480, 1959.

141. Ostergaard, E. and Starup, J. "Laparotomy Observations During Oral Contraception," *Proceedings 5th Conference of the Europe and Near East Region of the IPPF*, July 1966, p. 33.

142. Ozsoylu, S. and Corbacioglu, B. "Oral Contraceptives for Haemophilia," *Lancet,* II:1001, 1967.

143. Palitz, L. L., Milberg, I. L. and Kantor, I. "Enovid for Acne in the Female," *Skin, 3:*243, 1964.

144. Palva, I. P. "Oral Contraceptives and Liver Damage," *Brit. Med. J.,* II:688, 1964.

145. Peterson, W. F., Steel, M., Jr. and Coyne, R. "Analysis of the Effect of Ovulatory Suppressants on Glucose Tolerance," *Amer. J. Obstet. Gynec., 95:*484, 1966.

146. Phillips, L. L., Turksoy, R. N. and Southam, A. L., "Influence of Ovarian Function on the Fibrinolytic Enzyme System: Influence of Exogenous Steroids," *Amer. J. Obstet. Gynec., 82:*1216, 1961.

147. Pilgeran, L. O. "Blood Coagulability and Oral Contraception," *Brit. Med. J.,* I:883, 1964.

148. Pincus, G. "Control of Conception by Hormonal Steroids," *Science, 153:*493, 1966.

149. Pincus, G. "Frontiers in Methods of Fertility Control" *in* Greep, R. O., ed. *Human Fertility and Population Problems.* Cambridge: Schenkman Pub. Co., 1963, p. 188.

150. Pincus, G. *The Control of Fertility.* New York: Academic Press, 1965, p. 243.

151. Pincus, G., Bialy, G., Layne, D. S., Paniagua, M. and Williams

K. I. H. "Radioactivity in the Milk of Subjects Receiving Radioactive 19-Norsteroids," *Nature, 212:*924, 1966

152. Pincus, G. and Garcia, C-R "Long-Term Use of Progestin-Oestrogen Combinations," *in* Shearman, R. P., ed. *Recent Advances in Ovarian and Synthetic Steroids and Control of Ovarian Function.* Searle, High Wycombe, 1965, p. 111.

153. Pincus, G., Rock, J. and Garcia, C-R. "Effects of Certain 19-Norsteroids Upon Reproductive Processes in New Steroid Compounds with Progestational Activity," *Am. New York Acad. Sci., 17:*677, 1958.

154. Pincus, G., Rock J. and Garcia, C-R. "Field Trials With Norethinydrol as an Oral Contraceptive" (Chapter 6). *Preliminary Session: Oral Methods of Fertility Control. Proc. of 6th IPPF Conf. in New Delhi, India,* p. 216-30 (special discussion). Periodica Copenhagen, 1959.

155. Pincus, G., Rock, J., Garcia, C-R, Rice-Wray, E., Paniagua, M. and Rodriquez I. "Fertility Control With Oral Medication," *Amer. J. Obstet. Gynec., 75:*1333, 1958.

156. Plate, W. P. "Ovarian Changes After Long-Term Oral Contraception," *Acta Endocr.* (Kobenhavn) *55:*71, 1967.

157. Popper, H., Rubin, E., Cardiol, D., Schaffner, F. and Paronetto, F. "Drug-Induced Liver Disease: A Penalty For Progress," *Ach. Intern. Med., 115:*128, 1965.

158. Posner, N. A., Silverstone, F. A., Pomerance, W. and Baumgold, D. "Oral Contraceptives and Intravenous Glucose Tolerance: I. Data Noted Early in Treatment," *Obstet. Gynec.,* 29:79, 1967.

159. Posner, N. A., Silverstone, F. A., Pomerance, W. and Singer, N. "Oral Contraceptives and Intravenous Glucose Tolerance: II. Long-Term Effect," *Obstet Gynec., 29:*87, 1967.

160. Puga, J. A., Zanartu, J., Rodriguez-Bravo, R. Garcia-Huidobro, M., Pupkin, M. and Rosenberg, D. *Acta Ginec.* (Madrid). In press.

161. Pujol-Amat, P., Urgell-Roca, J., Esteban-Altirriba, J., Marquez-Ramirez, M. and Hernandez-Soler, J. "Studies of Ovarian Biopsies From Women Cyclically Treated With the Combination Ethynodiol Diacetate and Mestranol," *Acta. Endocr.* (Kobenhavn) *119:*151, 1967.

162. Pullen, D. " 'Conovid-E' as an Oral Contraceptive," *Brit. Med. J.,* ii:1016, 1962.

163. Reed, D. L. and Coon, W. W. "Thromboembolism in Patients Receiving Progrestational Drugs," *New Eng. J. Med., 269:*622, 1963.

164. Registrar General of England and Wales: *Statistical Rev. of England and Wales For the Year 1964,* (Parts I & II), H.M.S.O., London, 1966.

165. *Report on Survey of Experience with Oral Contraceptive Pills,* Committee on Public Education of the American College of Obstetricians and Gynecologists, October, 1967.

166. Rice-Wray, E. "Oral Contraceptives and Liver Damage," *Brit. Med. J.,* ii:1011, 1964.

167. Rice-Wray, E., Cervantes, A., Gutierrez, J., Rosell, A. A. and Goldzieher, J. "The Acceptability of Oral Progestins in Fertility Control," *Metabolism, 14:*451, 1965.

168. Rice-Wray, E., Correu, S., Gorodovsky, J., Esquivel, J. and Goldzieher, J. W. "Return of Ovulation After Discontinuance of Oral Contraception," *Fertil. Steril., 18:*212, 1967.

169. Rice-Wray, E., Gatelum, H. and de la Pena, F. "Steroidal Anti-fertility Agents, Long-Term Use," *Proc. of the 2nd Int. Cong. on Hormonal Steroids.* I.C.S. No. *132*, Excerpta Medica, New York, 1966, p. 852.

170. Rice-Wray, E. Goldzieher, J. W and Aranda-Rosell, A. "Oral Progestins in Fertility Control: A Comparative Study," *Fertil. Steril., 14:*402, 1963.

171. Rice-Wray, E., Schulz-Contreras, M., Guerrero, I. and Aranda-Rosell, A. "Long-Term Administration of Norethindrone in Fertility Control," *J.A.M.A., 180:*355, 1962.

172. Richman, G. "Thrombophlebitis and 'Enavid'" *Brit. Med. J.,* ii:729, 1962.

173. Richter, R. H. H. "Planning of Clinical Trials with Oral Contraception *in* Dukes, M N. G., ed. *Social and Medical Aspects of Oral Contraception,* Int. Cong. Series *130,* Excerpta Medica Foundation, Amsterdam, 1966, p. 53.

174. Robertson, G. S. "Serum Protein and Cholinesterase Changes in Association with Contraceptive Pills," *Lancet,* i:232, 1967.

175. Robinson, R. W. "Effect of Estrogen-Progestin Combinations on Clotting Factors," *Amer. J. Obstet.,* Gynec. *99:*163, 1967.

176. Rock, J., Pincus, G. and Garcia, C-R. "Effects of Certain 19-Norsteroids on the Normal Human Menstrual Cycle," *Science, 124:*891, 1956.

177. Rovinsky, J. J. "Clinical Effectiveness of a Low-Dose Progestin-Estrogen Combination," *Obstet. Gynec., 23:*840, 1964.

178. Rudel, H. W. and Kincl, F. A. "The Biology of Antifertility Steroids," *Acta Endocr.* (Kobenhavn), Suppl. 105, *51:*34, 1966.

179. Ryan, G. M., Craig, J. and Reid D. "Histology of the Uterus and Ovaries After Long-Term Cyclic Norethynodrel Therapy," *Amer. J. Obstet. Gynec., 90:*715, 1964.

180. Ryder, N. B. and Westoff, C. F. "Use of Oral Contraception in the United States, 1965," *Science, 153:*1199, 1966.

181. Sandberg, A. A. and Slaunwhite, W. R., Jr. "Transcortin: A Corticosteroid-Binding Protein of Plasma," *J. Clin. Invest., 38:*1290, 1959.

182. Satterthwaite, A. P. "A Comparative Study of Low Dosage Oral Contraceptives," *Appl. Ther., 6:*410, 1964.

183. Sawyer, C. H. and Kawakami, M. "Interaction Between the Central Nervous System and Hormones Influencing Ovulation," *in* Ville, C. A., ed. *Control of Ovulation.* Oxford: Pergamon Press, 1961.

184. Schatz, I. J., Smith, R. F., Breneman, G. M. and Bower, G. C. "Thromboembolic Disease Associated With Norethynodrel," *J.A.M.A., 188:*493, 1964.

185. Segaloff, A. *Cancer Chemother,* Rep. *11:*109, 1961. Progress Report: Results of Studies by the Cooperative Breast Cancer Group— 1956-60.

186. Semm, K. "Contraception and Lactation" *in* Dukes, M. N. G., ed. *Social and Medical Aspects of Oral Contraception.* Int. Cong. Series 130, Excerpta Medica Foundation Amsterdam, 1966, p. 98.

187. Shearman, R. P. "Amenorrhea After Treatment With Oral Contraceptives," *Lancet,* ii:1110, 1966.

188. Simkin, B. and Arce, R. "Prolactin Activity in Blood During the

Normal Human Menstrual Cycle," *Proc. Soc. Exp. Biol. & Med., 113:*485, 1963.

189. Sobrero, A. J., Fenichel, R. L. and Singher, H. O. "Effects of a Progestin-Estrogen Preparation on Blood Coagulation Mechanisms," *J.A.M.A., 185:*136, 1963.

190. Sotaniemi, E., Kreus, K. E. and Scheinin, T. M. "Oral Contraception and Liver Damage," *Brit. Med. J.,* ii:1264, 1964.

191. Spellacy, W. N. *et. al.* "Sedimentation Rate in the Normal Menstrual Cycle or With Oral Contraceptives," *Minn Med.,* 50:645, 1967.

192. Spellacy, W. N. and Carlson, K. L. "Plasma Insulin and Blood Glucose Levels in Patients Taking Oral Contraceptives. A Preliminary Report of a Prospective Study," *Amer. J. Obstet. Gynec.,* 95:474, 1966.

193. Spellacy, W. N., Carlson, K. L. and Schade, S. L. "Human Growth Hormone (HGH) Measurements in Subjects Taking Oral Contraceptives," *Clin. Research, 15:*330, 1967.

194. Spellacy, W. N., Carlson, K. L. and Schade, S. L. "Human Growth Hormone Levels in Normal Subjects Receiving an Oral Contraceptive." J.A.M.A. *202:*451, 1967.

195. Stadden, I. S. "Thrombophlebitis and 'Enavid.'" *Brit. Med. J.,* ii:857, 1962.

196. Stein, I. F. and Cohen, M. R. "Sperm Survival at Estimated Ovulation Time: Prognostic Significance," *Fertil. Steril., 1:*169, 1950.

197. Stevens, V. C., Vorys, N., Besch, P. K. and Barry, R. D. "The Effects of a New Oral Contraceptive on Gonadotropin Excretion," *Metabolism,* 14:327, 1965.

198. Stewart-Wallace, A. M. "Cerebrovascular Accidents and Oral Contraception," *Brit. Med. J.,* ii:1528, 1964.

199. Stoll, B. A. "A New Progestational Steroid in the Therapy of Endometrial Carcinoma—A Preliminary Report," *Cancer Chemother. Rep. 14:*83, 1961.

200. Stoll, B. A., Andrews, J. T. and Motteram, R. "Liver Damage from Oral Contraceptives," *Brit. Med. J.,* i:960, 1966.

201. Strauss, J. S. and Pochi, P. E. "Effect of Enovid on Sebum Production in Females: A Preliminary Report," *Recent Progr. Hormone Res. 10:*385, 1963.

202. Sturgis, S. H. and Albright, F. "Mechanism of Estrin Therapy in Relief of Dysmenorrhea," *Endocrinology, 26:*68, 1940.

203. Swaab, L. I. "Oral Contraceptives and Liver Damage," *Brit. Med. J.,* ii:755, 1964.

204. Szontogh, F. E. and Sas, M. "Effect of Orga-Steron (methyloestrenolon) on the Production of Chorionic Gonadotropin in Early Pregnancy," *Gynaecologia* (Basel) *154:*71, 1962.

205. Tait, J. F. and Burstein, S. "In Vivo Studies of Steroid Dynamics in Man," *in* Pincus, G., Thimann, K. V. and Astwood, E. B., eds. *The Hormones,* Vol. 5, New York: Academic Press, 1964, p. 441.

206. Tausk, M. "Discussion of paper by F. E. Hefnawi—Four years field study with oral contraception in Egypt *in* Dukes, M. N. G., ed. *Social and Medical Aspects of Oral Contraception,* Int. Cong. Series *130:*, Excerpta Medica Foundation, Amsterdam, 1966, p. 44.

207. Taylor, H. B., Irey, N. S. and Norris, H. J. "Atypical Endocervi-

cal Hyperplasia in Women Taking Oral Contraceptives," *J.A.M.A.,* *202*:637, 1967.

208. Thomson, J. M. and Poller, L. "Oral Contraceptive Hormones and Blood Coagulability," *Brit. Med. J.,* II:270, 1965.

209. Tietze, C. "Use and Effectiveness of Contraceptive Methods in the U.S." *in* Calderone, M.S., ed., *Manual of Contraceptive Practice.* Baltimore: The Williams and Wilkins Co., 1964, pp. 129-31 and 285-97.

210. Turksoy, R. M., Phillips, L. L. and Southam, A. L. "Influence of Ovarian Function on the Fibrinolytic Enzyme System: I. Ovulatory and Anovulatory Cycles," *Amer. J. Obstet. Gynec., 82*:1211, 1216, 1961.

211. Tyler, E. T. "Current Status of Oral Contraception," *J.A.M.A., 187*:562, 1964.

212. Tyler, E. T. "Eight Years' Experience with Oral Contraception and an Analysis of Use of Low-Dosage Norethisterone," *Brit. Med. J.,* II:843, 1964.

213. Tyler, E. T. "Sequential Mestranol-Chlormadinone Acetate as an Oral Contraceptive," *Obstet. Gynec., 28*:787, 1966.

214. Tyler, E. T. and Olson, H. J. "Fertility Promoting and Inhibiting Effects of New Steroid Hormonal Substances," *J.A.M.A., 169*:1843, 1959.

215. Tyler, E., Olson, H. J., Gotlib, M., Levin, M. and Behme, D. "Long-Term Usage of Norethindrone with Mestranol Preparations in the Control of Human Fertility," *Clin. Med., 71*:997, 1964.

216. Venning, G. "The Influence of Contraceptive Practice upon Maternal and Child Health," *Metabolism, 14*:457, 1965.

217. Vorys, N., Ullery, J. and Stevens, V. "The Effects of Sex Steroids on Gonadotropins," *Amer. J. Obstet. Gynec., 93*:641, 1965.

218. Wallach, E. E. and Garcia, C-R. "Psychodynamic Aspects of Oral Contraception," *J.A.M.A., 203*(11):927, 1968.

219. Walsh, H., Hildebrandt, R. J. and Prystowsky, H. "Candidial Vaginitis Associated with the Use of Oral Progestive Agents," *Amer. J. Obstet. Gynec., 93*:904, 1965.

220. West, J. and West, E. D. "The Electroencephalogram and Personality of Women with Headaches on Oral Contraceptives," *Lancet,* I:1180, 1966.

221. Whitelaw, M. J., Nola, V. F. and Kalman, C. F., "Irregular Menses, Amenorrhea, and Infertility Following Synthetic Progestational Agents," *J.A.M.A., 195*:780, 1966.

222. Williamson, H. O. "Thyroid Function in Oral Contraceptives" *in* Charles, D., ed. *Progress in Conception Control.* Philadelphia: Lippincott, 1967, pp. 11-21.

223. Winter, I. C. "The Incidence of Thromboembolism in Enovid Users." *Metabolism, 14*:422, 1965.

224. Wiseman, A. "Oral Contraception," *Brit. Med. J.,* II:55, 1963.

225. Woods, J. W. "Oral Contraceptives and Hypertension," *Lancet,* II:653, 1967.

226. *World Health Organization Technical Report Series No. 326* (Clinical Aspects of Oral Gestogens), 1966.

227. Wynn, W. and Doar, J. H. "Some Effects of Oral Contraceptives on Carbohydrate Metabolism," *Lancet,* II:715, 1966.

228. Wynn, V., Doar, J. W. N. and Mills, G. L. "Some Effects of Oral

Contraceptives on Serum-Lipid and Lipoprotein Levels," *Lancet*, II:720, 1966.

229. Young, C. C., Jr., Mammen, E. F. and Spain, W. T. "The Effects of Sequential Hormone Therapy on the Reproductive Cycle," *Pacif. Med. Surg.*, 73:35, 1965.

230. Zañartu, J. "Effect of Synthetic Oral Gestagens on Cervical Mucus and Sperm Penetration," *Int. J. Fertil.*, 9:225, 1964.

231. Zell, J. R. and Crisp, W. E. "A Psychiatric Evaluation of the Use of Oral Contraceptives: A Study of 250 Private Patients," *Obstet. Gynec.*, 23:657, 1964.

232. Ziegler, F. J. and Rodgers, D. A. "Vasectomy Ovulation Suppressors and Sexual Behavior," Orthopsychiatric Meeting, 1966.

233. Zilkha, K. J. "Cerebrovascular Accidents and Oral Contraception," *Brit. Med. J.*, II:1132, 1964.

234. Zondek, B. "Sperm Penetration of Cervical Mucus," *Fertil. Steril.*, 1:463, 1957.

235. Zussman, W. F., Forbes. D. A. and Carpenter, R. J., Jr. "Ovarian Morphology Following Cyclic Norethindrone-Mestranol Therapy," *Amer. J. Obstet. Gynec.*, 99:99, 1967.

BIOLOGICAL ASPECTS OF
FERTILITY REGULATION

Sheldon J. Segal

The Population Council; Rockefeller University

AMONG VERTEBRATES, the vast majority of somatic and behavioral expressions of sexuality, as well as the processes involved in the production of the gametes, are regulated by endocrine mechanisms. The range of hormonally controlled sexual characteristics in vertebrates extends from exotic courtship rites of salamanders to such majestic ornaments as the antlers of the deer or the mane of the lion. Under the influence of gonadal sex hormones male guppies develop a gonapod; thumbpads appear on the digits of male frogs. In the turtle, the three middle foreclaws, which are used to stimulate the female during courtship, begin to elongate. Voice changes, not unlike those of young boys approaching puberty, become apparent in such diverse vertebrates as the leopard frog, tree toad, prairie chicken, domestic duck, and the male mink. With the onset of testicular functions in the Virginia deer, antler growth begins. By the time these appendages are needed for fighting during courtship, they have shed the velvet and have grown hard in response to the hormones of the testis. The boar's tusks, the bull's horns and crest, the goat's odor gland, the ram's horns, and the rooster's comb and spurs are all well-known secondary sex characteristics that respond to the action of male sex hormones. Females are equally dependent upon hormonal stimuli to fulfill their capacity to reproduce. The thread-like oviducts of the female frog enlarge to fill most of the abdominal cavity, as the breeding season approaches. The female opossum's vicious resentment of the male's advances is replaced by eager acceptance as ovarian function becomes established. Indeed, in all sub-primate animals studied, the female's behavioral estrus corresponds to the peak in ovarian estrogen production. The female clawed-toad, Xenopus, externally undistinguishable from males as young juveniles, responds to ovarian hormone production by a typical feminine growth pattern just as the awakening ovary stimulates the development of feminine contours in the human female at puberty.

These somatic and behavioral characteristics are related directly to the process of reproduction. Even sex-specific characteristics which have no apparent association with fertility and reproduction are controlled by hormones of the reproductive system. This inexorable link between reproductive potential and endocrine function has established the guideline for modern scientific efforts to regulate fertility by controlled interference with physiological events. Almost without exception, experimental efforts to stimulate or inhibit fertility can be described as attempts to manipulate a key event in the endocrine control of reproduction. With the gradual elucidation of the normal hormonal requirements of the reproductive process, it becomes apparent that there are many steps in this sequence that are vulnerable to controlled interference.

Control of Ovulation

Oral contraceptives presently in use consist of estrogen and a progestin, either in combination tablets or administered sequentially. These preparations inhibit ovulation. The effect on ovulation is subsequent to suppression of pituitary gonadotropin release which, in turn, is the result of an action by the administered steroids at the hypothalamus or higher brain center. Sufficiently high doses of either the estrogen or the progestin alone can prevent ovulation in this indirect fashion. The combination is employed to assure ovulation suppression while maintaining an acceptable pattern of endometrial withdrawal bleeding in the course of cyclic tablet ingestion. There is now considerable evidence that the steroid-feedback system, controlling the release of gonadotropins, operates at the level of the central nervous system. Stereotaxic implants of tiny amounts of estradiol in the arcuate nucleus of the hypothalamus of the rat inhibit gonadotropic function and ovulation (20). Implants in the pituitary gland itself are ineffective. Progestins also interact at the level of the brain and not directly on the anterior pituitary. Implants of norethindrone in the rabbit hypophysis, for example, do not block copulation-induced ovulation whereas implants in the posterior median eminence prevent ovulation for periods up to 8 weeks (13). The experimental evidence suggests that norethindrone may inhibit the discharge of endogenous gonadotropin-releasing factors. Similar laboratory findings have been reported for another synthetic progestin, chlormadinone (9).

Ovulation suppression by means of a primary action at the level of the central nervous system can be achieved experimentally by a number of nonsteroidal pharmacologic agents including tranquilizers, anti-cholinergic and anti-adrenergic drugs (13). In spite of indirect evidence that morphine and the tranquilizers (6,45) interfere with ovulation in human and infra-human primates, a practical application of these observations for the purpose of controlling ovulation seems unlikely since there is no evidence that the antiovulatory effect can be isolated from the general pharmacologic effect of these compounds.

Considerable progress has been made in the last few years in our comprehension of the manner in which the neuroendocrine link at the hypothalamus operates. Hypothalamic-releasing factors, which regulate the release of follicle-stimulating-hormone and luteinizing hormone, have been identified (36). They appear to be dialyzable substances of relatively low molecular weight. The precise chemistry remains to be established, and until then, the possibility of using hypothalamic-releasing factors or analogues that may act as competitive antagonists as a basis for fertility control must remain conjectural. Of greater potential, perhaps, is the finding of Morrison and Johnson (30), confirmed by Pincus (33), that the hypothalamus may produce, in addition to gonadotropin-releasing factors, inhibitory substances which provide a physiologically normal means to suppress gonadotropin production. The inhibitor has been found in the hypothalamus of infants and prepuberal children, suggesting that it may play a role in holding the pituitary-gonadal circuit in check until puberty (7).

Direct suppression of gonadotropin production at the pituitary level, or interference with action of circulating gonadotropins, can be achieved by immunologic means. Antibodies to gonadotropins can be induced in experimental animals by immunization with homologous or isologous FSH or LH (38). Immunized animals, either male or female, have typical manifestations of gonadotropin deficiency (19). In the male, spermatogenesis is impaired; in the female, ovum maturation or ovulation is prevented. There remain, however, several important issues to be resolved; a practical application of these experimental findings in human subjects is not imminent. We cannot, for example, envisage now a means of imparting controlled reversibility to a method of fertility inhibition based on active immunization with gonadotropins. Also, our present inability to completely purify luteinizing hormone and follicle-stimulating-hormone makes it difficult to separate an immunologically induced interference with the gamete- producing function of the gonad from an undesirable interference with the gland's hormone-producing function.

Another approach to the inactivation of circulating gonadotropins has been the study of natural plant products. Most widely investigated has been the North American prairie grass, *Lithosper-*

mum ruderale. Inactivation of gonadotropin *in vitro* by alcoholic extracts of this plant was demonstrated convincingly (*32*) and a fairly stable powder containing in *vivo* activity has been prepared (*1*). Fractionation of extracts has led to the isolation of crystalline and non-crystalline constituents but until now, no stable, active constituent has been isolated. Another plant yielding an anti-gonadotropic extract is *Lycopas virginicas*, but this activity has not been separated from a strong anti-thyrotropic effect (*16*).

In general, the evaluation of plant extracts for antifertility action by means of gonadotropin inactivation or any other route of activity, has been discouraging and unrewarding. From time to time, a plant product is described that has a clear antifertility effect in laboratory rodents. Almost invariably these results can be ascribed to a mild estrogenic activity common in many legumes and other plants, an activity that has no practical significance for contraceptive purposes.

It appears, therefore, that control of fertility based on ovulation suppression will, in the foreseeable future, continue to depend on the action of synthetic hormones similar to those now in use as constituents of the widely used oral contraceptive agents. There are under study variations in the mode of administering steroidal antiovulants. For example, steroids with the capacity to be stored in body fat, following oral ingestion, provide the opportunity to develop a technique for one-pill-a-month contraception. Long-acting injections of steroids can give a depot effect which may last for many months. Each mode of administration has advantages and disadvantages; all have the same underlying mode of action.

The most widely studied procedure has been periodic injections of synthetic progestins in microcrystalline form. Several thousands of women have been investigated for over 20,000 woman-months of use of the synthetic progestin 6-alpha-methyl, 17-alpha-hydroxy-progesterone acetate. The regimen investigated most completely is 150 mg injected every 90 days, although studies are also in progress with semi-annual injections of 500 mg. With this procedure, ovulation is generally suppressed through an interference with mid-cycle LH peaking. Ovarian follicle development appears, nevertheless, to occur so that endogenous estrogen production is not completely obliterated. The endometrial pattern, however, reveals that the established estrogen-progestin balance is far from normal. As a result, uterine bleeding is totally unpredictable for women on this regimen. Women bleed on the average 3 out of 10 days for the first 3 months after an injection of 150 mg, and 1 out of 10 days (less bleeding than normal menstruation) after 5 or 6 tri-monthly injections. There is, of course, considerable patient variation, but by the end of a year, the majority of women have atrophic endometria and are amenorrheic. An extremely low pregnancy rate has been obtained with this procedure. There is, however, considerable delay in the restoration of ovulatory cycles when desired. Delays in ovulation from 12 months to 21 months are not uncommon and the time required for the establishment of a regular ovulatory pattern, post-treatment, is still not certain.

Tubal Transport of Ova

Ovarian steroid hormones have a major regulatory influence on the tubal transport of ova. Estrogens increase the rate of secretion of tubal fluid, stimulate ciliary growth and activity at the ostial portion of the tube, and increase the peristaltic activity of the tubal musculature (27,2). Progesterone generally has the opposite effect on each parameter. Upsetting the proper sequence of hormonal influences, therefore, can disturb the normal passage of cleaving ova in the fallopian tubes. Indeed, this has been demonstrated by many experiments, but no simple unifying concept can be synthesized from the reported observations. Nevertheless, the apparent liability of the regulatory mechanisms for normal tubal transport of ova provides tentative explanations for at least two highly significant contraceptive developments.

Much credit for focusing attention on this area is due to Mastroianni and his collaborators for their studies of tubal transport of ova in rhesus monkeys bearing intrauterine devices (26). Their investigations have shown that the antifertility action of an intrauterine device (IUD) may occur not only in the uterus, but at the tubal level as well. This finding is compatible with the extensive clinical data on intrauterine contraception which established that IUDs prevent both uterine pregnancies and ectopic tubal pregnancies (44). Mastroianni's work suggests that rapid expulsion of tubal ova occurs in gonadotropin-stimulated monkeys with intrauterine devices while gonadotropin-treatment itself does not have this effect. Ova cannot be found in the tubes of monkeys with IUDs within 24 hours following timed ovulations. Since gonadotropin-treated animals tend to have multiple ovulations, an elevated level of ovarian steroids may contribute to the acceleration of tubal ova. That this phenomenon in itself does not account for the rapid passage of ova is evidenced by the recovery of ova from gonadotropin-treated animals without IUD's. Subsequent experiments (25,8) establish that ova can be recovered from the tubes of normally ovulating monkeys, although the precise rate of tubal passage in this situation has not yet been established. The data suggest that while the additive effect of gonadotropin stimulation and the presence of an IUD may be required to demonstrate a dramatic tube-flushing effect within 24 hours, each stimulus alone may influence the tubal transport rate to some lesser extent. Careful timing of tubal transport rates in monkeys with IUDs and under different conditions of ovarian function will be required to elucidate this issue. Investigations by Malkani and Sujan (24) establish that sperm may reach the fallopian tubes, but whether fertilization occurs in women using IUD's effectively has not been established, and the recovery of several hundred human ova will be required before this important point can be clarified.

An influence on tubal transport of ova or zygotes may be involved also in the recent work of Morris and Van Wagenen (29). These investigators have reported the effectiveness of post-coitally administered hormonal agents in the prevention of nidation in subhuman primates. Pregnancy in the rhesus monkey can be prevented by the administration of an estrogen during the four-day period after mating when the fertilized egg is traversing the fallopian tube. Estradiol, stilbestrol, ethinyl estradiol, mestranol, or an experimental compound that is both anti-estrogenic and estrogenic were administered orally following over 300 matings in a colony of rhesus monkeys that normally achieves a 70 percent pregnancy rate after mating. When the estrogen was administered post-coitally, not a single pregnancy ensued.

In these experiments there were no direct attempts to ascertain the cause for the antifertility action. Accelerated tubal transport is implicated because, in other species, the relationship has been established between post-coital estrogen treatment and acceleration of tubal transport of ova. In 1958, Segal and Nelson reported that a synthetic compound with estrogenic activity prevents pregnancy in the rat if administered during the period of tubal transport of ova. In a subsequent experiment with a related compound (38), careful ovum counts revealed that accelerated passage of tubal ova had occurred. With other estrogens, this premature expulsion of the ova from the fallopian tubes has been demonstrated in rats (10), rabbits (11), and guinea pigs (5). The effect has now been reported with a variety of compounds, both steroidal and non-steroidal, but it becomes evident that the common feature of all is their estrogenicity. On the basis of his studies with a number of chemical classes of compounds in laboratory rodents, Chang (4) concluded, "One may deduce that any compound with estrogenic activity may have antifertility activity if taken at a particular time soon after mating." The data available on the application of this principle to human subjects are too few to permit an evaluation, although it has been reported that no pregnancies have occurred in a limited number of rape cases and volunteer subjects treated with 5 to 50 mg of stilbestrol, or 0.5 mg ethinyl estradiol on day 4 to 6 after mid-cycle insemination (29). A systematic analysis of the potential antifertility action of post-coital estrogen treatment in the human female has now been initiated so that ultimate resolution of this issue should be possible in the near future.

Sperm Capacitation and Fertilization
Mammalian spermatozoa may have complete morphological appearances of normalcy and normal motility without possessing the capacity to fertilize ova. This final maturation stage of sperm has been termed "capacitation" (3). Evidence for capacitation has been obtained in a number of mammalian species, including rabbit, rat, hamster, sheep, and cow. From the viewpoint of fertility control research, the intriguing extension of the capacitation concept is an understanding of the manner in which it can be inhibited. Sperm do not capacitate in the uterus of a rabbit injected with progesterone, or in the uterus of a rabbit in the pseudo-pregnant state (progestational condition) (3). In fact, it has even been suggested that fully capacitated sperm can lose their fertilizing capacity by exposure to a female reproductive tract under progestin domination (12). Although the process of capacitation has not been demonstrated as an essential element of sperm maturation in primates, the assumption that it does occur seems reasonable. With the greater availability of sub-human primates for reproductive research, this issue should be clarified before long. In any event, the evidence from other eutherian mammals suggests that interference with sperm capacitation may account for the contraceptive action of continuous low-dose progestin therapy that imparts an antifertility effect without the benefit of added estrogen and without inhibiting ovulation.

Attempting to evaluate the role of the progestin in contraceptive preparations of estrogen and progestin, Rudel *et al.* (35) made several important discoveries concerning the pharmacology of ovulation suppression. Of even greater significance perhaps was the observation that ". . . in the group receiving chlormadinone, 0.5 mg, even though the incidence of ovulatory cycles was high as evidenced by the endometrial histologic features, no pregnancies occurred." This was the first clear indication that the anti-fertility effect of a progestin could be completely independent of the anti-ovulatory effect. During the investigation of oral progestin-estrogen contraceptives, several investigators, on the basis of gonadotropin assays (21), and even corpora lutea visualization at laparotomy (28), concluded that ovulations were occurring in a significant percentage of cycles, even though the anti-fertility effect appeared to be absolute. Yet, it was not until 1965 that

Rudel *et al.* implied that ovulation suppression could be dispensed with entirely while still retaining a potent antifertility action. By 1967, their preliminary observations were extended to a substantial clinical trial of effectiveness and menstrual patterns (23). Chlormadinone acetate (6 chloro—6 dehydro—17 alpha-acetoxy progesterone) 0.5 mg daily was given, continuously, to a group of 945 menstruating women, and the women were seen at the clinic monthly during the period of investigation which covered 8091 cycles. Fourteen pregnancies occurred, 13 of which were ascribed to patient failure to take the medication regularly. Considering only the single so-called "method failure," a pregnancy rate of 0.2 can be calculated. However, when all unintended pregnancies are considered regardless of reason, the pregnancy rate is 2.1. In either event, this is highly effective contraception. With regard to menstrual patterns, between 60 percent and 74 percent of women, for any given month, had a cycle length of 25 to 35 days. However, 20.5 percent had breakthrough bleeding in cycle 1; this decreased to 11.9 percent by the fifth cycle. Approximately two-thirds of the patients had some cycle irregularity during the 20-month study period. With this particular compound, at the dosage employed, problems with cycle control appear to be a serious handicap, but the contraceptive effectiveness of the continuous progestin method seems clearly established. Meanwhile, at least six other synthetic progestins have been placed in clinical investigations at doses intended to replicate the experience reported by Rudel for chlormadinone acetate. Experience is sufficient with two of these compounds, megestrol acetate and norgestryl, to indicate confirmatory results.

The mechanism by which the uninterrupted daily administration of these progestational agents creates a state of infertility without inhibiting the hypothalamo-hypophyseal-gonadal axis remains uncertain, although the possibilities can be narrowed down considerably. That the therapy does not interfere with ovulation suggests that the mode of action may be on sperm or ovum transport, the fertilization process itself, transport of the zygote, or the preparation of the endometrium for nidation. Histologic evidence from biopsy material suggests that endometrial changes are not responsible for the antifertility effect. Sperm transport could be affected at the level of passage of sperm through the cervical mucus, or higher in the female tract. Although the preliminary reports tended to emphasize changes in cervical mucus which could create a barrier hostile to spermatozoa, it now appears that these changes are not necessarily correlated with the anti-fertility effect. Future investigations will be required to establish the effect of microdoses of progestins on such key factors as tubal transport rates of gametes and fertilization itself. As indicated earlier, the effect of progestins in preventing sperm capacitation in other mammals may very well reveal the mechanism behind the anti-fertility effect observed in clinical usage.

The discovery of this antifertility action, based on uninterrupted administration, opens for the first time the possibility of single-administration, long-term, reversible control of fertility by hormonal means, in a manner that would allow for maintenance of ovarian function and menstrual cycles. A possible application of this principle is suggested by recent experiments which demonstrate that steroid hormones may be released at low and constant rates from capsules made of various silicone polymers (37). One such material, Silastic, is already widely used in surgery and is found to be non-reactive when implanted sub-dermally in human subjects. Silastic capsules containing either estrogen or the synthetic progestin, megestrol acetate, have been inserted subdermally in female rats or rabbits, and biologic evidence of slow and constant release of the hormone has been obtained.

The experiments with estrogen-containing capsules are most advanced. The implantation of capsules into castrate female rats has resulted in persistent vaginal cornification for periods of nearly 2 years, the duration of our longest experiments. By calculating the daily amount of hormones absorbed, we can extrapolate that a capsule that could be inserted through an 18-gauge needle could theoretically maintain a hormonal effect in a rat for 20 years. Similar periods of reversible hormonal supplementation in the human male or female may very well be one of the next developments in contraceptive methodology.

Blastocyst Nidation and Corpus Luteum Function

The uterine environment is not essential for blastocyst survival, implantation, and development. In some species, ova can be fertilized and cultured *in vitro* (4). A human ectopic pregnancy is quite independent of the uterine environment. Nevertheless, in all species studied, a successful intrauterine pregnancy requires adequate progestational preparation and maintenance of the endometrium. It seems likely that the same situation prevails in the human female although, admittedly, this is difficult to prove in the absolute.

On this assumption, several investigators have sought steroid inhibitors of implantation by examining a variety of compounds for their anti-progestational effect. Pincus and his collaborators, for example, have tested nearly 200 steroid compounds for their ability to inhibit progesterone in a standard assay, based on the endometrial carbonic anhydrase content of the estrogen-primed female rabbit

(33). Of these compounds, a few have emerged that, in subsequent testing, appear to have implantation-inhibiting activity (in rats and mice while being virtually devoid of estrogenic (uterotrophic) activity. In the A-nor-androstane series of compounds, synthesized by Jacques and studied biologically by Pincus, at least one compound with an excellent record in biological assays has been carried to preliminary clinical trial with evidence for anti-progestational activity obtained. Extensive trials in sub-human primates will, however, be required before actual tests for antifertility potential of this and related compounds can be established. As mentioned earlier, Chang points out that the separation of estrogenic from antiprogestational activity may be more semantic than realistic so that the antifertility activity studied with this class of compounds in rodents may be the ovum-expulsion phenomenon associated with postcoital estrogen treatment, rather than a primary effect on the endometrium. A non-steroidal compound synthesized by Miguel and studied in Stockholm by Engstrom may fall in the same category. The compound is described in the lay press as an anti-progestational agent, but its chemical structure brings it in close relationship with a series of synthetic compounds known to be mildly estrogenic.

Another approach to the neutralization of the progesterone needed for nidation has been to interfere with the function of the corpus luteum by pharmacologic means. A series of amine oxidase inhibitors with phenyl hydrazine structure, when studied in the rat, appear to have this effect either directly or through a depressing effect on the pituitary production of luteotrophin (34). The oral administration of these compounds terminates pregnancy in the rat up to mid-term, the time when pituitary luteotrophin is no longer required for the maintenance of the corpus luteum of pregnancy. The role of the amine oxidases and their inhibitors in the reproductive process is as yet inadequately investigated. However, this could be one of the more important pharmacological approaches to the study of fertility regulation.

A similar luteolytic effect by means of inhibition of luteotrophic hormones release is believed to account for the antifertility activity of ergocornine, an antihistamine of the ergot series (41). The compound prevents implantation in the rat or mouse when administered during a limited period of tubal transport of fertilized ova. The fact that progesterone administration reverses the action of the drug suggests that a basic mechanism of the drug action is to suppress endogenous progestin production. It has been several years since the interesting biological activity of this compound was described. Unpublished clinical trials have revealed apparent toxicity at doses required to test effectiveness. Consequently, future development of this particular compound for contraception is not likely (*18*).

The present disappointments notwithstanding, anti-fertility action through a luteolytic effect is one of the more intriguing prospects on the research horizon. In theory, an oral preparation active in such a manner could be taken by a woman, either monthly, at the time of the expected menses, or only on the occasion of a suspected fertile cycle, as evidenced by delay in the onset of menstruation. Efforts along these lines will be stimulated by the growing evidence for the existence, in many species, of a humoral luteolytic substance, produced by the uterus and transmitted by tissue diffusion and common blood supply to the ovary. Partial purification of the luteolytic factor from sheep uterus has revealed the material to be a polypeptide that has adequate stability for further purification and testing.

Chemical Abortifacient Agents
It is not surprising that many of the compounds arising from the research for cancer chemotherapeutic agents are able to interfere with the growth of embryonic cells as well as cancer cells. Compounds that act as mitotic poisons, inhibitors of protein synthesis, or antimetabolites will cause resorption or abortion of implanted embryos. The more recent data on antimetabolites, including 6-thioguanine (*43*) suggest that it is possible to separate the abortifacient activity from the general toxic effects to the mother that may be expected with these potent cytotoxic agents. It is difficult to visualize the extension of these studies in the rat to the clinical level for any purpose other than carefully controlled tests.

Spermatogenesis
Because it has been difficult to separate the steroid-induced suppression of follicle-stimulating-hormone from suppression of luteinizing hormone, the use of steroid hormones to inhibit sperm production in the human male has not been practicable. With the complete suppression of the pituitary gonadotropin complex, testicular hormone production, as well as gamete production, will be suppressed. The resultant effect on libido and potentia would not be acceptable. There are, however, long-acting androgen esters now available that may provide long-term suppression of spermatogenesis while maintaining libido and general well-being. At the moment, this approach seems more encouraging than the search for compounds that act directly on the seminiferous tubules. There have been several such compounds studied which are able to suppress spermatogenesis in experimental animals, and even in the human male (*14*). Until now,

however, each has been associated with undesirable toxicity or associated reactions, so as to make their use impractical. One of the most promising of these, studied by Nelson (31) several years ago, is a dinitropyrrole compound which impairs spermatogenesis in the rat for as long as four weeks after a single oral dose. Nelson reported the maintenance of an infertile state indefinitely by administering single doses at intervals of four weeks. Sperm production recovered fully when treatment was finally stopped. Subsequent toxicologic finding resulted in the withdrawal of the compound from investigation, but it is possible that a related compound may be discovered which retains the antispermatogenic activity while being devoid of toxicity.

Attempts to isolate testicular antigens that could be used for specific immunization to prevent spermatogenesis have been reported (15). Indeed, even non-purified, crude testicular extracts can cause aspermatogenesis in the guinea pig and in the rat. An attempt has been made to immunize human males with testicular extract believed to be purified for the aspermatogenic factor, but the results have not been notable (22). Immunization with tissue extracts for the purpose of inducing sterility in either the male or female organism seems distant at this juncture. The basic problems of cross-tissue reactions, specificity of antigens, controlled reversibility of the immune reaction, and development of acceptable adjuvants still impede progress in this field.

More encouraging is the result of immunizing male animals with gonadotropins in order to neutralize endogenous FSH or LH (19). The objective of inducing specific suppression of the seminiferous tubules without interfering with Leydig cell function may be achieved by this procedure, particularly as more highly purified gonadotropins become available.

Conclusion

Finally, a consideration of the biological aspects of fertility regulation could not be complete without some mention of the great strides being made in our understanding of the basic biology and biochemistry of reproduction. Endocrinologists are now probing the molecular basis of hormone action and even suggesting gene-hormone interactions. Biochemists are unraveling entirely new concepts in steroidogenesis. Perhaps it is too soon to expect such new thoughts in biology to catalyze new directions of applied research. Yet, several new concepts in endocrinology appear to have been added to the list of events potentially vulnerable to controlled interference. Identification and partial purification of an estrogen receptor protein from uterine tissue (42) has been a great stride in our understanding of the mechanism of estrogen action. At the same time, this protein, when isolated, may provide the elusive antigen that will have the high degree of specificity lacking among the antigens now used in attempts to interfere with reproduction immunologically.

It seems likely that within the general field of endocrinology the next two humoral substances to be isolated, purified, and identified will be within the realm of reproductive endocrinology, i.e., gonadotropin releasing factors and the uterine luteolytic factor. Their availability will undoubtedly stimulate imaginative research to utilize them or their analogues for controlled interference with a step in the reproductive process.

In the realm of biochemistry, one of the more intriguing developments has been the recent appearance of compounds, currently of interest in the field of lipid biochemistry, that inhibit the synthesis of cholesterol by action on defined enzymatic steps in the biosynthesis of this steroid. The possibilities for the use of these compounds or related ones to inhibit progesterone production, for example, or in some other way to manipulate a key event in reproduction, have just begun to be evident. These are but a few examples drawn from a rapidly growing field of biological science. They are some of the future pathways; undoubtedly there will be others as well.

Synopsis

For the reader who may be less interested in "biologic aspects" and more concerned with "current status" of fertility control, the following synopsis is drawn from the body of this manuscript to provide a current report on contraceptive research.

1. "The Pill" (available)

Combination of estrogen and progestin that are orally active antiovulants. Presently, there are twelve commercial products available in the United States. They consist of a combination of one of six synthetic progestational agents with an estrogen—either ethinyl estradiol or its 6 methyl-ether. From the original preparations that use 10 mg of progestin, pills have now been evolved with only 1 mg of progestin. The estrogenic constituent has remained about the same.

2. "The IUD" (available)

At least six and probably twelve styles of IUD are available commercially in the United States. The major manufacturers have distributed to suppliers nearly three million IUD's in the United States as of September 1967. Several experimental designs are currently under investigation, as is the question of mechanism of action. Evidence continues to suggest a tubal effect as well as a uterine effect.

3. "The Minipill" (clinical investigation only)

(Continuous low-dose progestin, oral preparation.) Chlormadinone acetate, 0.5 mg, has been tested in over 1000 women for close to 10,000 cycles. The effectiveness is good but cycle control is not fully satisfactory. Two-thirds of the women have some bleeding irregularity. Other compounds are being studied for their performance in this type of regimen—at least six.

4. "The Time Capsule" (laboratory studies only)

(Continuous low-dose progestin-systemic preparation.) Laboratory work has been completed to establish the feasibility of sustaining long-term constant release of steroids from capsules of silicone rubber which can safely be implanted under the skin. It has also been established that the daily release rate with at least one synthetic progestin (megestrol acetate) is within the range required to exert an antifertility effect without inhibiting ovulation or menstruation.

5. "Swedish Abortion Pill" (laboratory studies only)

(Anti-implantation drug, non-steroidal, oral.) Referred to as "F-6103," this compound is viewed as a potential anti-progestational or luteolytic agent. If effective in the human female, drug would prevent completion of implantation if taken at the time of expected menses, or prevent maintenance of implantation site if taken later. There have been a few clinical trials but these were not meaningful. No systematic (if any) clinical study is now in progress.

6. "Morning-After Pill" (limited clinical investigation)

(Post-coital estrogen, oral administration.) Work with monkeys has established that virtually any estrogen, within a few days of copulation, will prevent pregnancy from being established. A small number of women—volunteers, including rape victims—have taken estrogen according to this schedule and none have become pregnant. The clinical trial is not yet meaningful.

7. "Once-A-Month Pill" (clinical investigation only)

(Fat-stored progestin and estrogen, oral.) This is a clever modification of the manner to use estrogen-progestin, antiovulant combinations. The steroids used are absorbed from the gastro-intestinal tract, stored in the body fat, and released gradually over a period of time (tablets are calibrated to last a month). Data not yet available for evaluation, but cycle control and bleeding irregularity are probable problems. In all likelihood, the "once-every-six-months" or "once-a-year" pills one occasionally hears about are extreme modifications of this principle, in which the problem of bleeding control is probably extreme as well.

8. "Long-Term Injectable" (clinical investigation only)

(Depot injection of progestin or progestin-estrogen combination,

systemic.) This is another modification of the manner for using estrogen-progestin combinations or large doses of progestin for anti-
ovulatory contraception. Essentially, it replaces daily pill-taking with
periodic trips for an injection. Published reports indicate troublesome
problems with unpredictable bleeding and with uncertainty as to the
restoration of ovulatory cycles.

REFERENCES

1. Breneman, W. R. and Carmack, M. "*In Vitro* and *in Vivo* Inactivation of Hormones by Lithosperm," *Anat. Rec., 131:* 538, 1958.
2. Brenner, R. M. "The Biology of Oviductal Cilia," *in The Mammalian Oviduct.*, eds. Blandau and Hafez. Springer Verlag. In press.
3. Chang, M. C. "Capacitation of Rabbit Spermatozoa in the Uterus with Special Reference to the Reproductive Phases of the Female," *Endocrinology, 63:* 619, 1958.
4. Chang, M. C. and Yanagimachi, R. "Effect of Estrogens and Other Compounds as Oral Antifertility Agents on the Development of Rabbit Ova and Hamster Embryos," *Fertility and Sterility, 16:* 281, 1965.
5. Deansley, R. "Further Observations of the Effects of Oestradiol on Tubal Eggs and Implantation in the Guinea Pig," *Journal Reprod. and Fertility, 5:*49-57, 1963.
6. De Feo, V. J. and Reynolds, S. R. M. "Modification of the Menstrual Cycle in Rhesus Monkeys by Reserpine," *Science, 124:*726-27, 1956.
7. De la Lastra, M. and Arrau, J. "Inhibitory Action of Extracts of Human Hypothalamus on Ovulation in Rats," *Proc. Eighth Intern. Conf. Int. Pl. Parenth. Fed.*, Santiago, Chile, pp. 453-57, 1967.
8. Eckstein, P. "Studies on the Effects of IUDs on Tubo-Uterine Motility in Rhesus Monkeys," *Proc. Eighth Int. Conf. Int. Pl. Parenth. Fed.*, Santiago, Chile, pp 440-42, 1967.
9. Gellert R. J. and Exley, D. *Proc. 48th Annual Meeting Endocr. Society*, Chicago, 1966.
10. Greenwald, G. S. 'The Antifertility Effects in Pregnant Rats of a Single Injection of Estradiol Cyclopentylpropionate," *Endocrinology, 69:* 1068-73, 1961.
11. Greenwald, G. S. "The Comparative Effectiveness of Estrogens in Interrupting Pregnancy in the Rabbit," *Fertility and Sterility, 10:*155-61, 1959.
12. Hamner, C. E., Jones, J. P. and Sojka, N. Y. "Influence of the Hormonal State of the Female on the Capacitation of Rabbit Spermatozoa," *Fertility and Sterility, 1968.* (In press).
13. Hilliard, J., Hayward, J. N. and Sawyer, C. H. "Blockage of Pituitary Ovulating Hormone Release by Norethindrone," *Proc. 2nd Int. Congress of Endocrinol.*, London, Excerpta Medica Congr. Series No. 83, p. 1275, 1964.
14. Jackson, H. *Antifertility Compounds in the Male and Female.* Chicago: Charles C. Thomas, 1966.
15. Katsh, S. "Adjuvants and Aspermatogenesis in the Guinea Pig," *Int. Arch. Allergy, 24:*319-31, 1964.

16. Kemper, F. and Loeser, A. "Lycopus—New Aspects of Actions Against Hypophyseal Hormones," *Acta Endocr., 38*:200-206, 1961.

17. Kirby, D. R. S. "Extra-Uterine Growth of Trophoblast," *Fetal Homeostasis*, vol. 2, ed. R. Wynn, New York Acad. Scis. p. 123, 1967.

18. Kobayashi, T. Personal Communication, 1967.

19. Laurence, K. A. and Ichikawa, S. "The Effects of Active Immunization with Bovine Luteinizing Hormone on Reproduction in the Female Rat," *Endocrinology, 82*:1190-99, 1968.

20. Lisk, R. D. "Estrogen-Sensitive Centers in the Hypothalamus of the Rat," *J. Exp. Zool., 145*:197, 1960.

21. Loraine, J. A., Bell, E. T., Harkness, R. A., Mears, E. and Jackson, M. C. N. "Oral Progestational Agents: Effects of Long-Term Administration on Hormone Excretion in Normally Menstruating Women," *Lancet II*, pp. 902-5, 1963.

22. Mancini, R. E., Andrada, J. A., Saraceni, D., Bachmann, A. E., Lavieri, J. C. and Nemirovsky. "Immunological and Testicular Response in Man Sensitized With Human Testicular Homogenate," *J. Clinical Endocrinology and Metabolism, 25*:859, 1965.

23. Martinez-Manautou, J., Giner, J., Cortez, V., Azner, R., Rojas, B., Guiterez, A. and Rudel, H. W. "Daily Progestogen for Contraception: A Clinical Study," *British Medical Journal, 2*:730-32, 1967.

24. Malkani, P. K. and Sujan, S. "Sperm Migration in the Female Reproductive Tract in the Presence of Intra-Uterine Devices," *Am. J. Obstet. and Gynec., 88*:963, 1964.

25. Mastroianni L. Jr. "Tubal Ovular Relationships," *Proc. Eighth Int. Conf. Pl. Parenth. Fed.*, Santiago, Chile, pp 369-70, 1967.

26. Mastroianni, L. Jr. and Rosseau, C. H. "Influence of the Intra-Uterine Coil on Ovum Transport and Sperm Distribution in the Monkey," *Am. J. Obstet. and Gynec., 93*:416-20, 1965.

27. Mastroianni, L. Jr. and Wallach, R. C. "Effect of Ovulation and Early Gestation on Oviduct Secretions in the Rabbit," *Amer. J. Physiol., 200*:815-18, 1961.

28. Matsumoto, S., Ito, T. and Inoue, S. Geburtsh. u. Frauenheilkunde, *20*:250, 1960.

29. Morris J. McL. and Van Wagenen, G. "Compounds Interfering with Ovum Implantation and Development. III The Role of Estrogens," *Amer. J. Obstet. and Gynec., 96*:804-13, 1966.

30. Morrison, R. L. and Johnson, D. C. "The Effects of Androgenization in Male Rats Castrated at Birth," *J. Endocrinol., 34*:117, 1966.

31. Nelson, W. O. "The Inhibitory Aspects on Gonads of the Male," In: *Human Fertility and Population Problems*, Cambridge, Mass., Schenkman Publishing Co., pp. 212-64, 1963.

32. Noble, R. L., Plunkett, E. R. and Graham, R. C. B. "Direct Hormone Inactivation by Extracts of Lithospermum Ruderale," *J. Endocrinol., 10*:212-27, 1954.

33. Pincus, G. "Experimental Studies of Fertility Control by Hormonal Steroids in Mammals," *Proc. 2nd Int. Congr. on Hormonal Steroids*, Milan, Excerpta Medica Congress Series No. 111, pp. 100-110, 1966.

34. Robson, J. M. "Effect of Drugs on Pregnancy," *Brit. Med. Abstracts, 6*:489-97, 1966.

35. Rudel, H. W., Martinez-Manautou, J. and Maqueo-Topete, M.

"The Role of Progestogens in the Hormonal Control of Fertility,"*Fertility & Sterility, 16:*158-69, 1965.

36. Schally, A. V., Bowers, C. Y. and Locke, W. "Neurohumoral Functions of the Hypothalamus" *Amer. J. Med. Sci., 248:*79, 1964.

37. Segal, S. J. and Croxatto, H. "Single Administration of Hormones for Long Term Control of Reproductive Function," *Fertility and Sterility,* in press, 1968.

38. Segal, S. J. and Davidson, O. W. "The Prolonged Antifertility Action of Chlomaphene in Delayed Implantation," *Anat. Rec. 142:*278, 1962.

39. Segal, S. J. and Nelson, W. O. "An Orally Active Compound with Antifertility Effects in Rats," *Proc. Soc. Exp. Biol. & Med.,* 98:471, 1958.

40. Segal, S. J. and Laurence K. A. Perlbachs M. and Hakim, S. "Immunochemical Analysis of Sheep Pituitary Gonadotropins," *Gen. and Comp. Endocr.,* Suppl. 1, pp. 12-21. 1961.

41. Shelesnyak, M. C. and Barnea, A. "Studies on the Mechanism of Ergocornine (Ergotoxine) Interference with Decidualization and Nidation: II Failure of Topical Application of Ergocornine to Reveal the Site of Action of the Alkaloid," *Acta Endocrinol. 43:*469, 1963.

42. Talwar G. P., Segal, S. J., Evans, A. and Davidson, O. W. "The Binding of Estradiol in the Uterus: A Mechanism for Derepression of RNA Synthesis," *Proc. Nat. Acad. Scis.,* 52:1059-66, 1964.

43. Thiersch, J. B. "Effect of Substituted Mercaptopurines on the Rat Litter *In Utero," J. Reprod. and Fertility,* 4:291-95, 1962.

44. Tietze, C. and Lewit, S. "Intra-Uterine Contraception: Effectiveness and Acceptability," *Proc. 2nd Int. Conf. on Intra-uterine Contraception,* Excerpta Medica Int. Congr. Series No. 86, 98-110, Amsterdam, 1965.

45. Whitelaw, M. J. "Chlorpromazine (Thorazine) in the Infertile Female," *International J. Fertility,* 5:175, 1960.

INDUCED ABORTION AS A METHOD
OF FERTILITY CONTROL

Christopher Tietze

The Population Council

CONTROL OF FERTILITY through induced abortion has been known to mankind since time immemorial, although the absence of records, which prevails to the present, makes any estimate of the extent of its practice almost entirely a matter of conjecture. Currently, comprehensive information on induced abortion is available for some of the countries that have provided by law for the interruption of pregnancy as a part of their medical services. Nevertheless, induced abortion— and particularly illegal abortion—constitutes one of the major areas of ignorance within the scope of public health and population studies.

So far as information on this subject is concerned, the United States is one of the underdeveloped areas of the world. In 1957, a committee of the Arden House Conference on Abortion reported that "a plausible estimate of the frequency of induced abortion in the United States could be as low as 200,000 and as high as 1,200,000 per year" (10). The group saw "no objective basis for the selection of a particular figure between these two estimates as an approximation of the actual frequency."

No new data on which to base a more reliable estimate have become available since. Although two nationwide surveys devoted to the growth of American families have furnished comprehensive information on the use of contraceptive methods and on surgical sterilization, no effort was made to obtain information on induced abortions. It has been contended that this type of data cannot be obtained by survey methods, at least not in the United States.

This negative view is not shared by all investigators. Harter and Beasley have made a determined attempt to obtain abortion data from a representative sample of 483 women of reproductive age in New Orleans who reported a total of 1536 pregnancies (27). Among these women, only three admitted attempts at abortion, two of which were unsuccessful. It is possible that the third attempt was successful, but the history suggests that the woman was not even pregnant. The authors state that "the small number of cases of admitted abortion attempts raises some doubt as to the reliability of this research methodology," but they also feel that they "have some reason to suspect that the number of attempted induced abortions in New Orleans is quite low."

Be that as it may, American demographers and sociologists appear to be more interested in the incidence of abortion now than at any previous time and are more willing to try harder to get the facts. A methodological study of several types of questionnaires is being sponsored by The Population Council. Field work on this study is now underway.

Outside of the United States investigators in several countries have been able to elicit information on induced abortions from respondents in house-to-house surveys and have reported frequencies which are at least high enough to be plausible.

In 1962, Armijo and Monreal interviewed a city-wide sample of 1890 women of reproductive age in Santiago, Chile (5). Among these women, 496 or 26 percent admitted 1394 induced abortions, or 74 per 100 women interviewed. Based on the entire life experience of the respondents, the total incidence amounted to almost 1.25 induced abortions per woman by the end of the childbearing period.

An even higher frequency of induced abortion has been reported by Requeña for a sample of 580 women drawn from one of the poor districts of Santiago (56). The total number of induced abortions in this group was 608, or 105 per 100 women interviewed. The total incidence was on the order of 2.5 induced abortions per woman.

From the other side of the world comes a report by Hong, based on the statements of 3204 married women interviewed in Seoul, Korea, in 1964 (31). Among these women, 805 or one in four gave a history of induced abortion. The number of induced abortions was 1498 or 47 per 100 women, suggesting a substantially lower incidence than in Santiago. Inspection of age-specific abortion rates reveals, however, that these rates are lower in Seoul than in Santiago during the first half of the reproductive period (15-29), but much higher after age 30. As a result, the total incidence for the Korean sample is 1.55 per woman reaching the end of the childbearing period.

In late 1965 Hong interviewed 2084 married women in a rural area of Korea (32). Among these women, only 102 or 5 percent admitted to a total of 142 abortions, or 7 per 100 women interviewed. The total incidence was 0.38 per woman, i.e., one-fourth of the comparable figure in the capital. The reported induced abortions were highly concentrated in the later part of the childbearing period.

It should be noted that the laws regulating abortion in Chile and in Korea are very similar to those in the United States, although attitudes are obviously more relaxed. For most other countries the available information on illegal abortion is as unsatisfactory as it is for the United States. It would serve no useful purpose to burden this report with a series of more or less—all too often less—informed guesses. The following discussion of abortion is, therefore, focused on legal abortion according to the laws of the countries concerned.

United States

In the United States, the laws of most states stipulate a threat to the life of the pregnant woman as the sole legal ground on which abortion may be performed. In a few states this permission is extended to cases where a serious threat to the woman's health is to be averted. Abortions performed under these laws are referred to as "therapeutic abortion."

A more liberal type of legislation has been proposed by the American Law Institute in its Model Penal Code. The relevant paragraph (230.3/2), first drafted in 1955, reads as follows:

"Justifiable abortion. A licensed physician is justified in terminating a pregnancy if he believes there is substantial risk that continuance of the pregnancy would gravely impair the physical or mental health of the mother or that the child would be born with grave physical or mental defect, or that the pregnancy resulted from rape, incest, or other felonious intercourse. All illicit intercourse with a girl below the age of 16 shall be deemed felonious for purposes of this subsection. Justifiable abortions shall be performed only in a licensed hospital except in case of emergency when hospital facilities are unavailable" (3).

Widespread popular support for the proposal of the American Law Institute is indicated by the findings of a survey conducted by the National Opinion Research Center in December, 1965 (58.) A representative sample of 1484 adults were asked their views on the conditions under which it should be possible for a woman to obtain a legal abortion. The percent distribution of the answers appears on the following page. It is equally clear that the respondents did not approve of legal abortion on socioeconomic grounds, let alone on demand.

During the first nine months of 1967, three states, Colorado, North Carolina, and California, enacted abortion statutes based more or less on the Model Penal Code of the American Law Institute. In all three states the new law stipulates unanimous approval by a board

	Percent		
	Yes	*No*	*Don't know*
If the woman's own health is seriously endangered by the pregnancy	71	26	3
If she became pregnant as a result of rape	56	38	6
If there is a strong chance of serious defect in the baby	55	41	4
If the family has a very low income and cannot afford any more children	21	77	2
If she is not married and does not want to marry the man	18	80	2
If she is married and does not want any more children	15	83	2

of three licensed physicians. North Carolina further requires the woman to be a resident of the state for four months before an abortion can be authorized. California has not authorized abortion on eugenic indication.

Abortion law reform was a highly controversial subject in a number of other states, including New York, during the past or current legislative session. Of the more than twenty bills introduced, some were defeated or died in committee, others are still pending. Continued agitation and legislative efforts are predicted for the coming year.

How deeply the tide of opposition to restrictive abortion laws is running may be judged from the fact that even the American Medical Association has joined the bandwagon, albeit with characteristic reluctance and caution. At its annual meeting in June, 1967, the House of Delegates approved a policy statement (4) listing the conditions under which the AMA is *not* opposed to induced abortion, to wit that:

(1) There is documented medical evidence that continuance of the pregnancy may threaten the health or life of the mother, or

(2) There is documented medical evidence that the infant may be born with incapacitating physical deformity or mental deficiency, or

(3) There is documented medical evidence that continuance of a pregnancy, resulting from legally established statutory or forcible rape or incest may constitute a threat to the mental or physical health of the patient;

(4) Two other physicians chosen because of their recognized professional competence have examined the patient and have concurred in writing; and

(5) The procedure is performed in a hospital accredited by the Joint Commission on Accreditation of Hospitals.

Available information on the frequency of therapeutic abortion in the United States is sketchy. In New York City, where the registration of all fetal deaths is required by law, the annual numbers of therapeutic abortions declined from about 700 in 1943-47 (68) to about 300 in 1960-62 (24); the ratio per 1000 live births fell from 5.1 to 1.8. This overall trend conceals a sharp and continuing decline in traditional medical indications and a slight increase in the incidence of abortion on psychiatric grounds. The proportion of therapeutic abortions in New York City performed for psychiatric indications has increased from about one tenth of the total to about one half.

A mail survey of sixty hospitals, covering mainly the years 1957-62, revealed 1039 therapeutic abortions and 522,600 deliveries, corresponding to a ratio of 2.0 abortions per 1000 deliveries (25). This ratio was confirmed by a more recent and still unpublished survey of several hundred hospitals throughout the country participating in the Professional Activities Survey of the Commission on Professional and Hospital Activities in Ann Arbor during the three-year period 1963-65 (71).

Accepting, then, a ratio of about 2 therapeutic abortions per 1000 deliveries, the corresponding estimate for the United States would be on the order of 8000 per year.

All statistics show clearly that in the United States therapeutic abortion is more readily available to well-to-do women than to the underprivileged. In New York City, for instance, the abortion ratio during the period 1960-62 was 3.9 per 1000 deliveries in proprietary hospitals, 2.4 on the private services of nonprofit hospitals, 0.7 on the ward services of nonprofit hospitals, and only 0.1 per 1000 in the municipal hospitals.

This socioeconomic differential was associated with an equally striking ethnic differential. The abortion ratio in New York City was 2.6 per 1000 deliveries for white women, 0.5 for Negroes, and 0.1 for Puerto Ricans.

In Canada, Latin America, western and southern Europe, and in most countries of Asia, Africa, and Oceania, the legal situation is similar to that prevailing in the United States. In these countries, legal abortion is permitted on medical indication only. In some countries, this exception from a general prohibition is written into the statutes; more often, it has been established through custom or judicial interpretation of the law. Generally, therapeutic abortion is done sparingly and with reluctance, but this is not universally true and in a few cities, e.g., in Switzerland the practice of the medical profession is extremely liberal (23, 41). Although reliable figures are lacking, illegal abortions are thought to be very common in many countries. However, certain widely quoted estimates, according to which the number of illegal abortions in some countries is equal to or greater than the number of births, are not supported by tangible evidence.

Germany (26, 42)

In Germany, abortion was proscribed by section 218 of the Penal Code of 1871 which is still the law of the land in the Federal Republic. A formal exception for abortion on medical indication was established in 1935 by section 14 of the Law for the Prevention of Offspring Suffering from Hereditary Disease. While the main provisions of the law relating to abortion and sterilization on eugenic grounds have been universally repealed, the provision with regard to medical indication has been retained in all but two of the states of the Federal Republic. In these two states, abortion to save the life of the mother is permitted under a general provision of the Federal Penal Code, which condones otherwise forbidden acts if they are performed to avert a danger to "life and limb." The draft of a new Federal Penal Code, which has been under consideration for several years, contains a paragraph (157) which defines and authorizes interruption of pregnancy on medical indication (8, 49). All therapeutic abortions must be authorized by the regional Chamber of Physicians on the basis of written opinions submitted by two experts selected by the Chamber. One of these experts must be a gynecologist or obstetrician, the other a specialist in the relevant field of medicine.

In the territory of the German Democratic Republic, section 218 of the old Penal Code was replaced after World War II by a series of state laws under which legal abortion could be performed on medical, eugenic, and humanitarian grounds, and to some extent also on social or economic grounds. These statutes were in turn superseded in 1950 by the Law for the Protection of Mother and Child, which permits abortion on medical and eugenic indication only. The decision lies with regional commissions which include among their members not only physicians but also representatives of the social services and the quasi-official Union of German Women.

During the first few years following World War II, unprecedented numbers of abortions were authorized not only in East Germany but also in the western Zones of Occupation. Many cases involved rape, actual or at least claimed. As the political situation stabilized and economic conditions improved, efforts were made to reduce the number of abortions. German medical literature of that period is replete with articles by leading obstetricians, urging the profession to adhere strictly to the traditional medical indications.

These exhortations were not in vain. In 1950 the number of therapeutic abortions in the Federal Republic was 9500 or 12 per 1000 live births (78). Four years later, these figures were halved.

Year	Number	Rate
1950	9500	12
1951	8000	10
1952	6500	8
1955	4600	6

According to fragmentary data, the decline continued for several more years. My own estimate for 1959, based on Harmsen's reports from four states, suggests a total of 3100 or 3.3 per 1000 births. Since then, the incidence of therapeutic abortion appears to have remained relatively constant (15, 60).

The overall trend in the German Democratic Republic was quite similar to that in the Federal Republic. From 1959 through 1962 the number of authorized abortions in East Germany averaged 800 or 2.7 per 1000 live births, with only minor fluctuations from year to year (45). In 1965, the regional commissions were authorized to extend the medical indication, taking into account the woman's circumstances of life. It has been reported that the number of legal abortions increased substantially in the following year.

France
In France, therapeutic abortion is regulated by the Code de la Santé Publique. According to the decree of May 11, 1955, a physician may interrupt a pregnancy only if the "life of the mother is gravely threatened." He must consult with two other doctors, one of whom must be selected from a list of experts attached to the Civil Courts. These doctors must certify that the danger to the mother's life cannot be averted in any other way and a copy of the certification must be sent to the president of the departmental Council of Physicians (16).

Statistical information is virtually nonexistent. In Paris, according to an official report, only 132 abortions were authorized during a 3-year period ending in mid-1950, corresponding to 0.5 abortions per 1000 live births (53). Extrapolation of this ratio to the entire country suggests an annual total of about 400 therapeutic abortions. Pulmonary tuberculosis accounted for one-half of the abortions authorized in Paris and cardio-vascular-renal disorders, for one-fourth. Only three pregnancies were interrupted on psychiatric indications.

United Kingdom

In the United Kingdom, the statute applicable until very recently was the Offences Against the Person Act of 1861 which made "unlawfully" induced abortion a felony punishable by life imprisonment. The Act did not define "unlawfully" and made no provision for the therapeutic interruption of pregnancy. However, in 1938, in the famous case of *Rex* vs. *Bourne,* Mr. Justice Macnaghten held it reasonable to read into the law an exception stipulated in the Infant Life (Preservation) Act of 1929 that abortion need not be unlawful if done in good faith to save the mother's life. "If the doctor is of the opinion . . . that the probable consequences . . . will be to make the woman a physical and mental wreck, the jury is quite entitled to take the view that the doctor . . . is operating for the purpose of preserving the life of the mother." Bourne, who had aborted a young girl who was the victim of a rape attack, was acquitted and a legal precedent was set. (*18*).

Nevertheless, the official attitude and practice of the British medical profession have remained conservative. Estimates based on a 10 percent sample suggest that about 1600 abortions were performed in the National Health Service Hospitals of England and Wales in 1958, rising to 3300 in 1964 (*59,74*). The latter figure corresponds to a ratio of 3.8 per 1000 live births.

Year	Number	Rate
1958	1600	2.2
1961	2300	2.8
1962	2800	3.3
1963	2600	3.0
1964	3300	3.8

A notable exception has been Sir Dugald Baird at the University of Aberdeen, whose liberal views have raised the incidence of therapeutic abortion in that city to about 20 per 1000 births (*6*). Outside the National Health Service, an estimated 10,000 so-called "West End legal" abortions are performed annually in private nursing homes or in their offices by a number of gynecologists and surgeons in private practice, mainly in London.

In October, 1967, after a long and bitter legislative struggle (*1*), Parliament enacted a liberalized abortion statute, authorizing abortion if two physicians ". . . are of the opinion, formed in good faith: that the continuance of the pregnancy would involve risk to the life of the pregnant woman or of injury to the physical or mental health of the pregnant woman or any existing children of her family greater than if the pregnancy were terminated or that there is a substantial risk that if the child were born it would suffer from such physical or mental abnormalities as to be seriously handicapped." The new law provides further that "in determining whether or not there is such risk of injury to health, account may be taken of the pregnant woman's environment both at the time when the child would be born and thereafter so far as foreseeable." An abortion may be performed. in National Health Service hospitals or in "a place" approved by the Minister of Health; the latter category presumably will include private nursing homes. Conscientious objectors are specifically excused from participating in abortion procedures. The law will come into force six months after enactment (75).

The most revolutionary innovation of the British Abortion Act of 1967 revolves around the seven words "or any existing children of her family." Couched in medical terms ("physical or mental health"), this clause constitutes a clear recognition of the fact that not only the mother but her entire family may be adversely affected by the birth of an unwanted child. Another important facet of the new law is that it does not establish any special apparatus to authorize the interruption of pregnancy. Any two physicians can do so if they feel that the required conditions are met.

The Abortion Act of 1967 has made British law more permissive than the laws which have been in force in, say, Sweden, for many years. It is, therefore, of interest to turn to the experience of northern Europe.

Northern Europe (69)

The first steps toward liberalization of abortion laws were taken during the 1930's in Iceland (1935), Sweden (1938), and Denmark (1939). After World War II, Sweden in 1946 and again in 1963, and Denmark in 1956 further liberalized their abortion laws. Quite recently the Swedish government appointed a new commission of experts to re-evaluate the abortion question with a mandate to recommend a further broadening of indications. Finland passed a liberal abortion statute in 1950 (21) and Norway, in 1960 (51). In the latter country, the new law merely codified what had long become accepted medical practice.

The range of acceptable indications is roughly the same in the four major countries. In each instance the law recognizes a medical indication, a eugenic indication, and a humanitarian (ethical, juridical) indication. The scope of the medical indication has been explicitly extended to include considerations of a mixed socio-medical character. The wording of the Danish statute of 1956 may serve as an example (14). Under this statute, abortion is permitted "if the induction of an abortion is necessary to avert a serious danger to the life or health of the woman. In order to evaluate this danger, an appreciation shall be made of all the circumstances of the case, including the conditions under which the woman will have to live, and consideration shall be given not only to physical or mental illness, but also to any actual or potential state of physical or mental infirmity."

In regard to the eugenic indication, the older statutes mention only the hereditary transmission of mental disease, mental deficiency, and other severe illness or defect. The Swedish Royal Medical Board has, however, authorized the interruption of pregnancy on medical indication in many cases of German measles and in at least one celebrated case of thalidomide poisoning (20). The 1963 amendment to the Swedish law (63) and the new Danish and Norwegian statutes have extended the traditional eugenic indication to cover damage or disease acquired during intrauterine life. The humanitarian indication applies to pregnancies resulting from offenses against the penal code, such as forcible and statutory rape, as well as incest.

With minor exceptions, the maximum period of gestation at which abortion is permissible is 5 months in Sweden, 4 months in Denmark and Finland, and 3 months in Norway.

Examination of the administrative machinery implementing the abortion statutes also reveals important differences among the four major countries. The procedure is most centralized in Sweden where until 1965 more than 85 percent of all legal abortions were authorized by the Royal Medical Board in Stockholm, which makes its decision on the basis of a written report by the physician who has examined the woman seeking abortion. The remaining 15 percent of the interruptions were performed on the authority of a certificate signed by two physicians. The latter type of authorization was chosen in one-fourth of all cases in 1966 and in about one-third during 1967, possibly indicating a greater willingness on the part of Swedish doctors to accept responsibility for the decision.

In Denmark, most legal abortions require authorization by a committee of three persons, attached to the local Mothers' Aid Institution, a publicly supported organization, which conducts a thorough medical and social investigation. Twenty such committees have been established throughout the country, including five in greater Copenhagen. Each consists of a psychiatrist, a gynecologist, and a social worker. An authorization for interruption of pregnancy must be unanimous. Abortions on purely medical indications, where the threat to life and health results from a disease and not from the conditions under which the woman lives, may be performed on the sole authority of the appropriate chief of service.

In Finland and Norway, the administration is relatively decentralized. In both countries, most legal abortions are approved by two physicians one of whom must be a gynecologist or surgeon on the permanent staff of a hospital. In Finland, the other physician is drawn from a roster of medical specialists established by the State Medical Board; in Norway, he is appointed by the county health officer and must be trained in psychiatry or social medicine.

Following the adoption of the Swedish law in 1938, the number of legal abortions in that country increased from about 400 to more than 6300 in 1951 (Table 1), and the ratio of abortions per 1000 live births rose from 5 to 57. A parallel development occurred in Denmark, pushing the number of legal abortions from about 500 in 1939 to 5400 in 1955 and the ratio per 1000 live births from 7 to 70. The trend was then reversed and the numbers of abortions dropped to about 2800 in 1960 in Sweden and 3600 in 1959 in Denmark. Thereafter the upward trend was reestablished, with totals for 1966 substantially exceeding the high points of the early 1950's. The corresponding ratio per 1000 live births was about 59 in Sweden and 67 in Denmark. A preliminary estimate places the number of legal abortions in Sweden in 1967 at about 9600, indicating an increase of almost one-third over the preceding year.

In Finland, the number of legal abortions rose from about 3000 in 1951 to 6200 or 75 per 1000 live births in 1960. Over the next five years, a moderate decline to 4800 was recorded. In Norway, two special surveys established the numbers of abortions performed in hospitals at approximately 2000 in 1949 and 3200 in 1954 (50). The latter figure equals 50 per 1000 live births. So far, no information has become available as to the numbers performed under the statute of 1960. In Iceland, according to unpublished data furnished by the Ministry of Health, legal abortions averaged slightly more than 50 per year during the decade 1954-63, without a discernible trend; this figure corresponds to 11 cases per 1000 live births (34).

The overwhelming majority of legal abortions in northern Europe are performed on medical indication and most often on psychiatric grounds. This category includes conditions described as "exhaustion" of the mother. The eugenic indication plays a very minor role and abortions on humanitarian grounds are even rarer.

One of the major goals of the liberalization of abortion laws in northern Europe was to reduce the incidence of illegal abortion. A further objective was to reduce the total number of abortions, legal and illegal combined, by establishing early contact with the pregnant woman and making available to her a broad range of social services. There is no agreement among Scandinavian authors to what extent the first of these objectives has been achieved in any of the countries concerned, and it is even less likely that the second goal has been realized. Whether the abortion laws have actually contributed to an "abortion mentality" has been a much debated question (2,30,36,55, 79).

A by-product of the liberal laws in northern Europe has been the compilation of nationwide statistics on mortality associated with legal abortion. The longest series is available for Sweden (39,64):

Period	Legal Abortions	Deaths	Rate per 100,000
1946-48	10,500	27	257
1949-53	28,000	27	97
1954-59	22,800	15	66
1960-66	30,600	12	39

Comparable figures have been reported from Finland in 1950-57 (18 deaths among 27,100 legal abortions or 66 per 100,000) (52) and Denmark in 1953-57 (16 deaths among 23,700 abortions or 68 per 100,000) (7).

While the decline of the risk to life over 20 years is marked and gratifying, mortality associated with legal abortion in northern Europe has remained substantially above the levels achieved in Japan and in eastern Europe. These higher death rates may be attributed to the fact that a substantial proportion of legal abortions in northern Europe is performed after the third month of gestation: 35 percent in Sweden (1949) (62) and 25 percent in Denmark during the two years 1955 and 1957 (22). These late abortions contribute heavily to the total numbers of deaths. In addition, many women undergoing legal abortion in northern Europe are ill or at least in poor physical condition while in Japan and in eastern Europe the overwhelming majority are in good health.

The somatic and emotional sequelae of legal abortion in Sweden have been carefully studied by Lindahl and Ekblad, respectively (40,17).

While laws and practices relating to abortion are much more liberal in northern Europe than in western and southern Europe, abortion has, in fact, been "legalized" on limited grounds only. Japan and most of the socialist countries in eastern Europe have adopted far more radical policies, and it is to these countries that we shall now turn our attention.

Japan

In Japan, the Eugenic Protection Law of 1948 authorized interruption of pregnancy for economic as well as for medical reasons (47). The crucial passage is contained in article 14 of the law and permits the interruption of pregnancy in a woman "whose health may be affected seriously from the physical or economic viewpoint by the continuation of pregnancy or by confinement." The subsequent interpretation of this paragraph by the medical profession, by the authorities, and by the public has been tantamount to making abortion available on request.

As shown in Table 2, the reported numbers of legal abortions in Japan rose from 246,000 in 1949 to 1,170,000 in 1955. Since 1955, the number has declined by more than one-fourth and the rate per 1000 population by about one-third. The numbers reported are believed to fall short of the actual totals by several hundred thousand, owing (it has been alleged) to the reluctance of physicians to pay income taxes on their full earnings (48,66).

Some light has been shed on this question by the experience of 1966. In that year a precipitous drop occurred in the number of births and in the birth rate, followed by a compensatory rise in 1967. The decline is generally attributed to the fact that 1966 was the "Year of the Fire and Horse," a combination which occurs every 60 years according to the traditional Chinese calendar still widely used in Japan. Girls born in such a year are believed to be very stubborn and it is difficult to find husbands for them.

In this situation one would expect a rise in the number of abortions in the later part of 1965 and in the first half of 1966. Unfortunately, monthly data on legal abortions are not available, but the reported annual totals continued to decline. This would suggest that the deferment of births was achieved mainly by contraception and poses the dilemma that either the most tradition-bound segment of Japanese society practiced contraception successfully or the reported decline in abortions is, at least in part, a statistical artifact.

Deaths attributed to abortions performed on medical or legal grounds are shown separately in the annual volumes of vital statistics (37). The following mortality rates are based on these data and the reported numbers of legal abortions:

Period	Legal Abortions	Deaths	Rate per 100,000
1950-53	2,994,000	253	8.5
1954-58	5,723,000	334	5.8
1959-63	5,138,000	210	4.1

If the deaths are correctly attributed but the numbers of legal abortions are larger than the numbers reported, as has been suggested, the mortality rates shown above would be proportionally overstated.

Eastern Europe (*43,44,70,72*)

In eastern Europe, abortion policy has undergone several major changes since November 8, 1920, when interruption of pregnancy at the request of the pregnant woman was legalized in the U.S.S.R. by a joint decree of the Commissariats of Health and Justice. On June 27, 1936, another decree restricted legal abortion to a list of specified medical and eugenic indications. On November 23, 1955, the policy was once more reversed and the restrictive decree of 1936 repealed by the Presidium of the Supreme Soviet (*19*).

Following the example of the U.S.S.R. all the socialist countries of eastern Europe, except East Germany and Albania, adopted similar liberalizing legislation (*9,12,33,54,81*). The stated aims of this legislation, in the words of the preamble to the Soviet decree, are "the limitation of the harm caused to the health of women by abortions carried out outside of hospitals" and to "give women the possibility of deciding by themselves the question of motherhood."

Throughout eastern Europe, official concern with overpopulation or rapid population growth is proscribed by Marxist philosophy. Moreover, several of the countries concerned have very low birth rates, and none has a high birth rate by global standards. At least two countries (Czechoslovakia and Hungary) pursue an active population policy by means of family allowances for third and later children.

Within the overall pattern of legal abortion, considerable variation between individual countries is apparent. Abortion at the request of the pregnant woman is currently permitted in Bulgaria, Hungary, and the U.S.S.R. In Poland, the law of 1956 stipulates a "difficult social situation" as an acceptable reason for the interruption of pregnancy and makes the physician responsible for the determination of its existence.

In Czechoslovakia, the law permits abortion for reasons "which deserve special consideration" among which the Ministry of Health listed in 1957: (a) advanced age, (b) numerous children, (c) loss or disability of husband, (d) broken home, (e) predominant economic responsibility of the woman for the maintenance of the family or the child, (f) difficult circumstances of an unmarried woman resulting from her pregnancy, and (g) pregnancy due to rape or other offense. In late 1961, a new regulation restricted voluntary abortions on the ground of multiparity to women with three or more living children, and also required a threat to the level of living in cases of predominant economic responsibility of the woman (*13*). In Yugoslavia, interruption of pregnancy may be authorized if the birth of the child would result in a serious personal, familial, or economic situation for the pregnant woman which cannot be averted in any other way.

Romania legalized abortion on demand in 1957 but reversed her position in October, 1966, restricting abortion to women over 45 years of age and to mothers supporting four or more living children, in addition to the usual medical, eugenic, and humanitarian (rape, incest) indications (57). The medical indication is narrowly defined as a threat to the woman's life.

The preamble of the decree of 1966 refers to the "great prejudice to the birth rate and the rate of natural increase" resulting from the practice of abortion as well as to "severe consequences to the health of the woman." In the absence of any reports from Romania on mortality or morbidity associated with legal abortion in that country, one may conclude that the primary reason for the repeal of the law of 1957 was concern over the decline of the birth rate, which, by 1965, had dropped to 14.6 per 1000 population, the second lowest in Europe.

Commissions for the authorization of abortion, consisting of physicians and representatives of the social services, have been established in Czechoslovakia and Yugoslavia. Medical boards also exist in Hungary, but their function has become purely formal since they must now assent if the applicant insists on having her pregnancy interrupted. In Poland, abortion is authorized by a certificate from a single physician.

Throughout eastern Europe abortion is prohibited in cases of pregnancy of more than 3 months' duration, except for medical reasons, and also if the applicant had undergone an induced abortion during the preceding 6 months. In some countries, such as Czechoslovakia and Hungary, the operation must be performed in an appropriately equipped and staffed hospital, where the typical period of stay is two or three days, followed by sick leave if the woman is a wage earner. In Poland and Yugoslavia, however, many legal abortions are done on ambulatory patients. In recent years, the method of vacuum extraction, originally developed in China (80), has been used on an increasing scale throughout eastern Europe. According to reports, it is technically easier, faster, and less traumatic than the traditional dilatation and curettage (38,76).

Abortions for medical reasons are performed free of charge. Those done on request or on social indications must be paid for by the applicant. The charges cover only part of the cost of the operation and hospitalization.

The new legislation has resulted in spectacular increases in the incidence of legal abortion throughout eastern Europe. Table 3 summarizes the available information, along with data on live births and on "other abortions," i.e., women admitted to hospitals for the treatment of incomplete abortion or of complications. The table also shows the corresponding rates per 1000 population.

The most comprehensive and trustworthy statistics are those for Czechoslovakia and Hungary. Coverage is almost certainly incomplete for Poland, Yugoslavia (except in Slovenia), and Romania. No statistics have been published for the U.S.S.R. and attempts to "reconstruct" them by the manipulation of "bits and pieces" have not produced convincing results (28).

In Hungary strong efforts were made in 1952 and 1953 to enforce existing laws against criminal abortion. These efforts were followed by an increase in births in 1953 and 1954. At about the same time, medical boards for the authorization of therapeutic abortions were established. The growing numbers of legal abortions since 1953 indicate the progressive liberalization of the policies of these boards (29). After the decree of June 3, 1956 had introduced interruption of pregnancy on request, the number of legal abortions increased rapidly until it reached 186,600 in 1966, exceeding the number of live births by more than one-third.

In Czechoslovakia, legalization of abortion for nonmedical reasons was preceded by almost two years of public discussion. Moderate increases in therapeutic abortions in 1956 and 1957 reflect the changing attitude of the medical profession (77). Promulgation of a new and liberalized abortion law in December 1957 was followed by a steep rise in legal abortions in 1958, which continued at a decelerating pace until 1961, when 94,300 were registered. The trend was then reversed with a drop to 70,500 in 1963, followed by a renewed upward movement two years later.

The reported numbers of "other abortions" shown in Table 3 include criminal as well as spontaneous abortions. These figures, based on hospital admissions, have not changed drastically in any of the six countries during the period under consideration. There is little doubt that the number of criminal abortions has declined substantially throughout the region but it appears that these declines have been masked by increased hospitalization after spontaneous or illegal abortion, resulting at least in part from the fact that women no longer fear prosecution. Nevertheless, criminal abortions have not entirely disappeared even in countries where abortion is available on request. It has been suggested that this stubborn survival of illegal abortion is associated with the relative lack of privacy of the official procedure.

Mortality associated with legal abortion has been exceedingly low in eastern Europe. For Hungary, Hirschler's thorough investigation reported 15 deaths following 269,000 abortions during the 2-year period 1957-58, corresponding to a mortality rate of 5.6 per 100,000 legal abortions. More recent figures, for the 4-year period 1960-63 yield a mortality rate of 3.1 per 100,000, based on 21 deaths among 670,000 cases (65). In Czechoslovakia, a mortality rate of 6.8 per 100,000 was reported for 1957-60; there were 16 deaths among 236,000 legal abortions (11). By 1961-64, mortality had dropped to 1.2 per 100,000 cases, based on 4 deaths and 325,000 abortions. In Yugoslavia, according to Mojić, 8 deaths occurred in 1960-61 among 177,000 legal abortions, corresponding to a rate of 4.5 per 100,000 cases (46). It is almost certain that the low level of mortality in eastern Europe reflects primarily the restriction of legal abortion to the first three months of pregnancy except in cases with a medical indication.

Developing countries
Abortion on request, without reference to family size, was legalized in Mainland China by the Ministry of Health in May, 1957, against the advice of the Chinese Medical Association (67). According to an unpublished report by a well-qualified Japanese visitor, abortion was freely available in 1964 and no change in policy is known to have occurred since that time.

Several of the developing countries outside the Communist orbit have given consideration to the possible legalization of abortion as a part of their national family planning programs. So far, none of these countries has accepted legal abortion as a major policy. While this restraint doubtless reflects religious beliefs and traditional medical attitudes, it is probably reinforced by the severe shortages of medical personnel and facilities in most of the developing countries.

In 1964, the government of India appointed a committee to study the question of Legalization of Abortion (35). A questionnaire survey sponsored by this committee produced responses from 570 individuals and groups, mainly health officers (127) and other physicians (235) and welfare organizations, including family planning groups and women's associations (140). According to the committee's report, 96 percent of the respondents favored a legal abortion to avert a serious threat to the mother's life or physical or mental health and 82 percent in cases of rape, while 57 percent supported abortion for socioeconomic reasons. On all questions the position of the welfare organizations was more liberal than that of the other respondents.

The committee, more conservative than the persons and groups responding to the questionnaire, recommended a modest liberalization of the type represented by the Model Penal Code of the American Law Institute and by the Termination of Pregnancy Bill then being discussed in Britain. In making its recommendations, the committee made it clear that it considered not only "the more metaphysical or ethical considerations" but also "the lack of sufficient medical facilities for operative work" in India.

In Tunisia abortion on request was legalized in 1965 for women with five or more living children (73). However, this legislation has not been widely publicized and the number of women who have taken advantage of it appears to be relatively small.

In Singapore, the Health Minister announced in August, 1967 that a bill "legalizing" abortion would be presented to parliament at its next sitting (61). So far, no details of the proposed legislation have been made public but the Minister said that in the future "every child born in Singapore would be a wanted child." According to newspaper reports, "women with three children will find the least trouble getting abortions for subsequent pregnancies." A nominal fee of $5 (U.S. $1.67) is to be charged for each abortion.

No one can say what the future will bring. Current restraints may well be abandoned if contraceptive methods, including the IUD's and the "pill," and surgical sterilization fail to bring down birth rates fast enough and far enough to avert the economic and social consequences of rapid population growth. In that case, health authorities in developing countries may ask for technical assistance wherever they can find it. It appears to me that a well-planned program of research in safe and simple methods of inducing abortion should at least be started before these requests are made. Such a program must be international in scope, since clinical research requires access to large numbers of healthy women undergoing induced abortion in a hospital environment. This condition cannot be met in countries such as the United States, where the indications for legal abortion are narrowly defined. However, even in the United States there is no need to be idle until the abortion laws are repealed or radically changed. This may take a long time, in view of the generally conservative nature of political institutions and of what is known about the attitudes of our electorate. In the interim, laboratory research on other mammals and especially on infra-human primates could and should be initiated without delay and pursued energetically.

Table 1. Legal abortions in Sweden, Denmark, and Finland: 1939-1966

| Year | Number | | | Ratio per 1000 live births | | |
	Sweden	Denmark	Finland	Sweden	Denmark	Finland
1939	439	484	—	5	7	—
1940	506	522	—	5	7	—
1941	496	519	—	5	7	—
1942	568	824	—	5	10	—
1943	703	977	—	6	12	—

Table 1.—Cont.

| Year | Number | | | Ratio per 1000 live births | | |
	Sweden	Denmark	Finland	Sweden	Denmark	Finland
1944	1088	1286	—	8	14	—
1945	1623	1577	—	12	17	—
1946	2378	1930	—	18	20	—
1947	3534	2240	—	28	24	—
1948	4585	2543	—	36	30	—
1949	5503	3425	—	45	43	—
1950	5889	3909	—	51	49	—
1951	6328	4743	3007	57	62	32
1952	5322	5031	3327	48	65	35
1953	4915	4795	3802	45	61	42
1954	5089	5140	3699	48	67	41
1955	4562	5381	3659	43	70	41
1956	3851	4522	4090	36	59	46
1957	3386	4023	4553	32	53	52
1958	2823	3895	5274	27	52	65
1959	3071	3587	5773	29	48	69
1960	2792	3918	6188	27	51	75
1961	2909	4124	5867	28	54	72
1962	3205	3996	6015	30	51	74
1963	3528	3971	5616	31	48	68
1964	4671	4527	4919	38	54	61
1965	6208	5188	4783	51	60	61
1966	7254	5726	—	59	67	—

Sources: Sweden. Medicinalstyrelsen. *Allmän Hälso—och Sjukvård.* Various years.
Denmark. Sundhedsstyrelsen. *Medicinalberetning for kongeriget Danmark.*
Various years.
Finland: Lääkintohallitus. *Yleinen terveyden—ja sairaanhoito.* (Suomen
Virallinen Tilasto, XI: 67) pp. 154-56. Helsinki, 1966.

Table 2. Live births and legal abortions in Japan: 1949-1966

| | Number in 1000's | | Rate per 1000 population | |
Year	Live births	Legal abortions	Live births	Legal abortions
1949	2696.6	246.1	33.2	3.0
1950	2337.5	489.1	28.2	5.9
1951	2137.7	638.4	25.4	7.6
1952	2005.2	798.2	23.5	9.3
1953	1868.0	1068.1	21.5	12.3
1954	1769.6	1143.1	20.1	13.0
1955	1730.7	1170.1	19.4	13.1
1956	1665.3	1159.3	18.5	12.9
1957	1566.7	1122.3	17.2	12.3
1958	1649.8	1128.2	18.0	12.3

Table 2.—Cont.

Year	Number in 1000's		Rate per 1000 population	
	Live births	Legal abortions	Live births	Legal abortions
1959	1622.8	1098.9	17.5	11.9
1960	1603.0	1063.2	17.2	11.4
1961	1586.4	1035.0	16.9	11.0
1962	1613.1	985.4	17.0	10.4
1963	1657.4	955.1	17.3	10.0
1964	1714.7	878.7	17.7	9.1
1965	1821.8	843.2	18.6	8.6
1966	1356.4	808.4	13.7	8.2

Source: Japan: Ministry of Health and Welfare. *Report of Statistics on Eugenic Protection.* Various years.

Table 3. Births and abortions in Eastern Europe: numbers and rates

Year	Number in 1000's			Rate per 1000 population		
	Live births	Legal abortions	Other abortions*	Live births	Legal abortions	Other abortions*
Hungary						
1950	195.6	1.7	34.3	20.9	0.2	3.7
1951	190.6	1.7	36.1	20.2	0.2	3.8
1952	185.8	1.7	42.0	19.6	0.2	4.4
1953	206.9	2.8	39.9	21.6	0.3	4.2
1954	223.3	16.3	42.0	23.0	1.7	4.3
1955	210.4	35.4	43.1	21.4	3.6	4.4
1956	192.8	82.5	41.1	19.5	8.3	4.2
1957	167.2	123.3	39.5	17.0	12.5	4.0
1958	158.4	145.6	37.4	16.0	14.7	3.8
1959	151.2	152.4	35.3	15.2	15.3	3.5
1960	146.5	162.2	33.8	14.7	16.2	3.4
1961	140.4	170.0	33.7	14.0	17.0	3.4
1962	130.1	163.7	33.9	12.9	16.3	3.4
1963	132.3	173.8	34.1	13.1	17.2	3.4
1964	132.1	184.4	34.3	13.1	18.2	3.4
1965	133.0	180.3	33.7	13.1	17.8	3.3
1966	138.5	186.8	33.6	13.6	18.3	3.3
Czechoslovakia						
1953	271.7	1.5	29.1	21.2	0.1	2.3
1954	266.7	2.8	30.6	20.6	0.2	2.4
1955	265.2	2.1	33.0	20.3	0.2	2.5
1956	262.0	3.1	31.0	19.8	0.2	2.3
1957	252.7	7.3	30.2	18.9	0.5	2.3

*Hospital admissions

Table 3.—Cont.

| Year | Number in 1000's | | | Rate per 1000 population | | |
	Live births	Legal abortions	Other abortions*	Live births	Legal abortions	Other abortions*
Czechoslovakia						
1958	235.0	61.4	27.7	17.4	4.6	2.1
1959	217.0	79.1	26.4	16.0	5.8	1.9
1960	217.3	88.3	26.3	15.9	6.5	1.9
1961	218.4	94.3	26.0	15.8	6.8	1.9
1962	217.5	89.8	26.1	15.7	6.5	1.9
1963	236.0	70.5	29.4	16.9	5.0	2.1
1964	241.1	70.7	28.5	17.1	5.0	2.0
1965	231.6	79.6	26.2	16.4	5.6	1.8
1966	222.5	90.0	25.4	15.6	6.3	1.8
Poland						
1954	778.1	72.3		29.1	2.7	
1955	793.8	1.4	101.6	29.1	0.1	3.7
1956	779.8	18.9	101.9	28.0	0.7	3.7
1957	782.3	36.4	85.4	27.6	1.3	2.9
1958	755.5	44.2	82.2	26.3	1.5	2.9
1959	722.9	79.0	82.9	24.7	2.7	2.8
1960	660.9	150.4	73.4	22.3	5.1	2.5
1961	627.6	143.8	72.8	20.9	4.8	2.4
1962	599.5	140.5	70.4	19.8	4.6	2.3
1963	588.2	135.4	68.5	19.2	4.4	2.2
1964	562.9	133.5	67.1	18.1	4.3	2.2
1965	546.3	124.8	65.1	17.3	4.0	2.1
Yugoslavia (Total)						
1959	424.3	54.5	57.3	23.3	3.0	3.1
1960	432.6	76.7	56.6	23.5	4.2	3.1
1961	422.2	104.7	59.8	22.7	5.6	3.2
Yugoslavia (*Slovenia*)						
1955	32.1	0.4	5.0	21.0	0.3	3.3
1956	31.5	0.8	4.6	20.4	0.5	3.0
1957	30.1	2.2	5.6	19.4	1.4	3.6
1958	28.2	4.7	6.0	18.1	3.0	3.8
1959	28.4	6.4	5.2	18.2	4.1	3.3
1960	27.8	8.2	5.5	17.6	5.2	3.5
1961	29.0	9.3	5.6	18.2	5.8	3.5
1962	29.0	9.5	5.6	18.1	5.9	3.5
1963	29.2	9.4	6.1	18.1	5.8	3.8
1964	29.2	9.4	6.0	17.9	5.8	3.7
1965	30.7	9.9	6.1	18.6	6.0	3.7

Table 3.—Cont.

Year	Number in 1000's			Rate per 1000 population		
	Live births	Legal abortions	Other abortions*	Live births	Legal abortions	Other abortions*
Bulgaria						
1953	153.2	1.1	16.3	20.9	0.2	2.2
1954	149.9	1.1	17.5	20.2	0.2	2.4
1955	151.0	19.1		20.1	2.5	
1956	147.9	40.0		19.5	5.3	
1957	141.0	31.7	14.5	18.4	4.1	1.9
1958	138.3	38.1	17.4	17.9	4.9	2.3
1959	136.9	45.6	18.2	17.6	5.8	2.3
1960	140.1	54.8	19.3	17.8	7.0	2.5
1961	137.9	68.8	19.9	17.4	8.7	2.5
1962	134.1	76.7	21.1	16.7	9.6	2.6
1963	132.1	83.3	20.5	16.4	10.3	2.5
Romania						
1958	390.5	112.1	17.4	21.6	6.2	1.0
1959	368.0	219.1	16.7	20.2	12.0	0.9

Sources:　1. Mehlan K-H. "National Programs, Achievements and Problems: The Socialist Countries of Europe," *Family Planning and Population Programs* (B. Berelson, R. K. Anderson, O. Harkavy, J. Maier, W. P. Mauldin, S. J. Segal, eds.), pp. 207-26. Chicago: University of Chicago Press, 1966.

2. Hungary: Kŏzponti Statisztikai Hivatal. *Magyarország népesedése: demográfiai évkönyv* (Statisztikai idŏszaki kŏzlemények). Various years.

3. Vojta M. "Die Abortsituation in der Tschechoslowakischen Sozialistischen Republik," *Internationale Abortsituation Abortbekämpfung Antikonzeption* (K-H. Mehlan, ed.), pp. 107-13. Leipzig: Thieme, 1961.

4. Srb V., Kučera M. "Potratovost v Československu v letech 1958-1962," *Demografie*, 5:289-307, 1963.

5. Czechoslovakia: Ministerstvo Zdravotnictvi. "Potraty 1965," *Zdravotnická Statistika ČSSR*, 2:1-76, 1966.

6. Srb V. "Pohyb obyvatelstva v roce 1966," *Demografie*, 9:168-74, 1967.

7. Poland: Ministerstvo Zdrowia I Opieki Spolecznej. "Opieka nad matka i dzieckiem," *Biuletin Statistyczny*, Nr. 2, 1964.

8. Yugoslavia. Slovenia: Zavod Za Zdravstveno Varstvo. *Zgodnja Fetalna Smrtnost v SR Sloveniji, 1955-1964*. Ljubljana, 1966.

9. Yugoslavia. Slovenia: Zavod Za Zdravstveno Varstvo. *Splav in Njegovo Preprecevanje v SRS v Letu 1965*. Ljubljana, 1966.

10. Starkaleff I., Papasoff B., Stoimenoff G. "Die Abortsituation in der Volksrepublik Bulgarien," *Internationale Abortsituation Abortbekämpfung Antikonzeption* (K-H. Mehlan, ed.), pp. 26-31. Leipzig: Thieme, 1961.

REFERENCES

1. Abortion Law Reform Association. *Alra Newsletter,* No. 19. Summer, 1967.

2. Aldén, T. "Om de illegala abortenas antal och geografiska fördelning," *Abortfrågan* (Sweden: Inrikesdepartementet), pp. 222-34. Stockholm, 1953.

3. American Law Institute. *Model Penal Code,* pp. 189-92. Philadelphia, 1962.

4. American Medical Association: Committee on Human Reproduction: "AMA Policy on Therapeutic Abortion," *J.A.M.A., 201:*544, Aug. 14, 1967.

5. Armijo, R., Monreal, T. "Epidemiology of Provoked Abortion in Santiago, Chile," *Population Dynamics* (M. Muramatsu, and P. A. Harper, eds.) pp. 137-60. Baltimore: Johns Hopkins Press, 1965.

6. Baird, D. "A Fifth Freedom?" *Brit. Med. J.,* 2:1141-48. Nov. 13, 1965.

7. Berthelsen, H. G and Østergaard, E. "Komplikationer og mortalitet ved legal abortus provocatus baseret på 23,666 anmeldelser til sundhedsstyrelsen i årene 1953 til 1957," *Ugeskrift for laeger, 120:*1005-9, July 31, 1958.

8. Breitenecker, L., and Breitenecker, R. "Abortion in the German-Speaking Countries of Europe," *Westrn. Resv. Law Rev.,* 17:553-68, Dec. 1965.

9. Bulgaria: Laws, Statutes, Etc. "Interruption of Pregnancy," *Intern. Digest Hlth. Legislation, 8:*605-7, 1957.

10. Calderone, M. S. *Abortion in the United States,* p. 180. New York: Hoeber, 1958.

11. Černoch, A. "Les autorisations d'interruptions de grossesse en Tchécoslovaquie: étude de ses effets et conséquences," *Gynaecologia 160:*293-99, 1965.

12. Czechoslovakia: Laws, Statutes, Etc. "Interruption of Pregnancy," *Intern. Digest Hlth. Legislation, 10:*283-92 1959.

13. Czechoslovakia: Laws, Statutes, Etc. "Interruption of Pregnancy," *Intern. Digest Hlth. Legislation, 13:*491-92, 1962.

14. Denmark: Laws, Statutes, Etc. "Interruption of Pregnancy," *Intern. Digest Hlth. Legislation, 8:*377-81, 1957.

15. Döring, G. K. "Aktuelle forensische Probleme in der Geburtshilfe und Gynäkologie: Empfängnisverhütung, Schwangerschaftsunterbrechung und Sterilisation," *Deutsche Zeitschrift für die gesamte Gerichtliche Medizin, 55:*194-200, Sept. 1, 1964.

16. Dourlen-Rollier, A-M. *La verité sur l'avortement,* pp. 33-35. Paris: Maloine, 1963.

17. Ekblad, M. "Induced Abortion on Psychiatric Grounds: A Follow-up Study of 479 Women," *Acta Psychiatrica et Neurologica Scandinavica*, suppl., 99:1-238, 1955.

18. Ferris, P. *The Nameless: Abortion in Britain Today*, pp. 42-48. London: Hutchinson, 1966.

19. Field, M. G. "The Re-Legalization of Abortion in Soviet Russia," *New England Journal of Medicine*, 255:421-27, Aug. 30, 1956.

20. Finkbine, S. "The Lesser of Two Evils," *The Case for Legalized Abortion Now* (A. F. Guttmacher, ed.), pp. 15-25. Berkeley, California: Diablo Press, 1967.

21. Finland: Laws, Statutes, Etc. "Interruption of Pregnancy," *Intern. Digest Hlth. Legislation*, 2:559-61, 1951.

22. Frandsen, E., Mosbech, J., Mølgaard, B. "Abortus provocatus i Danmark i 1955 og 1957," *Ugeskrift for laeger*, 121:1538-43, October 1, 1959.

23. Geiser, M. "Zahlen und Gedanken zur legalen Schwangerschaftsunterbrechung in der Schweiz und im Ausland," *Schweizerische medizinischen Wochenschrift*, 86:1006-10, Sept. 8, 1956.

24. Gold, E. M., Erhardt, C. L., Jacobziner, H., and Nelson, F. G. "Therapeutic Abortions in New York City: A 20-Year Review," *Amer. J. Public Hlth.*, 55:964-72, July 1965.

25. Hall, R. E. "Therapeutic Abortion, Sterilization, and Contraception," *Amer. J. Obstet. Gynec.*, 91:518-32, Feb. 15, 1965.

26. Harmsen, H. "Die Abortsituation in der Duetschen Bundesrepublik," *Internationale Abortsituation Abortbekämpfung Antikonzeption* (K.-H. Mehlan, ed.) pp. 41-51. Leipzig. Thieme, 1961.

27. Harter, C. L. and Beasley, J. D. "A Survey Concerning Induced Abortions in New Orleans," *Amer. J. Public Hlth.*, 57:1937-47, Nov. 1967.

28. Heer, D. M. "Abortion, Contraception, and Population Policy in the Soviet Union," *Demography*, 2:531-39, 1965.

29. Hirschler, I. "Die Abortsituation in der Volksrepublik Ungarn," *Internationale Abortsituation Abortbekämpfung Antikonzeption* (K.-H. Mehlan, ed.) pp. 114-22. Leipzig: Thieme, 1961.

30. Hoffmeyer, H., and Nørgaard, M. "Konceptionshyppighed og svangerskabsforløb: undersøgelser og beregninger af den illegale aborthyppighed siden 1940," *Ugeskrift for laeger*, 126:355-71, Mar. 12, 1964.

31. Hong, S. B. *Induced Abortion in Seoul, Korea*, p. 26. Seoul: Dong-A, 1966.

32. Hong, S. B. "Induced Abortion in Rural Korea: Based on the Survey in Yongi-Gun, Chungchongnamdo," *Korea Journal of Obstetrics and Gynecology*, 10:275-304, June 1967.

33. Hungary: Laws, Statutes, Etc. "Interruption of Pregnancy," *Intern. Digest Hlth. Legislation*, 9:536-40, 1958.

34. Iceland: Ministry of Health, *Personal communication*.

35. India: Ministry of Health and Family Planning. *Report of the Committee to Study the Question of Legalization of Abortion*. New Delhi, 1967, pp. 143.

36. Ingelman-Sundberg, A. "Om de illegala aborternas antal och geografiska fördelning," *Svenska Läkartidningen*, 50:2386-92, Nov. 13, 1953.

37. Japan: Ministry of Health and Welfare. *Vital Statistics.* Published annually.

38. Kerslake, D. and Casey, D. "Abortion Induced by Means of the Uterine Aspirator," *Obstet. Gynec., 30:*35-45, July 1967.

39. Klintskog, E. "Operationsriskerna vid legal abort." *Abortfrågan* (Sweden: Inrikesdepartementet), pp. 252-61. Stockholm, 1953.

40. Lindahl, J. M. *Somatic Complications Following Legal Abortion.* Stockholm: Svenska bokförlaget, 1959, pp. 182.

41. Marr, S. "Abortion á la Suisse," *New Statesman,* April 7, 1967.

42. Mehlan, K.-H. "Die Abortsituation in der Deutschen Demokratischen Republik," *International Abortsituation Abortbekämpfung Antikonzeption* (K.-H. Mehlan, ed.) pp. 52-63. Leipzig: Thieme, 1961.

43. Mehlan, K.-H. (ed.). *International Abortsituation, Abortbekämpfung, Antikonzeption.* Leipzig: Thieme, 1961.

44. Mehlan, K.-H. "National Programs, Achievements and Problems: The Socialist Countries of Europe," *Family Planning and Population Programs* (B. Berelson, R. K. Anderson, O. Harkavy, J. Maier, W. P. Mauldin, S. J. Segal, eds.) pp. 207-26. Chicago: University of Chicago Press, 1966.

45. Mehlan, K.-H. and Falkenthal, S. "Der legal Abort in der Deutschen Demokratischen Republik: Statistik der Jahre 1953 bis 1962," *Deutsche Gesundheitswesen. 20:*1163-67, June 24, 1965.

46. Mojić, A. "Abortion as a Method of Family Planning: Experiences of the Yugoslav Health Service," *Proceedings of the Third Conference of the Region for Europe, Near East and Africa* (International Planned Parenthood Federation), pp. 77-79, 1962.

47. Muramatsu, M. (ed.). *Japan's Experience in Family Planning—Past and Present,* pp. 107-14. Tokyo: Family Planning Federation of Japan, 1967.

48. Muramatsu, M. "Effect of Induced Abortion on the Reduction of Births in Japan," *Milbank Memorial Fund Quarterly, 38:*153-66, Apr. 1960.

49. Muth, H. and Engelhardt, H. *Schwangerschaftsunterbrechung und Sterilisierung in neuerer Sicht,* pp. 5-9. München: Urban & Schwarzenberg, 1964.

50. Norway: Justisdepartementet. *Innstilling fra straffelovrådet om adgangen til a avbryte svangerskap,* p. 74. Trondhieim, 1956.

51. Norway: Laws, Statutes, Etc. "Interruption of Pregnancy," *Intern. Digest Hlth. Legislation. 16:*148-54, 1965.

52. Olki, M. "Die Abortsituation in Finnland," *International Abortsituation Abortbekämpfung Antikonzeption* (K.-H. Mehlan, ed.), pp. 64-69. Leipzig: Thieme, 1961.

53. Piédelièvre, M. R. "L'avortement thérapeutique dans le départment de la Seine," *Bulletin de l'Académie National de Médecine, 134:*577-84, Oct. 17, 1950.

54. Poland: Laws, Statutes, Etc. "Interruption of Pregnancy," *Intern. Digest Hlth. Legislation, 9:*319-23, 1958.

55. Quensel, C. E., and Genell, S. "Ha de illegala aborterna minskat under de senare åren?" *Svenska Läkartidningen, 50:*2784-92, Dec. 24, 1953.

56. Requena B., M. "Social and Economic Correlates of Induced Abortion in Santiago, Chile," *Demography, 2:*33-49, 1965.

57. Romania: Laws, Statutes, Etc. "Interruption of Pregnancy," *Intern. Digest Hlth. Legislation, 18*:822-37, 1967.

58. Rossi, A. S. "Abortion Laws and Their Victims," *Trans-action, 3*:7-12, Sept.-Oct., 1966.

59. Royal College of Obstetricians and Gynaecologists. "Legalized Abortion: Report by the Council of the Royal College of Obstetricians and Gynaecologists," *Brit. Med. J., 1*:850-54, Apr. 2, 1966.

60. Schubert, G. "Erfahrungen eines Frauenklinikers bei Anträgen zu Schwangerschaftsunterbrechungen im norddeutschen Raum," *Internist, 4*:124-31, Apr. 1963.

61. *Straits Times.* August 12, 1967.

62. Sweden: Inrikesdepartementet. *Abortfrågan. Betänkande avgivet av 1950 års abortutredning.* (Statens Offentliga Utredningar 1953-29), p. 221. Stockholm, 1953.

63. Sweden: Laws, Statutes, Etc. "Interruption of Pregnancy," *Intern. Digest Hlth. Legislation, 17*:152, 1966.

64. Sweden: Medicinalstyrelson. *Allmän Hälso-och Sjukvård.* Published annually.

65. Szabady, E. and Miltenyi, K. "Abortion in Hungary: Demographic and Health Aspects" *Sex and Human Relations: Proceedings of the Fourth Conference of the Region for Europe, Near East and Africa* (International Planned Parenthood Federation), pp. 84-88, 1965.

66. Taeuber, I. B. *The Population of Japan,* p. 276. Princeton: Princeton University Press, 1958.

67. Tien, H. Y. "Induced Abortion and Population Control in Mainland China," *Marriage and Family Living,* 25:35-43, Feb. 1963.

68. Tietze, C. "Therapeutic Abortions in New York City, 1943-1947," *Amer. J. Obstet. Gynec., 60*:146-52, July 1950.

69. Tietze, C. "Legal Abortion in Scandinavia," *Quarterly Rev. Surg. Obstet. Gynec., 16*:227-30, Oct.-Dec. 1959.

70. Tietze, C. and Lehfeldt, H. "Legal Abortion in Eastern Europe," *J.A.M.A., 175*:1149-54, Apr. 1, 1961.

71. Tietze, C. "Therapeutic Abortions in the United States, 1963-65," *Amer. J. Obstet. Gynec.* (in press).

72. Tietze, C. "The Demographic Significance of Legal Abortion in Eastern Europe." *Demography, 1*:119-25, 1964.

73. Tunisia: Laws, Statutes, Etc. "Interruption of Pregnancy," *Intern. Digest Hlth. Legislation, 17*:406, 1966.

74. United Kingdom. House of Commons: "Abortion Admissions in N.H.S. Hospitals," *Lancet, 1*:516, Mar. 4, 1967.

75. United Kingdom: Laws, Statutes, Etc. *An Act to Amend and Clarify the Law Relating to Termination of Pregnancy by Registered Medical Practitioners. (27th October 1967).* London: Her Majesty's Stationery Office, 1967, p. 4.

76. Vojta, M. "A Critical View of Vacuum Aspiration: A New Method for the Termination of Pregnancy," *Obstet. Gynec., 30*:28-34, July 1967.

77. Vojta, M. "Die Abortsituation in der Tschechoslowakischen Sozialistischen Republik," *Internationale Abortsituation Abortbekämpfung Antikonzeption* (K.–H. Mehlan, ed.) pp. 107-13. Leipzig: Thieme, 1961.

78. Von Rohden, F. "Die Entwicklung der legalen Schwangerschaft-

sunterbrechung im Bundesgebiet im ersten Nachkriegsjahrzehnt," *Schleswig-Holsteinisches Ä'rzteblatt, 9:*196-208, 1956.

79. Wahlen, T. "De illegala aborternas antal: en kommentar till abortbetänkandets bilaga II," *Svenska Läkartidningen, 51:*248-50, Jan. 29, 1954.

80. Wu, P. C. "The Use of Vacuum Bottle in Therapeutic Abortion: A Collective Survey," *Chinese Med. J., 85:*245-48, Apr. 1966.

81. Yugoslavia: Laws, Statutes, Etc. "Interruption of Pregnancy." *Intern. Digest Hlth. Legislation, 12:*619-22, 1961.

IV. PUBLIC PROGRAMS FOR FAMILY PLANNING

NATIONAL FAMILY PLANNING PROGRAMS: WHERE WE STAND

Bernard Berelson

The Population Council

THIS IS A REVIEW of where we stand with regard to national family planning programs: What has been the experience? What have we learned from it? What does it come to? Accordingly, this paper is not limited to scientific research on the one hand nor, I hope, is it merely a set of personal impressions on the other: the first would be incomplete as a guide to action, the second not necessarily helpful. Rather, this is an effort to pull together research results, operational data, and informed observations into one overall summary of "where we stand." It is only right to stress at the outset that this is only one person's view of the present situation.[1] Someone else might see the situation differently, but at the least I would hope that he would want to take into account all of the following topics even if he did not agree with all of the propositions.

This paper deals with large, organized, more or less official programs that bring family planning information, services, and supplies to mass populations in the developing world in order to promote effective family planning practices, for the welfare of the individual family and/or the national community. As a framework for the subsequent discussion, what does such a family planning program look like? What are the major steps that need to be taken, from first consideration to full implementation? Although such programs vary widely in their specifics, as is only to be expected from the variety of local circumstances, there is a characteristic progression of events:

> The pressure for family planning policy typically originates in the planning board or its equivalent, as economists come to appreciate what the current rate of population growth means for their development plans—or, in fewer countries, it originates in medical circles with concern over the high incidence of induced abortions and their personal and social costs. (The ground had often been prepared by the local, private family planning asso-

341

ciation; and its relationship to the governmental effort sometimes makes for the natural tensions of organizational rivalries.) Someone in a high position who wishes to promote the policy invites a foreign mission of experts to review the population situation and make recommendations, which then call for adoption of a family planning policy. Even after the policy is formally proclaimed, however, there often remains some ambivalence at high levels based on political sensitivities, actual or perceived.

When the effort does begin it is placed under medical auspices: the official program becomes the responsibility of the Ministry of Health, it is closely tied to maternal and child health services and health centers, and a medical man with experience in public health is usually named director of the program. He begins by designating family planning as another health service, to be administered through the existing network, and/or by setting up family planning clinics wherever possible. These approaches typically fail and slowly the responsible officials (who by now are likely not to be the ones who started in charge) come to recognize that more vigorous efforts are needed in the form of special staff, materials, and supplies, and in ways to reach people rather than waiting for them to come in.

Meanwhile, the medical people are reviewing available contraceptive methods and doing clinical tests to see which will be approved for use in their country; communications specialists are only slowly developing informational and educational materials and campaigns, partly because of some reluctance at high levels to allow full publicity; and the bureaucracy—particularly finance and, where they exist, relations between the center and regional units—takes its inevitable toll.

Sooner or later, information, services, and supplies are brought to the attention of the target population, usually through female field workers specially trained for the purpose; and contraceptive methods are offered free of charge on a voluntary basis and as a so-called cafeteria choice of techniques, though with particular emphasis on the IUD as presumably the most effective method. Incentive payments for medical and paramedical personnel are provided and often finder's fees as well—for which a rather elaborate scheme for administration needs to be developed. An evaluation unit is set up to guide the program and measure its results, and it does either job only with some difficulty and delay. Throughout this period the program has received external assistance in both funding and expertise. By this time, it is a few years after the policy decision was taken, an organization to do the work is just coming into effective operation, and any effect on the birth rate is yet to be demonstrated if not actually brought about.

That brief summary contains references to the several aspects of family planning programs that require attention in this review, having to do with the establishment of programs, their operation, the target population, the contraceptive technology, the program's impact and guidance. Against this background I shall report "where we stand" in the following propositions, with accompanying discussion, elaboration, qualification, observation, and evidence.

The Establishment of Programs

1. *A substantial and increasing number of developing countries now have favorable policies on family planning: all either established or revitalized in the 1960's and on all three developing continents but mainly in Asia. Adoption of such a policy is associated mainly with size of population and level of education, then with per capita income, partly with density and rate of growth, and inversely with the birth rate and the death rate.*

The recency of this movement is striking:[2] within the last five years or so, over 20 countries have taken a favorable position on family planning programs, have sharply invigorated their existing programs, or have major governmental involvement (Table 1). In the entire developing world today, about 65 percent of the people live in countries with such favorable policies (over 50 percent if Mainland China is omitted from both numerator and denominator). Moreover, all these countries have put governmental funds into family planning efforts (although, as we shall see, the vigor of implementation has varied widely).

Another 10-15 countries are now doing something in the family planning field—more than a private association but less than a national policy—and the record shows that once a country moves in this direction it rarely turns back, and then not for long. So the "population problem" has taken root in governmental policy in the developing world in a remarkably few years (as well as in the United States and the United Nations). It is, in fact, difficult to think of another movement of such combined delicacy and magnitude that has made similar headway, and especially so when the apparent political, religious, and cultural obstacles are taken into account.

The movement began in Asia and has made most headway there. Approximately 80 percent of the developing population in Asia lives in favoring countries (again, as above, 70 percent without Mainland China) as against only 20 percent in Africa (mainly in the northern tier) and 15 percent in Latin America. This disproportion testifies, perhaps, to the relative power of the cultural obstacle in Asia as against the religious in Latin America and the political in emerging

Africa. In Asia and Africa the movement is mainly based on the effect of population growth upon social and economic development and was mainly promoted by planning boards and their equivalent, i.e., largely economic considerations. In Latin America it is based more on medical and humanitarian concern with the prevalence of induced abortions and has mainly been promoted by medical schools, i.e., largely medical considerations. In virtually all cases, however, the programs themselves come under medical administration and are tied to maternal and child health out of both substantive and political concerns.

What predisposes a developing country toward a favorable position on family planning (as represented by columns 2 and 3 of Table 1)? Size of population and level of education appear to be most

Table 1. The place of family planning in developing countries*

Size of population (in millions) (1)	Have an official family planning policy and/or program, or major governmental involvement (2)	Are doing something official in family planning, or limited governmental involvement (3)	Are doing nothing official in family planning (4)
400 & more	China (1962?) India (1952, reorganized 1965)		
100-400	Pakistan (1960, reorganized 1965)	Indonesia	
50-100			Nigeria Brazil
25-50	Turkey (1965) United Arab Republic (1966) South Korea (1961)	Mexico Philippines Thailand	Burma
15-25	Iran (1967) Colombia (1967) North Vietnam (1964)†		Ethiopia Congo South Vietnam Afghanistan
10-15	Morocco (1966) Taiwan (1964) Ceylon (1967)	Peru Nepal	Sudan Algeria Tanzania North Korea
Less than 10	Malaysia (1966) Kenya (1966) Chile (1966) Tunisia (1966)	Venezuela Cuba Nicaragua Costa Rica	Africa—31 countries Asia—12 countries

Table 1.—Cont.

Size of population (in millions) (1)	Have an official family planning policy and/or program, or major governmental involvement (2)	Are doing something official in family planning, or limited governmental involvement (3)	Are doing nothing official in family planning (4)
Less than 10			
	Hong Kong (c1960) Dominican Republic (1967) Honduras (1965) Singapore (1966) Jamaica (1966) Trinidad & Tobago (1967) Mauritius (1965)	Barbados	Latin America 9 countries

*Due to the complexity of the situation in several countries, this classification is not easily applied in all cases. However, I believe this is essentially the present picture. The middle category is mixed: for example, the first encouragement of family planning activities under the new government in Indonesia, governmental support of research projects in Thailand, municipal and hospital programs in the Philippines, follow-up of a technical assistance mission in Nepal, population divisions within the health ministries in Peru and Venezuela.

†I enter this country here on the basis of the following paragraph from the November 25, 1967, issue of *Le Monde,* from an interview with the North Vietnamese Minister of Public Health by a French physician:

"The population of North Vietnam was in 1960 17 million inhabitants. The population is at present between 19 to 20 million inhabitants. Three years ago we had an important population increase which reached 34 percent (presumably: 3.4 percent) in Hanoi. We therefore started a national campaign to limit births which brought results since the birth rate came down very rapidly to approximately 20 percent (presumably: 20 per 1000). We are pursuing this campaign and the Prime Minister Pham Van Dong attaches great importance to it since he himself presides over the Committee for the Protection of Motherhood and Children which is in charge of organizing this campaign. The goal of this action is essentially the protection of the health of mothers and babies. Vietnamese mothers had on the average of 4 to 5 children some years ago and we wish to limit this number. We are essentially carrying out this program through a vast national information campaign, by mobilizing the minds. We counsel and distribute all traditional simple methods (withdrawal, prophylactics, etc.). We do not use the pill."

NOTE: After listing the above material, I received the following information from Mr. Vu-dinh-Dinh who is doing a paper on family planning in South Vietnam to be submitted to the faculty of the School of Public Health, University of Hawaii:

North Vietnam has never proclaimed a population policy. However, unofficial efforts have been made to make birth control devices available to the public and contraceptive methods have been discussed freely in a leading women's magazine. A 'Marriage and Family Law' promulgated in 1960 set the marriage-

important, then per capita income, then density, and only then the growth rate (Table 2). The birth rate and the death rate themselves actually show a negative relationship, due largely to the large number of small African states with high birth and death rates (and essentially the same distribution appears for the infant mortality rate).

Of the thirteen largest developing countries (those with over 25 million population), only three are now doing nothing officially: one is a Catholic country (Brazil), one has nationalistic problems leading to political instability (Nigeria), and one has isolated itself from international contacts (Burma). Of the next category in size (15-25 million), the Congo and South Vietnam have been engaged in warfare; and in Ethiopia, where population data are largely lacking, it would appear that the death rate is still very high and the growth rate accordingly low for a developing country (i.e., under 2 percent).

The experts base their recommendations for a family planning policy mainly upon growth rates, both demographic and economic. However, the policy-makers move to adopt population programs mainly when the rates of population growth are coupled with density and especially with education and absolute size (not to mention the special cases of Catholic countries and countries with political instability). In fact, the two factors of absolute size and level of education go far in differentiating countries with and without a favoring stand on family planning. The three-way classification used in Table 2 yields this striking breakdown (for all countries where data on both factors are available):

	Favorable	Not
High—High	2	0
High—Medium	9	1
High—Low & Medium—Medium	10	9

able ages for men and women at 20 and 18, respectively. So far as we know, family planning in North Vietnam is a voluntary movement in the sense that the state does not have a direct hand in the administration of the program. Neither pills nor IUDs are apparently used in the country. The traditional methods are available as well as vasectomy, ligature, and abortion, with the latter methods falling under the responsibility of the Ministry of Health. Family planning methods seem to be applicable only to highly motivated groups—primarily factory workers, governmental employees, and cooperative members who are readily committed to the regime and well organized. The rural inhabitants who constitute the bulk of the population have not been offered the benefits of family planning.
I am indebted to Mr. Vu-dinh-Dinh for this additional information.

	Favorable	Not
Medium—Low	8	26
Low—Low	0	18

(To read: High—High means those countries with 25 million population or more *and* with 75 percent school enrollment or more; High—Medium means the high category on one factor and the middle category on the other; and so on. Favorable refers to columns 2 and 3 in Table 1.)

Although the experts typically do not base major policy recommendations upon density (except in the special case of closed, extractive economies), the policy-makers take it more seriously: of all the countries in column 2 of Table 1 with 10 million population or more, the average density is about 350 per square mile; of those in column 3 (doing something) about 125; and of those in column 4 (doing nothing) about 85.

Finally, why do the smaller countries move in this direction? It may not be irrelevant to observe that of all the countries in column 2 of Table 1, not one with more than 15 million population is an island whereas below that figure 8 of 14 are islands (including Hong Kong), and have an average density of over 3000 per square mile. "Being pushed into the sea" by population pressures apparently carries some psychological weight.

But the major impact of Table 2, beyond absolute size, is the indication that the favoring countries have at least started on the road to modernization—that is, they have more popular education and higher per capita incomes and their birth and death rates tend to be low. This picture is part of the general story that development moves faster where the old has already begun to be superseded: when, for example, income starts up and people begin to appreciate what that can mean for the better life; or when death rates and infant mortality go down, and people begin to appreciate what that implies for their fertility. In this sense, the countries that may theoretically need family planning most—those with the highest birth rates and the lowest income—are still too far behind the trend of history to catch up, so to speak, all at once. From this standpoint, family planning programs contribute to those countries already moving toward modernization—indeed, are part of that movement.

2. *A favorable policy does not automatically lead to an effective program: the political and intellectual leadership is often ambivalent on the new policy, and in any case incorporation of a major new program into a bureaucracy is never easy on organizational, fiscal, and personnel grounds.*

Table 2. Policy position on family planning among developing countries*, by size, level of education, per capita income, density, population growth rate, birth rate, and death rate

	Number of countries with Favorable policy, program, or some official activity	No official activity
By Size		
25 million or more	10	3
10-25 million	7	9
Under 10 million	17	50
By Level of Education		
(Percentage enrolled in		
school, 1st & 2nd levels, adjusted)		
75 percent and over	11	3
30 percent-75 percent	19	28
under 30 percent	1	24
By Per Capita Income		
Over $250 per year	11	6
$100-$250 per year	15	17
Under $100 per year	5	28
By Density		
200 and over per square mile	13	9
50-200 per square mile	15	16
Under 50 per square mile	6	35
By Population Growth Rate		
(*natural increase*)		
3 percent per year and over	11	12
2.5 percent to 2.9 percent per year	13	12
Under 2.5 percent per year	9	16
By Crude Birth Rate		
Under 40 per 1000 per year	12	3
40-44 per 1000 per year	13	13
45 and over per 1000 per year	9	27
By Crude Death Rate		
10 and under per 1000 per year	14	5
11-20 per 1000 per year	15	13
21 and over per 1000 per year	3	19

*The total number of countries differs from one sub-table to another because of differential availability of data. The sources are the *United Nations Demographic Yearbook*, 1965; the *United Nations Population and Vital Statistics Report,* January 1967; the *United Nations Yearbook of National Accounts Statistics*, 1965; the *United Nations Population and Vital Statistics Report*, April 1967; and the *UNESCO Statistical Yearbook*, 1965.

A governmental policy (or at least governmental acquiescence) is necessary but it is never sufficient. Some countries listed above with favoring policies do not yet have even moderately effective programs, but at the same time one of the most successful efforts (in Taiwan) has gone forward without a formal policy statement at the highest levels of government, but has had quasi-governmental funding and official support at the level of the Provincial Health Department. What are the organizational problems?

To begin at the top, many high governmental officers come to this policy (as probably to any other of consequence) with misgivings and doubts. At the bottom this attitude may be based upon the residual feeling that national size means national power. But there are other questions involved too: Is there a domestic political liability in this policy that opponents can exploit with the mass of people? Is the developed world helping out of good motives or is their interest merely a new form of colonialism to be applied to the non-white peoples? Will neighboring countries continue to grow, and thus perhaps upset the military balance? Is the slowing of population growth an admission that national goals for development cannot otherwise be reached, and thus an admission of defeat that political opponents can capitalize? It is thus quite understandable why the decision to embark upon population control is not an easy one for a government to make, even in the absence of church-state complications, and why it is not made "all of a piece" with immediate and full implementation. In a sense, the people are often ahead of their leaders: they want contraception more than the leaders are prepared to provide it.

Consider the large countries in the list above. Mainland China apparently changed policy at least twice in the past decade (we really do not know much about the situation today). India had a policy for nearly 15 years before it had a program relatively free of bureaucratic restrictions and administered by a fully committed leadership. Pakistan has had strong support from the very top but a change to strong administrative leadership occurred only after four years of unsuccessful efforts. The United Arab Republic has support at the top but has not been able to get itself organized to run an effective program. Shortly after Turkey changed its law in order to accommodate a family planning program, the opposition came to power with the result that the program has moved only slowly in the perceived absence of high-level support. Similar situations are in effect elsewhere, and on this list only South Korea is a major exception. In consequence—and a point of deep significance—national programs of family planning across the world, young as they are, have had even fewer years of secure operation, where "secure" is defined as clear and firm support from the top plus reasonably smooth bureaucratic procedures.

Once organized, such programs are subject to personnel turnover. India changed directors of family planning twice within a year and not long after changed ministers. Pakistan set up a new commissionership and appointed a new commissioner. In the UAR, the top administrative posts have gone unfilled about as long as filled, and then by different people. In Turkey, there have been five ministers since the first technical mission and two undersecretaries. Again, South Korea is the exception, and its programmatic success is not unrelated to the stability (and the same would go for Taiwan). The moral is that like any other large effort, a family planning program needs not only strong but also continuous leadership for a period of years if it is to make an impact.

The progress of such programs often rests substantially upon the leadership of a very few key people, often a single man. That has been the case over a crucial period of years in Taiwan, in South Korea, in Turkey, and in Pakistan. In each instance, an able man in a key position inaugurated, guided, protected, and developed activities that in his absence might not have been undertaken—certainly not so early or so well. This represents a thin and hence risky line of leadership but it seems to be a fact of life in this field—and, one suspects, in others and in the developed world as well, since effective leadership seems always to be in short supply. The more general point, particularly important in view of the organizational analysis to which the programs are often subjected, is that personalities have a great deal to do with success and failure in this field. And already we are witnessing what sociologists call "the routinization of charisma"—the shift from charismatic to administrative leadership.

The Operation of Programs

3. *Any form of administrative organization will do that can exercise leadership and initiate policy; recruit, train, assign, and supervise personnel; deliver funds and supplies; and keep track of the consequences.*

Whether theoretically there is "one best way" to organize and administer family planning programs in the developing countries, in practice there apparently is not. Local circumstances, not to mention local personalities, take over, and a variety of organizational forms emerges.

Typically, the family planning program is set down in the health ministry, alongside or as part of maternal and child health. But the full organization is not usually so neat or simple as that. In South

Korea the program is the responsibility of the health ministry but the Planned Parenthood Federation of Korea has been closely involved in training and as a funding channel, and the universities have undertaken research projects intended to guide the national effort. In Taiwan, the Provincial Health Department provides information and education on family planning as part of its maternal and child care program, but in the absence of an official policy did not provide services or supplies; they were handled through an independently established Maternal and Child Health Association that administers the well-known Taiwan coupon system, and the Joint Commission on Rural Reconstruction serves again as a channel for funds. In Hong Kong, the entire program is run through the private Family Planning Association, with some governmental support, and that was the case in Singapore, too, until 1966. In Pakistan, the national leadership of the program in its latest reorganization was taken out of the health division and vested with a non-medical Commissioner of Family Planning, but the program operates largely through the health services of the two wings. In India, the center must work through the health programs in the states and it has taken considerable time and ingenuity to make those relations reasonably workable. In Colombia and Chile, the leadership comes from the medical schools with acquiescence from national health officials but no direct participation. In the United Arab Republic, a commission arrangement was set up because of jurisdictional problems at the departmental level. In Tunisia, the informational responsibility was vested in a different department from the service responsibility, and that split delayed the informational program for years.

In view of all this diversity among nations, it is impossible to correlate success of a program directly with organizational form. Setbacks and failures are more often attributable to actual or perceived ambivalence at the top, to funding difficulties, to administrative incompetence or inexperience, and to sheer personality problems than to organizational form itself. Short of being made a completely autonomous agency within the government, located at the highest level and removed from fiscal and administrative restrictions—and even that state of affairs could be readily sabotaged in operation by bypassed bureaucrats—the program must make do within the present system. And programs differently organized have done so: that is the main point. As a distinguished observer and advisor has succinctly remarked in this connection: "The main problems are how to get the money and how to get the work organized."[3]

It remains to note that in all the pressure to get governmental programs underway and keep them going, the potential contribution of the private sector appears to have been overlooked or neglected. Where efforts have been expended to make profitable the spread of contraception through commercial channels, they seem to have been worthwhile. Even in the poorer countries of the developing world, some network of commercial distribution usually exists, and could be exploited for the sale of condoms (as in a promising Indian plan now in process of development) and perhaps, in time, oral contraceptives as well. Certainly, in some countries (notably in Latin America), the commercial distribution of contraception has had a much larger impact than organized programs. Has the whole advertising/marketing approach been underplayed to date because the efforts have been guided by public officials and academic scholars?

4. *Thus far, information on family planning has apparently been more effective than education; person-to-person contact more effective in implementation than the mass media; and informal diffusion through trusted associates supplementary in an important degree to the formal program.*

By "information" I mean straightforward statements about what is available to control births, how and how well it works, what the side effects are, what the costs are, and where to get it: that is, statements that accept present norms of family size and simply seek to satisfy the existing interest. By "education" I mean statements designed to persuade people to different norms of family size or child spacing, to an appreciation of their own responsibility with regard to the population problem, to an acceptance of the concept of family planning against the drag of traditional belief. The one is an attempt to change behavior, the other to change attitudes.

So far in mass programs, it appears that the former has been more effective in bringing people to the practice of family planning than the latter. This does not say that education is unnecessary or worthless, or that better educational campaigns might not be quite effective, or that they may not be critically effective over the long run (particularly in view of the widely held belief that the first stages of a program "skim the cream" of the highly motivated and that the program must then replenish the demand through persuasion). But to date it does seem that communications bringing out the latent interest in the community and exposing the pluralistic ignorance are the best received and the most influential.

Nor is that surprising when considered against the resistance of strongly held beliefs to "mere arguments" and the demonstrated inability of communications to move them very much (in the developed world, among the highly educated, and on far less central topics, as well as in this connection). After all, the content of the family planning message is not particularly sophisticated or subtle, and no amount of "cleverness" on a matter so intimate and personal is likely to be very effective. So, in the short run, the power of persuasion seems to be severely limited by life circumstances.

As on marketing matters in general, person-to-person contact is often more effective in "making the sale" than messages through the impersonal media. At the same time, it must be added that in the nature of the case, given the illiteracy of many developing countries and the limited communication networks there, the mass media have not been largely utilized in family planning programs. They have not been given a full trial yet, which is partly why I say "thus far." Where they have been, as in the Hooghly experiment near Calcutta and in the city of Seoul, they have made an important contribution to the spread of family planning and/or of favorable attitudes. In Hooghly District, various media—radio, newspapers, films, posters, etc.—were utilized over a two-month period and measurably increased the awareness of family planning in that limited time.[4] In Sungdong Gu, a district of Seoul, where the family planning message was carried for about 18 months via radio spot announcements (about one a day), television spots (2 a week), newspaper announcements (one a week), and posters, about 50 percent of the women coming to the health stations for service attributed their visit, directly or indirectly, to the media program.[5] So it appears that the media can affect practice as well as knowledge and attitudes.

The most notable program to date in continuous use of the mass media has been South Korea's, and although there is little hard evidence as yet, there is a general belief among the responsible administrators that radio announcements and magazine advertisements—both informational rather than "persuasive"—have indeed contributed to the positive results of that program. The introduction of television into the developing countries, just beginning, should make the media even more effective, as has been demonstrated elsewhere. A well-organized and long-term media campaign, with large inputs at the start and carefully planned reinforcing messages subsequently, on the commercial model, has hardly been carried out anywhere.

Actually, from what we know in other circumstances, the persuasive effects of the mass media are more likely to be middle- and long-run than immediate. That is, the media can be importantly influential in determining the climate of discussion about family planning even when they do not promptly convert. They can get family planning "in the air"; make it a familiar, "natural," respectable topic of concern; get it "taken for granted"; support and reinforce the advocates with testimonials from the top. That in itself is a major contribution to long-term prospects for family planning, including spacing, not to mention the shorter-run contribution as well. And that is something a mass media campaign can do, and hence a direction or emphasis that national programs might adopt—something between "straight information" on the one hand and "hard-sell persuasion" on the other.

Testifying to the incipient interest in family limitation, word-of-mouth diffusion of the message has made a major contribution to every program where some measurement of the matter has been possible—diffusion from people in direct contact with the program out to neighbors, relatives, friends, and acquaintances. The Taichung experiment was designed to test the effect of diffusion among areas with different proportions of neighborhoods covered by field workers (a half, a third, a fifth) and its results are now well known: for example, during the first year of the program about three out of every four acceptors came *without* benefit of direct contact with field workers, and at the end of that year about one-quarter of the acceptors were coming from *outside* the city, where no programmatic effort was undertaken.[6] In Pho-tharam, Thailand, "52 percent of all acceptances, over the entire 32-week period (of the study), came from women who were led to visit the clinics as the result of conversations with friends who themselves had become contraceptive users."[7] Also in Thailand a service begun in a single hospital in Bangkok, *without* a formal informational effort, secured 12,000 IUD acceptors in a year: "Of greatest interest was the finding that women from three-fourths of the nation's provinces came to Bangkok to obtain IUDs the first year, with no inducement except information passed informally person-to-person."[8] In Sungdong Gu, in Seoul, half of the women coming to the clinics reported that they had heard of the service from friends, neighbors, and relatives.[9] In the post-partum program, located in 25 delivery hospitals throughout the world, nearly half the acceptors came from the community at large although the informational effort was limited to obstetrical patients.[10] Even in national programs, a large part of the clientele reports that it is recruited in this way: in Taiwan, for example, "it appears that about half of all referrals come as a result of hearing about the loop from friends, neighbors, and relatives,"[11] and in South Korea about 28 percent.[12]

There are two important implications of this process of diffusion. The first is that bad news diffuses as well as good news, perhaps even faster than good news. Thus, every IUD program from Taichung to India has been subjected to both truthful and untruthful reports of unsatisfactory performance, from simple bleeding to cancer promotion. There appears to be no better antidote than full and frank information—from the field worker at first contact, from the doctor at time of insertion, in the follow-up activities, and in the media wherever possible.

The second implication is a favorable one. Hardly any country can afford a sufficient cadre of field workers to reach every married woman of reproductive age within a reasonable time, or perhaps ever. Accordingly, it is fortunate that word-of-mouth can do a large part of the job—and, unit for unit, no doubt a more effective one in view of the personal trust involved. So programs can capitalize on diffusion by trying to reach only every Nth person or area in the target population, where N differs by local circumstance but probably, from Taichung experience, is of the order of 2 to 5, maybe more depending upon the need for efficiency as against effectiveness. And finally, the importance of capitalizing on diffusion is one of the reasons for concentrating at the outset of a program on the more highly motivated couples, in order to develop a network of support as soon as possible.

5. *Most operating programs provide fees for service by medical doctors, most provide finder's fees for official and unofficial field workers, and some provide subsidies for commercial sales of contraceptive products and incentive payments to the clients themselves (beyond free service and supplies, given everywhere but Taiwan).*

In short, national programs have found that the profit motive is a useful way to support the family planning motive. Fee for service has increased the collaboration of the medical community and perhaps its support of family planning; in some cases, revenue from induced abortion and non-program contraception had to be taken into account in developing ways to secure cooperation. Similarly for native midwives: they are quick to appreciate how the family planning program threatens their revenue from deliveries and they are in position to sabotage the work. Accordingly, for example, Pakistan has made a special effort to solicit their collaboration, on the "if-you-can't-beat-them-join-them" principle, by making them into "organizers" for the program and paying them a salary plus referral fee plus commission from sales of traditional contraceptives. And the practice extends to non-program agents as well. For example, in Comilla, in East Pakistan, traditional contraceptives were distributed by enlisting commercial sources in the villages through liberal subsidies; in Taiwan, IUD insertions were promoted by loop wearers, traveling sales persons, beauticians, *et al.*, made into referral agents for a fee; in South Korea, 35 percent of all insertions in Seoul in the first quarter of 1967 were referred by ban and tong chiefs, druggists, beauticians, and housewives for the finder's fee.

Most national programs employ fees and incentives in one way or another (Table 3). Thus field experience demonstrates, if it was not already known, that the program goes better if participants make money out of it. To date, most of the money has been made by doctors and field workers—and as the arithmetic shows, both groups can do very well indeed if they are located in a favorable situation and exert some effort. For example, in Pakistan a native midwife can make 40 rupees a month with only about 15 referrals for IUD insertion—alone about the monthly per capita income in that country; and a private doctor can make about 250 rupees a month by doing only two insertions a working day (the equivalent of one-third to one-fourth the salary of a government doctor); and both can still do their regular jobs at the same time.

The natural extension is to the client. Perhaps the most notable instance is the vasectomy program in Madras, India, in the early 1960's, which provided 40 rupees for travel and loss of working time as well as a liberal finder's fee to the already vasectomized. While that program was in effect it accounted for a large proportion of the vasectomies in all India, and the number was reportedly cut by a large proportion when the finder's fee was discontinued, only to recover when the fee was reestablished (with some men, again reportedly, making this their major occupation, with a network of "subcontractors").[13]

Whether people should be paid directly or indirectly to practice family planning, as a good investment for a national economy striving for development, is a question for each country that carries ethical and political overtones. All that is necessary here is to note that the concept exists now and that it may grow in the next years in those places where the population problem is given high priority and where the present effort does not promise to reach targets. As an instance, India has a high-level committee at work on incentives. Already, some critics of the present effort—critics who are for the effort but pessimistic as to its prospects of success—are beginning to suggest that some further measures may be necessary beyond the present acceptance of complete voluntarism,[14] and in 1967 the then Minister in India suggested preparing legislation authorizing compulsory sterilization for men with three or more children.

There is, of course, a substantial range between full freedom of choice as to contraception and full compulsion by the state, and it is hardly likely that any government could move the whole way very quickly. There is a large difference between positive incentives (bonuses to practice family planning effectively)[15] and negative incentives (economic or educational deprivations imposed on "too large" families or on the Nth child). In sum, the whole matter of incentives

Table 3. Fees and incentives in national programs, spring 1967

	Medical doctors	*Others*
India	$1.45/IUD insertion, private MD ($0.30 to government MD) $4.00/vasectomy, private MD ($0.70) $5.35/salpingectomy ($1.40)	$0.70/IUD insertion fee to client $1.70/vasectomy fee to client $3.50/tubal ligation fee to client Various small referral fees
Pakistan	$1.20/IUD insertion $3.00/sterilization	$0.60/insertion for paramedical workers $0.50/referral fee for *dais* (midwives) $0.40/referral fee for others $4.40/sterilization fee to client
South Korea	$1.30/insertion $3.30/vasectomy	$0.19/insertion for field worker $0.38/vasectomy for field worker or other finders $2.95/vasectomy fee to client
Taiwan	$1.50/insertion (half paid by client)	$0.25/referral fee for midwives Variable group incentives for field workers
Turkey	$1.10/insertion	$0.55/referral fee
U.A.R.	$0.70/insertion	$0.70/referral fee for IUD $0.70/client at time of IUD follow-up

is likely to secure more attention in the next years as some programs, forced by population pressures, seek further ways to success.

6. *In the efforts to date, the costs of national family planning programs are low as compared to the presumed benefits and well within the calculated economic value of a slower rate of population growth.*

At the present level of operation, the costs of family planning programs to national governments are low—low in absolute terms, quite low as a per caput figure, very low in relation to presumed socio-medico-economic returns. Up to the past year or so, the successful programs in South Korea and Taiwan have operated at the level of about US $0.05 per caput per year—a little higher in Korea, a little lower in Taiwan. The new five-year budgets for India and Pakistan included larger investments in family planning, but it remains to be seen how much will actually be spent. (The earlier budgets in both countries averaged only about one cent per caput per year, and even that was not fully spent.) In the major national programs in operation in spring 1967, the total cost averages about 6¢ per caput, or about 35¢ per married woman of reproductive age (MWRA), the usual target[16] (Table 4).

But that puts costs only against people or target members. What do the results cost? Here the best data probably come from South Korea and Taiwan. In those cases, each initial acceptor costs about $5.00; each acceptor continuing effective contraception for a year costs about $7-10; each prevented birth costs, say, $20-$30 (at three years of protection per averted birth); and each point off the birth rate at its present level costs approximately $750,000 in South Korea and $300,000 in Taiwan (or about $25,000 per million population). Even if these figures increase over time, as the program allegedly has greater difficulty by having to recruit a larger proportion of acceptors from the lesser motivated; or even if less advantaged countries need larger amounts for the same return; or even if an advantageous but expensive contraceptive method emerges—even so, there is still a good deal of room for increase before the cost approaches even half of what economists agree is the economic value of a prevented birth— that is, one to two times the annual per caput income (which in 1964

Table 4. Annual national budgets (authorized) for family planning programs— Spring 1967* (approximate figures)

	Total budget	Per caput	Per MWRA
India	$60,000,000	$.12	$.72
Pakistan	12,000,000	.11	.66
South Korea	2,150,000	.07	.42
Taiwan	425,000	.035	.21
Turkey	851,000	.028	.16
U.A.R.	2,300,000	.077	.45
Tunisia	500,000	.10	.60
Morocco	200,000	.015	.09
Malaysia	140,000	.016	.10
Singapore	120,000	.063	.38

*These data come from official plans, pro-rated to a single year, and/or from local representatives of technical assistance agencies. They are probably not precisely correct in every individual case but they are accurate in general order of magnitude. The MWRA figure, by rule of thumb, is 6 times the per capita figure.

was about \$140 in South Korea and \$180 in Taiwan). Indeed, any large-scale increase in funds would almost certainly be incapable of effective expenditure, or would meet political obstacles, or face bureaucratic difficulties over the preferential allocation of funds, or be simply unavailable (or unavailable in foreign exchange) long before it reached the point of economic inutility.

The Target Population
7. *There is interest in family planning among the people of the developing world: approval of the concept of family planning, desire for a substantially smaller family than present fertility will produce, interest in learning about family planning, desire for no more children now. And the major correlates of differential interest are virtually everywhere the same: education, parity and age, interval since last birth, but not particularly religion.*

If there has been one welcome surprise in the various surveys conducted on fertility matters over the past several years—welcome to family planning administrators and surprising to demographers— it has been the finding that there is more expressed interest in family planning than the experts had expected (or, in some cases, are yet willing to accept).[17]

In survey after survey from Asia to Latin America, a substantial proportion of respondents have indicated their desire to do something about fertility:[18]

"The most significant fact about the situation, therefore, was the large number of persons, both male and female, in the city as well as in the non-city area, who said that they would welcome information on the subject of family limitation and the substantial number among them who voluntarily said that they would immediately adopt the methods in practice. Positive opposition to family planning or limitation was surprisingly small in both the city and the non-city samples . . ."[19]

"There are strong indications that in general, women are not prejudiced against measures addressed to reducing their fertility.[20]

Now that we have the evidence of the surveys it is not hard to rationalize, or to understand, why the people of much of the developing world are interested in family planning (that is, at least in those parts of the developing world, as Table 2 suggests, where some betterment in the standard of living, some advance in education, and some decline in mortality have occurred). Having children is close to the heart of life, and it would be strange indeed if intelligent people did not see its relationship to life chances once some improvement in life's conditions comes about and is appreciated. After all, the single most cited reason for interest in family planning, in the developed as well as the developing world, is economic welfare of the family, including educational and occupational opportunities for the children. Nor is it hard to recognize that high fertility rates could in some part have been due to lack of suitable family planning information, services, and supplies rather than simply to traditional high fertility attitudes.

Nor, on the other side of the coin, is it hard to appreciate why such interest is not translated at the first opportunity into continuous, effective family planning. There is some natural ambivalence at the adoption of any important innovation, especially when the whole community is not simultaneously moving in the same direction—a proposition that applies to educated people in the developed world as well as to illiterate peasants. But beyond that is a lesson that the field has only gradually learned, and not yet completely: namely, that the realization of expressed interest is closely tied to the acceptability of the contraceptive technology available at the time. The greater the interest, the more will effective contraception be practiced at a given level of technology. The better the technology ("better" for the given population in convenience, cost, effectiveness, safety, etc.), the more will effective contraception be practiced at a given level of interest.

This basic relationship is of critical importance. In every society at a particular time there is a range of interest in family planning— from the people who desperately want a child *now* to the woman who will risk a non-medical induced abortion rather than have another child. And there is a curve of interest in between. The interest curve for different countries varies with respect to some conceivable absolute curve of interest: thus, there is more interest in family planning in the highly developed countries than in the developing, but the curves overlap, as depicted schematically in Figure 1.[21] The point is that a better technology cuts further down into any curve of interest than a poorer one, even though the very highly motivated can make do with the latter; and, hence, a given level of interest will be translated into actual practice more fully with a better technology. So an expression of interest is still an expression, but one of the main elements in turning it into behavior is the available technology (of which more later).

The same curves, drawn for various segments of the community (e.g., educated and uneducated), would show some (but less) distribution within segments and substantial differentiation between them, but still with some overlapping. This is to say that some parts of the community are readier for family planning than other parts—notably,

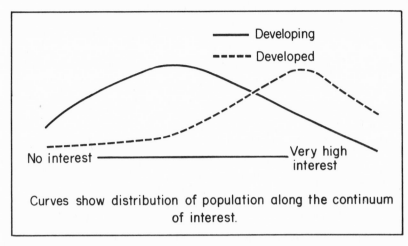

Figure 1. Schematic Curves of Interest in Family Planning: Developing and Developed Countries

the better educated, the higher parity (including sons) and hence the somewhat older, and the recently delivered (illustrative data on actual acceptances in Table 5; similar information is available on expressed interest and even on IUD termination rates[22]). The first of these can

Table 5. Personal characteristics and acceptance of family planning

	Percentage of each group accepting IUD (approx.)*	
	South Korea	*Taiwan*
By number of living children		
None or one	2%	4%
Two	7%	16%
Three	18%	26%
Four	29%	24%
Five or more	37%	21%
By age		
Under 25	3%	8%
25 - 29	14%	20%
30 - 34	29%	28%
35 - 39	29%	23%
40 - 44	23%	12%
By date of latest birth		
Over 30 months	8%	11%
Within 30 months	43%	24%

*Korean data from Ministry of Health & Social Affairs, *National Intra-Uterine Contraception Report,* June 1966. Taiwan data kindly provided by Ronald Freedman of Population Studies Center, University of Michigan.

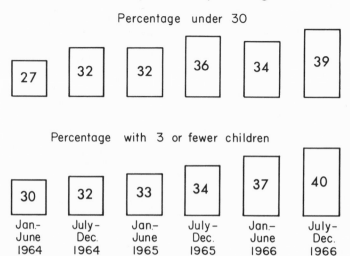

Figure 2. Age and Parity of IUD Acceptors in Taiwan

be considered responsive to modernization—what will happen as the developing countries extend popular schooling and move toward a modern social establishment in general. The others demonstrate that demographic factors are more influential in the mass population than social or psychological factors—influential, that is, in response to an intensive and deliberate effort to spread family planning as against response to the general trend toward modernization, in which case educational and social status is the most important factor.[23]

In these respects, the present pattern in the developing countries follows that of the West decades earlier, as it also does with respect to stopping as against spacing: the former is the first expression of family planning within a society and the latter follows only later. How much later is not really known but there are at least two favorable indications. In the advantaged situation of Taiwan, the average age and average parity of acceptors in the national program have been slowly declining even in this brief period (Figure 2). So the program there has not been "running out" of acceptors, in absolute figures, and the practice of family planning has filtered down the demographic pyramid by 10 percentage points in only 3 years. This is an important counter, and so is the Korean situation, to the widely held position that a program "skims the cream" of the highly motivated in its first efforts and then slows down. The opposite position, that the social appetite grows by what it feeds on, seems more likely at this stage, certainly so far as these two programs are concerned. Similarly, the Population Council's postpartum program, designed to reach women through hospitals at the time of delivery and directly thereafter, is beginning to show that young and low parity women will start family planning under those conditions, as can be seen by comparison with the national programs of South Korea and Taiwan (Table 6).[24]

There is, finally, a very practical factor, namely, proximity to the service. Every director of marketing knows that it is wasteful to develop an interest in his product if he cannot satisfy that interest—i.e., if the product is not on a convenient shelf. Similarly with family planning: it must be nearby as well as acceptable in principle. The difference that availability can make has been demonstrated recently with regard to the non-publicized program at Chulalongkorn Hospital in Bangkok, Thailand. Within twelve months after the hospital opened an IUD clinic, it had served 12,000 women, many of them from far out into the provinces of Thailand (as noted above, one or more acceptors had come from 54 of Thailand's 71 provinces). Still, the major impact was made close at hand: 19.8 acceptors per 1000 married women 20-44 from Bangkok itself as against 14.5 in "near" provinces, 4.1 in "intermediate", and 0.3 in "distant."[25] The administrative message is clear: availability is a variable too, and proximity to services is important along with other variables.

Those are characteristics of the individual. What of religion? To begin with, the major religious controversy over family planning in the world today, within the Catholic Church, seems to involve the doctrine of the leaders rather more than it does the behavior of the adherents. In Western Europe, the Catholic countries have quite low

Table 6. Comparison of age & parity distributions of initial acceptors from national programs and post-partum program

	Age distribution: percentages						
	24 & under	25- 29	30- 34	35- 39	40 & over	Total	Median
Korean & Taiwan programs	5%	23	34	26	12	100%	33.2
Post-partum program (direct acceptors)	35%	29	22	10	4	100%	26.5

	Parity distribution: percentages					
	2 or fewer children	3	4	5 & more	Total	Median
Korean & Taiwan programs	11%	19	25	45	100%	4.8
Post-partum program (direct acceptors)	40%	18	13	29	100%	2.6

birth rates—Italy 19.2, Spain 21.3, Austria 17.9, France 17.7—that almost certainly reflect the use of non-licit contraception; and, indeed, a Catholic country now has what is probably the highest ratio of legal abortions to births (Hungary, with 1.4 legal abortions for every birth).[26] In the United States, the latest survey shows that just over half of all Catholic women were using contraceptive methods not approved by Church doctrine.[27] In Latin America, major studies have concluded that Catholic belief is not a substantial barrier to the use of modern contraception:

> "The behavior of Catholic women toward this subject does not seem to be very different from that of other women."[28]

> "We may conclude . . . that (the Catholic) religion is no real impediment to realization of low-fertility ideals."[29]

Liberalization in the official Catholic position, should it ever come, might affect the practice of Catholics more indirectly than directly: that is, more by releasing the inhibitions of governmental elites with regard to sponsoring family planning programs than by releasing the conscience of the laity.

Actually, the Moslems are the religious community of world dimension with the highest fertility.[30] But here, too, most experts believe that Moslem fertility is based less on theological doctrine than on the traditional subordination of women in Moslem culture. Similarly, any inhibition to family planning among Hindus in India is probably attributable more to philosophical fatalism than to religious doctrine.

In short, it seems clear that formal religious considerations are of greater importance to the elite than to the masses; and that the broad social trends that everywhere affect the conditions of life— like industrialization, urbanization, popular education, and mortality rates—have more impact on fertility behavior.

The Contraceptive Technology

8. *The contraceptive technology is a key element in the spread of effective family planning: almost certainly, over the short run, an acceptable innovation in method results in more family planning than change in attitudes.*

The schematic curves shown above are on a long historical trend in the developing countries toward the acceptance of family planning as a way of life—the whole curve is, so to speak, moving to the right. Even if the technology remains fixed, there will be a larger proportion of family planners 10 or 25 years from now. But it does appear to be easier to reach larger proportions through changes in the technology than through shifts in attitudes. The major evidence for this viewpoint is provided by the IUD (and to a much lesser and just emerging extent, the oral pill). Of the new acceptors of family planning in the developing world in the past 5 years, as a result of national programs, of the order of 60-65 percent are accounted for by the IUD—and fully 80 percent in the more successful efforts in South Korea and Taiwan. Despite the recent discouragement with the IUD in some circles, in the light of allegedly low retention rates, it is still true that a great deal of whatever progress has been made since 1962 is attributable to that device.[31]

The contribution of the IUD has been both direct and indirect. Directly, in the developing world, it has provided protection to no fewer than four million women (estimated as of June 1967)—on the average protection of about 3½ or 4 years in duration. That has prevented, say, 2.5 million births.[32]

Indirectly, by giving national programs some hope of success, the IUD stimulated a wholly new level of effort, improved the morale of family planning workers from the top down, and, most importantly, brought about the development of family planning organizations in a form and magnitude not previously known. Whatever new contraceptive method emerges over the next years will benefit from the network of doctors, administrators, and field workers now in existence thanks largely to this device.

But the IUD is not without its difficulties. At the outset it faced the obstacle natural to any innovation within the medical community: it had to make its way again and again as different national committees came to test its effectiveness in their own countries. More than that, however, the IUD has had to contend with the inevitable disappointment once the honeymoon of first enthusiasm was over—that is, when "high" termination rates due to expulsion and removal became apparent.[33]

The history of the device to date, indeed, is an excellent case study of the innovation from which a very great deal is expected: too much optimism over the promise, too much pessimism over the performance. The fact is that despite the usual termination rates the IUD remains the best contraceptive method for mass programs available today: no other contraceptive can make its claims. Ironically, the disappointment over performance is due to the thorough follow-up to which the IUD has been subjected: we simply have more information on continuation rates with that device than with any other contraceptive method in mass use. In this sense, it has been a casualty of its own thorough research and the resulting knowledge.

However useful the IUD has been, and is, it is clear that it will not do the whole job by itself. Or, to put the matter more positively, the field needs several contraceptive methods of equivalent value or better. What of the other major contraceptive innovation of recent years, the oral pill? To date, largely due to costs, the pill has been used far more in the developed countries than the developing (used by about 25 percent of women in some of the former compared to not over 4 percent in any of the latter, or an estimated total of about 10 million users to about 2.9 million).[34] In the developing world, the pill is used almost entirely by the better-off people in the cities. Now that costs have come down considerably, a few programs are beginning to test acceptability and particularly continuity of the regimen under field conditions.

The results are not yet in: perhaps it is only fair to add that this is one of the field's major failures in evaluation, that we do not know what place the pill can fill in a mass program. One national effort based on the pill, in the United Arab Republic, has been so plagued by organizational and personnel difficulties (not to mention national problems) that no sound conclusions can be drawn. The pill programs in Singapore and Malaysia seem to be making progress. Where the pill is being tried experimentally, in South Korea and Taiwan, the findings to date seem to be that initial acceptance is equivalent to the IUD but that continuation is rather worse.

One might say, on the basis of experience to date, that any method that can be satisfactorily used by, say, 15 percent of the target population is a useful method. The 15 percent criterion does not at all rule out some traditional pre-IUD methods, notably the condom and sterilization (and, for that matter, coitus interruptus, though no national program has yet found a way to promote its use). Especially when subsidized, the condom is still a useful adjunct to family planning programs almost everywhere—and, again almost everywhere, despite "informed" beliefs to the contrary.

Sterilization is a contributory method in some countries though limited by the availability of medical personnel (and by custom: male sterilization in India, female in Taiwan). Of the impact to date, about 8 percent in South Korea but as much as 40 percent in India is attributable to sterilization. The major advantage of sterilization as a contraceptive method is its effectiveness. The major disadvantage is the other side of the same coin: its irreversibility limits it to stopping (as against spacing) and hence to clients of quite high parity. (Even in India, where sterilization has been most widespread as a contraceptive method, we have only fragmentary data on the relative parity of sterilized men as against IUD wearers. But what data there are suggest that the parity distributions are quite similar: a median of 5.3 for IUD wearers in the Punjab compared to 5.0 for sterilized cases in Trichur district in Trivandrum.)[35] Given equivalent parity, what is more valuable: the greater effectiveness of sterilization or the greater applicability of the IUD or the pill to the practice of spacing, later on?

It remains to mention what at least one leading observer has characterized as possibly "the most widely used single method (of family limitation) in the world today,"[36] namely, abortion. Induced abortion is legal in some countries (though nowhere as a measure of population control), illegal but openly tolerated in others, illegal and not tolerated in still others—and common everywhere. Estimates are not very reliable, for obvious reasons, but it would seem that a significant proportion of all conceptions in the developing world are terminated by induced abortion: no one knows the figure but in South Korea and Chile it is reported to be of the order of one-third to one-fourth.[37]

That abortion is now an important method of family limitation there can be no doubt. That it would make a significant contribution to family planning programs if utilized wherever there are medical doctors in any number—there can be little doubt of that either. The place of abortion within moral systems should of course be left to the various societies for local decision. At this time, at least three countries in Asia (South Korea, Singapore, and India) are reviewing their own legal position with regard to abortion, and with regard to its use as a method of family limitation; and Tunisia now allows abortions if the pregnancy is less than three months, if the request is made in writing, and if the parents have at least five living children (and from July 1965, when the law went into effect, to March 1967 there were nearly 2000 "social abortions").

To repeat, for deliberate emphasis, the contraceptive technology is of critical importance in national family planning programs.[38] Almost certainly, more effective contraception will result over a 5-10 year period from a major advance in technology than from information and persuasive efforts—that is, from a lower cut in the interest curves illustrated above than from moving the curves.[39] National family planning programs now need a great many things, but they particularly need advances in the technology of birth control—advances perceived as substantial improvements by the people for whom they are intended.[40] Aside from its other advantages, the new method also benefits from informal diffusion—it is the *new* method that is spread by word of mouth.[41]

The Impact of Programs
9. *Any reasonable form of delivering family planning services to the people will have some worthwhile, measurable effect—perhaps about as much effect as any other reasonable form.*

With a given contraceptive technology and a given level of interest in family planning—and both *are* given at a particular point in time—any way of bringing the one to the other may be as good as any other way. This is, then, a testimony to the strength of those two factors, and a signal that efficiency becomes particularly important when effectiveness is roughly equivalent.

It is still too early to be sure of this, but at least one can say that a variety of ways of taking modern (i.e., post-IUD) family planning to the people has worked, most of them to roughly the same extent. In addition to the typical effort of field workers in contact with women individually or in groups, several other means have been used and have yielded worthwhile results—worthwhile both in effectiveness and in efficiency (Table 7). The situations in Table 7 are widely different, both in approach and in geographical and cultural setting, but in every case a worthwhile impact was made. It would appear that even with the present state of the art in contraceptive technology, a rea-

Table 7. Various "special" ways of bringing family planning to people, and the results[43]

The Effort	The Result
India: Use of community leaders in 59 villages to inform and to distribute traditional contraceptives (Gandhigram)	7-fold increase of condom use over average of one-year period to about 1000 per thousand population per year, or say 150 eligible couples; and 6-fold increase of vasectomies to rate of 8.5 per thousand population—together achieving an approximate 12 percent of contraceptors as against approximately 2 percent at the outset
Pakistan: Use of local shopkeepers for sale of traditional contraceptives, in village population of 150,000 (Comilla)	In 3 months 111 shops selling 1000 dozen contraceptives per month; a year later, 250 shops and 2000 dozen per month. Estimate: approximately 15 percent of eligible couples reached
Turkey: Mobile teams bringing family planning services to rural district with total population of 59,500	Acceptance of contraception (mostly IUD, some pills) by 8-10 percent of MWRA in five weeks of service by 4 professionals
Tunisia: Group meetings on family planning by local workers of the political party, as part of regular party meetings; in one region before mobile IUD team comes to village and in the other in preparation for transport of clients to central hospital for IUD insertion	Acceptance by 6-7 percent of MWRA in the experimental areas, over a period of 10 months

Table 7.—Cont.

The Effort	The Result
Taiwan: Free offer for a limited time only given in 2 rural townships with 50,000 population	Acceptances from 20 percent of MWRA in first 3 months
Referral fee instituted for people in personal contact with community (mainly salespeople) in township with 45,000 population	IUD acceptances by 18 percent of target population in 18 months
Korea: Differentiated program featuring mass media, in district of Seoul with total population of 370,000 (45,000 MWRA)	Acceptances of family planning by 19 percent of the total MWRA or 58 percent of the "immediately eligible" in first 18 months
Thailand: Short-run field program featuring IUD in rural district (Photharam) of about 10,000 households, with intensive face-to-face educational program	"Acceptors of contraception" in before-and-after survey increased from 1 percent to 18 percent of MWRA in over 26 months. In addition, acceptors from outside the district outnumbered those from inside by more than 2 to 1.
Post-partum program: Family planning information offered at time of delivery, service provided then or at postpartum visit in 25 hospitals in 14 countries	Average of about 350 acceptors per hospital per month; one in every 4-5 obstetrical patients and an equivalent number from the community at large; acceptors of relatively low age and parity.

sonably energetic and systematic approach will at least start family planning with one segment of the community.

Thus, the lower limit is beginning to be visible; the upper limit surely varies by "modernization" of the society but is not yet really known. But it now seems clear that a market of more than insignificant size exists wherever a programmatic effort has been vigorously applied. In point of fact, every effort to spread family planning that has been carried out with thoroughness, energy, and continuity— with only one or two doubtful exceptions—has yielded promising results in actual acceptances. If it *is* done, it can be done: that is a finding whose importance is hard to overstate. The question then becomes: Can a given country or district sustain such an effort?

By the same token, a purely clinical service will not do. The program needs to take information and service to the people and cannot expect them to take the full initiative. To this end field workers are needed. In South Korea, there are 2377 full-time field workers, or one per 5000 married women of reproductive age in urban areas and one per 1500 in rural areas; in Taiwan, about 300, or one per 6500; in Pakistan, about 33,000 "organizers" (native midwives who work part-time for the program on both salary and fee).[42]

In marketing any new product, sales personnel are important—and no less here. It is no coincidence that the more successful programs to date, like Korea and Taiwan, have not only recruited a substantial core of such workers that give them a ratio of one worker to 1500-2000 of the target population, but have trained and retrained them and have given reasonably close supervision to their activities. And there is evidence from Taiwan that such input is directly correlated with results: the decline in fertility by district is correlated with the number of field workers operating in the district, as well as with the availability of doctors for IUD insertion.[44] So setting up clinics for family planning, as formerly in India and now in Turkey, will secure some acceptors from the immediate clientele but will not have the necessary mass impact. Field work in some form is apparently needed.

10. *A few national programs under favorable conditions have kept up with ambitious targets and have probably lowered the birth rate in the process. But over the short run (say, five to ten years), there is a natural limit on how much can be done, and only in the advantaged situations is the take-off point likely to be approached.*

The key question on the impact of a national program is clear: has it brought down the birth rate and, if so, by how much? That question cannot be answered unequivocally at the present time. Among other things, it must be qualified by programmatic, technical, and temporal considerations.

Let us begin with targets. Several of the active programs have established five- or ten-year targets—targets stated in birth rate, growth rate, and/or (sometimes derivatively) acceptances of contraceptive methods (Table 8). By and large, within a short period of years, the programs seek to lower the birth rate by 10-15 points and the growth rate by one percentage point—targets which require the program to make about 25-30 percent of the population into effective family planners. Targets are arbitrary, so can easily be met if set low enough. If anything, however, targets for acceptances have been put on the high side in most programs in order to "push" the personnel. The trick is to set a target that is just beyond the reach—enough to stimulate effort but not so much as to depress morale over anticipated failure. By and large, developing countries are now aiming at the birth rates of Western Europe 75 years ago or the United States 50 years ago.

Such goals have not yet been met anywhere—but active pro-

Table 8. Targets set for national family planning programs

	In birth rate	*In growth rate*	*In acceptances*
India	40 to 25 in 10 years		Current year: 2 million IUD's, 1 million sterilizations, 1.5 new users of conventional contraceptives
Pakistan	50 to 40 by 1970		
South Korea		2.9 in 1962 to 2.0 in 1971	1,000,000 IUD wearers 150,000 vasectomies 150,000 users of traditional contraceptives by 1971
Taiwan	36 in 1963 to 24 in 1973	3.02 in 1965 to 1.86 in 1973	600,000 IUD's in 5 years
Tunisia			120,000 IUD's in 2 years
Ceylon	33 to 25 in 8-10 years	1.6 in 1976	550,000 practicing couples by 1976
Singapore	30 to under 20 in 5 years		
Turkey		3.0 to 2.0 by 1972	5 percent of MWRA per year or 2 million by 1972
Malaysia		3.0 to 2.2 in 20 years	
Dominican Republic	48 to 40 in 4 years to 28 in 10 years	3.4 to 2.7 by 1972	2.5 million acceptors in 10 years; 1.5 million IUD's, one million other
Morocco	50 to 45 by 1973		600,000 IUD acceptors; 200,000 other acceptors
Trinidad & Tobago	38 to 19 in 10 years		

grams of national scope have not yet existed anywhere for as long as five years.[45] Where national programs have been vigorously prosecuted in the past few years, notably in the IUD program of South Korea and Taiwan, some indications are beginning to emerge that demonstrate a movement of the birth rate toward the target. In South Korea, the child-woman ratio (i.e., children up to age 5 per 1000 women age 15-44) of 851 in 1960 has steadily declined to 658 in 1965 as acceptances have risen—not proof, of course, but substantial evidence when put together with the results of KAP surveys in that country showing the sharp increase of contraception.

In Taiwan, where long-term fertility decline is in process, the Taichung effort appeared to affect the birth rate in that city: in the subsequent period, allowing for the proper lag, the birth rate in Taichung declined by 9 points as against only 6 points in other Taiwan cities. More recently there are two additional pieces of evidence, both provided by the exemplary evaluation conducted there by the Taiwan and Michigan Population Studies Centers. In the one case, the fertility of women who ever had an IUD inserted "has been reduced by from 56-80 percent over pre-insertion fertility levels."[46] In the other case, the urban townships with the highest and the lowest acceptance rates show not only a significant shift in fertility but also the importance of proximity to doctors:[47]

	10 townships with highest acceptance rates	10 townships with lowest acceptance rates
Fertility rate in 1963	5313	5286
Percent change before program, 1961-1963	−6.7	−6.9
Percent change after program, 1963-1965	−12.6	−5.3
Effort index for:		
field workers	19	13
doctors	71	31

Beyond such comparative evidence, there are inferences from recent analyses of births averted by IUD insertions, in the articles by Potter and Mauldin *et al.* previously referred to, which begin to show an effect on the birth rate equivalent to a reduction of the order of 3-5 points (given plausible assumptions about alternative practices).[48] If this result holds up under further inquiry, this is a notable first in the history of mankind: the first time a birth rate has declined under deliberate programmatic effort.

As everyone acknowledges, South Korea and Taiwan are favorable situations: compact geographically, high literacy, well served by medical resources, rising standard of living and of popular education, not too large. What of India and Pakistan? It is too early to say how those large programs are doing in their revised form, yet it is clear that family planning must succeed on that sub-continent (and in Mainland China) if the world's population problem is to be, not solved, but significantly ameliorated. Unfortunately, good detailed information on program results in India and Pakistan does not appear to be currently available, although the general reports are more encouraging in the past two years than previously. What can be said is that both programs face tremendous difficulties on almost every score; that Pakistan appears to be making progress under the current reorganization; and that India can show encouraging results to date mainly in a few states and in national figures for sterilization.

Leaving aside birth rates for the moment and dealing only with acceptances, it does appear that national programs have been able to double existing levels of contraception within the first few years of an active program—from under 9 percent to over 20 percent in South Korea in two years, from about 19 percent to about 40 percent in Taichung in three years, perhaps from 3-4 percent in Pakistan and India to double that in the first two years of the revitalized programs. And as we noted above, virtually every demonstration project carried out in a limited area, regardless of the mode of approach, has resulted in a substantial increase in family planning practice.

In any case, the question of impact on birth rates, with one exception, is now incapable of a direct answer because of technical difficulties, and that will probably be true for the next five years as well. Outside of Taiwan in the developing world, the system of vital statistics will not provide the necessary data; and even there a definitive answer is hard to come by because of analytic technicalities (particularly, how to determine what would have happened to fertility in the absence of the program).[49] Accordingly, program impact for the next period will rest mainly on acceptance figures and what flows from them: e.g., Pakistan's measure of "couple years of protection against pregnancy" or efforts to infer births prevented from use. In the absence of the direct measure, difficult at best, the indirect will have to do.

All of which raises a central question about a program's impact: what is "success"? Is a program "successful" if it reduces the birth rate by 10 points in three to five years? If it meets a predetermined target? If it secures 10 percent of the married women of reproductive age as initial acceptors in its first year of operation? If it secures 10 percent of the married women of reproductive age as continuing acceptors in its first year of operation? If it institutionalizes family planning within a society in the sense that it is now institutionalized in Western Europe or the United States? These and other definitions of "success" can be given, and such a list is useful if only in demonstrating how arbitrary the term can be.[50] So long as the specifics are known, the term itself adds little but propaganda value, one way or the other.

What is important, however, is to have some notion about natural limitations on a program's achievement. In any period of a few years —and the history of this field in the past five years shows how rapidly events have moved—there are some crucial "given's" in the situation, notably the level of popular interest, the contraceptive technology, and, to a lesser degree, the capacity of the family planning organization. These factors impose limits on what any program can do in the short run.

Program impact in that period, then, can thus be seen as a race toward two points: which will be reached first? One is the saturation point: the proportion of family planners beyond which a program can reach only with special difficulties and extra efforts. The other is the take-off point: the proportion of family planners within a society that is large enough to disseminate the practice without major input from a governmental program. The United States today can illustrate both points: family planning reached the take-off point decades ago and produced an essentially controlled fertility for about 85-90 percent of the society, the other segment being outside the mainstream of the society in other respects as well, as members of the ethnic poor. For them, special governmental programs need to be devised and are in process at this time.

In the developing countries, what is the take-off point? South Korea and Taiwan have already, in only a few years, brought family planning to well over 20 percent of the married women of reproductive age, and the programs are still in full swing. We do not know what the take-off point is for any reasonably large interacting population, though in my judgment it is not likely to be lower than 50 percent. Whatever it is, will it be reached before the program loses momentum? We do not know that either, though one can guess that the answer is favorable in the advantaged sites and doubtful in the others.

The Guidance of Programs
11. *The evaluation of family planning programs is not easy in principle, and in practice the record is mixed.*

The objective of evaluation is to contribute to the effectiveness and the efficiency of family planning programs by determining what in fact is happening among the several segments and sub-targets of the program and by suggesting better ways of operation. To date that objective has been continuously met in only one national program (Taiwan), though partial approaches have been successful elsewhere (notably in Korea), and in one international effort (the postpartum program).

The major problem is the technical difficulty of establishing sound data on increasingly complicated matters. It may not seem hard to collect good statistics on the services offered and/or accepted, by type and characteristics of recipients, but even that is not easy to do in a systematic and timely way and from a large number of sources (field workers, clinics, doctors, health stations, etc.) Beyond that, the conduct of a good survey requires a high degree of applied expertise, in sampling, interviewing, coding, and analysis. Still more difficult is a population growth estimate study designed to secure valid data on vital events (birth and death rates, mainly); to date, such studies have not been a typical feature of family planning programs as such, though they are in progress under different auspices in Pakistan and Turkey. Given the importance of these several measures, and particularly with the growing scope of the effort, there is an increasing body of work on the technical apparatus that promises to put the field in a better methodological position within the next few years.[51]

Furthermore, there are conceptual and/or administrative difficulties in determining just what is to be measured, along the continuum of potential measures: meetings held, messages distributed, clinic visits, expressed interest, initial acceptances, continuing acceptances, births prevented, birth rate, health of mothers, educational achievement of the children, economic status of the family . . . development of the society. Evaluating the consequences of a deliberate program of family planning is not hard at the top of such a list, but it quickly becomes so as one moves along. In general, the evaluational efforts so far have dealt mainly with initial acceptances, in the better ones with continuation data, and only recently with birth data—and that largely on an inferential basis. As noted, only in Taiwan can a more direct measure be expected in the next period of years, because of the absence elsewhere of a proper system of vital statistics.

The range of possibilities itself raises a central question: should research and evaluation be conducted primarily for administrative ends or for scientific ends? True enough, these ends are by no means incompatible—certainly not in the long run—but a question of emphasis often arises, out of competitive claims on resources if nothing else.[52] The needs of administrative guidance and of scientific knowledge are not identical,[53] and only in the unusual case (again Taiwan) are they both satisfied adequately, thanks to the invention of the coupon system that serves both administrative and research purposes, to the availability of vital data and to the exemplary collaboration of the Taiwan and Michigan Population Studies Centers.

Partly, proper evaluation has been slow to get underway because the programs have been slow: there needs to be something to evaluate. Partly it has been the scarcity of skilled personnel, and partly the indifference of the top administrators. But surely the need for good figures on program progress, for monitored demonstrations, for clues to better tactics, for cost-benefit analysis, and the like is increasingly recognized by responsible administrators as programs mature; and hopefully a corresponding recognition is growing among research scholars of the need for attention to short-run administrative relevance. Indeed, a case can be made that the "operations research" studies of the Taiwan program (as reported, for example, in *Studies in Family Planning*, No. 13, August 1966) have contributed more to the national program than several formal research projects in other countries. And, of course, suggestions on how to improve the programs come directly from non-research, operating field personnel.

Finally, the contribution of research to what might broadly be termed political purposes should not be underestimated. A survey may be more important, strategically, in demonstrating public interest to a handful of influential politicians than in advancing knowledge or identifying targets. A demonstration effort may be more important in showing the government that professed interest can be met with no political liabilities than in showing the informed administrator anything he did not already know. A research program in demography can begin to involve the university, and one in reproductive physiology the medical community. In short, there are, as we have been reminded, several "non-research uses of research."[54]

12. *Family planning on the one hand and general socioeconomic development on the other both require greater application, but the range of opportunities in between needs more attention in the next years.*

On a problem of this magnitude and importance, even if everything reasonable and possible is done, will that be "enough"? In the abstract, the answer is "No": on any great social problem we can never do "enough." But the question does alert us to review the whole continuum of conditions related to fertility decline, especially by way of anticipating the alternatives of the near future.

Think of such a continuum bounded on one end by contraception and on the other by those broad, historical trends that have stimulated fertility decline in the past, like industrialization, probably urbanization, popular education, and the like. The former is what national programs now deal with, almost exclusively; the latter are what development or modernization programs in general are aimed at, and they both require and will effect basic shifts in the social structure. Any movement on the latter front will have a favorable impact on the spread of contraception—and indeed has already done so, without doubt, in the two successful efforts now underway in South Korea and Taiwan. Still, direct effort on contraception is worthwhile in itself, as a contribution to the speeding-up of this element in the overall development equation: we need not wait until everything is done before doing something.

But there is a range of opportunities, along the continuum between contraception and development, that need to be considered by the makers of policy in the light of their own situations. I do not intend here to be either comprehensive or systematic about them, but only to call attention to a set of considerations usually cast in shadow by family planning activities on the one hand and general development on the other. Here are some possibilities, starting with where we now are:

Contraception: temporary (IUD, pill, condom, rhythm, etc.)
Contraception: permanent (sterilization)
Induced abortion
Institutionalization of maternal care, as a means for promotion of family planning, and particularly spacing, among other benefits
Inclusion of population material in all primary and secondary school programs
Development of an anti-natalist system of social services (e.g., pensions to couples reaching age 45 with fewer than N children)
Development of a system of negative incentives (e.g., tax burdens for over N children, educational benefits for the first N only, bonuses for child spacing)
Legal increase in minimum age at marriage and/or bonuses for delayed marriage
Promotion of light industry deliberately to attract a female labor force; legislation providing equal labor force benefits for women
Extension of popular education, and equivalently for girls
Establishment of a national system of television, for both direct use for family planning and indirect use for modernization programs in general
General development

Contraception and abortion have already been discussed. The institutionalization of maternal care, to bring some skilled attention to every pregnant woman in the developing world, is of obvious desirability on health and humanitarian grounds, quite aside from its contribution to population concerns. It seems feasible on all considerations except perhaps costs, and even there, a case can be made for its being an economic venture when the consequences are fully taken into account. The position has been put,[55] and careful studies are now being proposed.[56]

Including material on population in the school curriculum—on population, note, not on family planning—seems similarly valuable simply for its educational impact. The job just needs to be done, and here again the case has been made and materials are available.[57]

The next two possibilities can be considered together, since they tend to merge at the edges. The historical evidence appears to be that pro-natalist policies were not particularly effective—again testifying, incidentally, to the strength of fertility attitudes. Perhaps anti-natalist policies would do no better under prevailing conditions, but in view of the tenacity of such notions as the need for sons in India in lieu of social security system, the idea dies hard. Some thought and perhaps experimentation on the utility of such social intervention seem desirable.[58] As for negative incentives, the danger is that their burden will fall upon the children themselves, and that should of course be avoided. But there, too, some ingenuity seems both possible and needed.

Delaying age of marriage would have an important demographic effect through shifting to later fertility patterns and thus lengthening the generational span. A major analysis of this matter concluded "that postponement of marriage can contribute substantially to reduction in birth rates and population growth even when completed size of family is *not* reduced, and that this contribution is potentially greatest in those countries which have the highest fertility and low average age of marriage."[59] However, even in this hypothetical case, a 20 percent decline in fertility from 1956 to 1966 would have accounted for significantly fewer births in India over the next decades, and increasingly with time, than an age shift in fertility patterns bringing Indian practice into correspondence with that of the Singapore Chinese—a shift of about 2.5 years. The problem is, of course, how to bring about such a shift: changing the law, as is now under consideration in India, may help but will certainly not do the job in itself. Will social arrangements or educational campaigns to raise age of marriage be more effective than the effort to spread contraception? How is age of marriage to be raised in the absence of reinforcing social changes?[60]

The incorporation of women into the labor force has tended to lower fertility wherever it has occurred, as it may now be doing in South Korea. Here too, we do not know what the direct fertility effect over the short run would be, and hence what is the equivalence in contraception. Given the difficulties in promoting this shift in tradition, the promotion of light industry or labor force benefits for this purpose appears to hold promise only in countries already moving quite rapidly toward development. But again the appropriate question is: Which is easier to effect?

As for popular education and television their contributions would seem to be obvious, but the difficulties and costs are of course great. Fortunately, there are now some serious studies of what it would take —in facilities and costs—to develop an operating network of television for, say India; and with satellite transmission some of the technical problems can now be met.[61] It would seem highly likely that substantial benefits toward modernization in general and family planning in particular would accrue if every Indian village had two or three functioning television sets with a variety of educational and informational programming along with entertainment. At the very least, here would be an effective way of reaching the people in the countryside.

There may be several other plans that would effect some decline in fertility, directly or indirectly, beyond present efforts and short of full-scale transformation of the society.[62] This list only suggests some forward consideration of additional possibilities beyond those now in operation, including the practical problems of administration. To the extent that present efforts fall short of the goal, what are we prepared to do? It would seem that some such consideration of middle-range opportunities would be useful both for those who feel that contraception itself is sufficient and for those who feel that birth control is impossible in the absence of basic institutional change and unnecessary in its presence. But a key question is: How do the supplementary or additional proposals compare with family planning itself, given the realities? It is not obvious that they are automatically preferable.

By Way of Conclusion
13. *National programs of family planning have made considerable progress in the past few years, but still have a long way to go.*

Note, in capsule form, how much improvement has occurred in this field in a short period of years, essentially since 1960 and, even more, toward this end of this period. The field has moved from expressing alarm over the population problem to setting up organized and staffed efforts to do something about it—from the prophets to the operators[63]; from thinking that the people of the developing world were uninterested in family planning to learning that large proportions are interested; from complaining about the inappropriateness of the available methods to having one, perhaps two, much better methods, with others perhaps not far off; from worrying that only a very few would accept programmed contraception to finding out that good numbers would, when it was properly offered; from worrying that programs would quickly "skim the cream" of the highly motivated and then collapse to seeing that acceptances themselves tend to create a new situation of social support and thus work toward sustaining the effort in a dynamic way; from believing that cultural and social-psychological factors were dominant barriers to recognizing the importance of the couple's own demographic situation; from working hard on change of attitude (the small-family norm) to working hard on change of behavior (contraceptive practice); from citing the lack of ideas to citing the lack of implementation; from despairing about imperfect knowledge to appreciating how deficient we are in simply doing what, if done, would make a worthwhile difference.

And, not to lose sight of a notably worthwhile difference, the field has been instrumental in only the past few years in bringing voluntary family planning to something over 4 million couples. Leaving aside the population problem, that in itself is a worthy contribution to personal freedom and family welfare.

But, of course, the population problem cannot be left aside. If we are, as we say we are, working on one of the world's great problems, we must suit our actions to the claim. At least in my view—and it is only appropriate for me to repeat my warning at the outset, that this is one observer's view of the stage and what is happening thereon— the progress made on national family planning programs in a brief period of time is indeed impressive; the field promises to speed fertility decline by a number of decades over what would otherwise be the case; and the judgment of these recent years, despite all the disappointments, should on balance be favorable.

The challenge has just begun to be met—and partly with the distinctive contribution of The University of Michigan. When this great university was founded, the population of the world was about 900 million; today it is about 3.5 billion. Then the growth rate was about .5 percent; today it is over 2 percent. In the very nature of the problem, the next decades are crucial. When this university is 160 years old, or 175, what will the record show then: *fully* or *only*?

Notes

1. I am greatly indebted to Mrs. Dorothy Nortman, my colleague at The Population Council for her capable assistance in bringing together some of this material. Without her help, this paper would be the poorer, though I remain solely responsible for the views expressed.

2. My colleague James Fawcett makes this good observation: "In the same way that acceptance of family planning by *individuals* has been facilitated by a visible core group of users and by open discussion via mass media, acceptance by *nations* has been facilitated by the emergence of a group of developing countries with national programs and by spread of

information about national programs via news media and particularly international exchange visits and conferences among high government officials. What other countries are doing is a very persuasive element in moving countries toward a national family planning program."

3. S. M. Keeny in *Report to the Ministry of Health, Government of Iran, on Population Growth and Family Planning in Iran*, August, 1966.

4. T. R. Balakrishnan and Ravi J. Matthai, "India: Evaluation of a Publicity Program on Family Planning," *Studies in Family Planning*, no. 21, June 1967, p. 5-8.

5. Seoul National University, *Sungdong Gu Action-Research Project on Family Planning: A Progress Report for Period July 1964-December 1965. School of Public Health*, April 1966, p. 33, 62-63.

6. *Family Planning in Taiwan*, 1965-66, p. 126.

7. "Thailand: Family Growth in Pho-Tharam District," *Studies in Family Planning*, no. 8, Oct. 1965, p. 6.

8. "Thailand: An Analysis of Time and Distance Factors at an IUD Clinic in Bangkok," *Studies in Family Planning*, no. 19, May 1967, p. 12.

9. Seoul National University, *op. cit.*, 1966.

10. "International Post-Partum Family Planning Program," *Studies in Family Planning*, no. 22, Aug. 1967.

11. *Family Planning in Taiwan, 1965-1966*, p. v.

12. Ministry of Health and Social Affairs, *National Intra-uterine Contraception Report*, June 1966, p. 112.

13. I am indebted to personal communications from Dr. Moye Freymann and Dr. Ronald Freedman for this information. The substance has been "common knowledge" in the field but until very recently I had never seen any documentation of this highly important matter. Now, however, there is an important analysis of the experiment, in economic terms, and with a good deal of detailed information, in Chapter 5, "Time and Development Administration: A Case Study in Family Planning," in a Ph.D. dissertation by Robert Repetto, submitted to the Department of Economics of Harvard University, entitled "Temporal Elements of Indian Development." For an abridgement see *Studies in Family Planning* No. 31, May 1968, pp. 8-16.

14. For example, to cite two prominent U.S. demographers, the talks in the spring of 1967 by Kingsley Davis at the National Research Council and by Joseph Spengler at a conference on population at Indiana University. The former considers freedom of choice as "an article of faith" that is "ideologically self-limiting" and seems to be advocating economic penalties for too-large families (later published in *Science*, Nov. 10, 1967). The latter suggests "imposing tax and other economic burdens upon those producing more than three live births though in such wise as not to penalize the children." ("Agricultural Development Is Not Enough," p. 30).

15. Even if bonuses were accepted in principle, that is a far cry from finding an efficient mode of administration. To that end, my colleague Dr. Marshall Balfour in 1962 prepared a memorandum setting forth a practical scheme for providing bonuses to birth-free Indian women through use of postal savings certificates: "A Scheme for Rewarding Successful Family Planners," June 1962. On the general rationale, see Julian Simon, "The Role of Bonuses and Persuasive Propaganda in the Reduction of Birth Rates," forthcoming in *Economic Development and Cultural Change*; and the

remarks of Michael Young, Director of the Social Science Research Council in Britain, on the arrangement of social services for anti-natalist purposes, presented at a conference on "Behavioral Sciences and Family Planning Programs" held in June 1967 at the National Institutes of Health, in *Studies in Family Planning*, no. 23, Oct. 1967.

16. Which compares to 23-45¢ per capita to run large-scale malaria programs, according to John A. Ross, "Cost of Family Planning Programs," in Bernard Berelson et al., eds., *Family Planning and Population Programs*, (University of Chicago Press, 1966), p. 774. The costs are also low as a proportion of health budgets, except in South Korea and Pakistan, but even there the family planning funds are extra and do not come from the regular health budget.

17. One thrust of the "new wave" of criticism of present efforts is to question the validity of such reports: do the respondents mean what they say—or perhaps if so, do they *really* mean it? Now there are only two ways to find out what people believe: listen to what they say and watch what they do. Beyond the responses to direct questions in surveys, now under attack (e.g., in Philip Hauser's review of the Geneva Proceedings, *Demography*, 1967), various refinements to direct questions have been used, like projective-type questions (Jamaica), intensity questions (Turkey), hypothetical questions (Turkey), motivation scales (Thailand). Such refinements generally support the original responses but, at least in my opinion, do not add much of administrative utility. As for the direct question, Ronald Freedman makes the good point that to the extent responses are made just to please the investigator, at least respondents know what side the respected others take, and that in itself may be the first step (in Berelson et al., op. cit., p. 813).

The final test, of course, is behavior. In Korea, as an example, a highly sophisticated analysis showed that the respondent's answer to a simple question on desire for contraception was the single most differentiating factor in subsequent acceptance of contraception: 42 percent accepting of those who said "yes" as against 14 percent of those who said "no" (John Ross "Predicting the Adoption of Family Planning," *Studies in Family Planning*, No. 9, Jan. 1966, p. 8-12). These figures, incidentally, may help to clarify the issue: not every *individual* response is valid in the sense that everyone who says "yes" will adopt whatever means of family planning is offered and everyone who says "no" will not. But the *collective* response is valid in the sense that significantly more of those who say "yes" will do so than of those who say "no," and thus the total magnitude is of interest to policy-makers and administrators. Moreover, there are repeated surveys, as in Korea and Taiwan. And beyond the survey one would have thought that on broad policy grounds the diffusion material reported above as well as acceptance rates would serve as a valid indicator of women's interest in family planning, not to mention the incidence of induced abortions throughout the developing world.

18. Since I have recently reviewed the so-called KAP surveys from this point of view ("KAP Studies on Fertility," in Berelson et al., op. cit., p. 655-68), I forebear from doing so again here.

19. Kumudini Dandekar, "Family Planning Studies . . . etc. . . . .", in Clyde V. Kiser, ed., *Research in Family Planning*, (Princeton University Press, 1962), p. 5, reporting on one of the first Indian studies, in 1951.

20. Carmen A. Miro, "Some Misconceptions Disproved: A Program of Comparative Fertility Surveys in Latin America," in Berelson *et al., op. cit.,* p. 633.

21. A good view of the ambivalence among urban residents of a country situated at the left end of the interest continuum is provided in Thomas E. Dow, Jr. "Attitudes Toward Family Size and Family Planning in Nairobi," unpublished manuscript, 1967?, which concludes: "There is a paradox between the elements favorable to control and the attitudes and actions necessary to achieve it. This was particularly evident in the present study, in that people know of but did not use family planning; considered it good but did not practice it; recognized the general liabilities of large family size but expected and idealized a completed family size of six children. All this seems contradictory, but is actually evidence of a process that is simply not yet complete. These respondents, in their simultaneous endorsement of large family size and contraception, stand between two cultures, recognizing the advantages of control while at the same time holding family size ideals of a traditional character. Obviously, this position is not a stable one. Those who hold it are increasingly influenced by the requirements of modern urban life, and at the same time ever more aware of the consequences of large numbers. Under these circumstances, one would expect a gradual readjustment in desired family size, and hence a favorable resolution of this marginality. Indeed, in the presence of broad-based interest, knowledge and approval, one would be overly pessimistic not to anticipate a final stage of fertility control" (p. 15).

22. See L. P. Chow, R. Freedman, R. G. Potter Jr., and A. Jain, "Correlates of IUD Termination in a Mass Family Planning Program," in *Studies in Family Planning,* Fall 1967.

23. This point, made by Ronald Freedman, will be fully documented in his and John Takeshita's forthcoming monograph of the Taichung Study, and is supported by Korean data as well.

24. I have averaged the similar distributions of these two programs for ease of comparison with the hospital-based program. In the post-partum program, "direct acceptors" are those women who received some obstetrical service within the preceding 3 months. As an important additional point, the indirect acceptors, from the community at large, are of only slightly higher age and parity (medians of 28.5 and 3.0). The post-partum program operates in 19 cities in 14 countries; for fuller information, see *Studies in Family Planning,* No. 22, Aug. 1967.

25. *Op. cit., Studies in Family Planning,* No. 19, May 1967, p. 11.

26. K.-H. Mehlan, "The Socialist Countries of Europe," in Berelson *et al.,* eds., *op. cit.,* p. 211.

27. Charles F. Westoff and Norman Ryder, "U.S.: Methods of Fertility Control, 1955, 1960, 1965," *Studies in Family Planning,* No. 17, Feb. 1967, p. 5.

28. Miro, *op. cit.,* p. 633.

29. Reuben Hill, J. Mayone Stycos, and Kurt Back, *The Family and Population Control* (University of North Carolina Press, 1959), p. 202.

30. For a thorough review, see Dudley Kirk, "Factors Affecting Moslem Natality," in Berelson *et al., op. cit.,* p. 561-79.

31. And this despite the notion, and in some places the fact, that the IUD required female attendants in view of women's sensitivities about the

matter. In Taiwan this notion has proved unfounded. In Pakistan the need has given rise to the recruitment and training of a wholly new cadre of Lady Family Planning Visitors—high school graduates with a year's course in reproductive physiology and family planning, including a practical apprenticeship. There are now a few hundred such women at work in the field. On the technical side of operations, it begins to appear that paramedical personnel can do IUD insertions satisfactorily. (For an empirical study, see Henry W. Vaillant, G.T.M. Cummins, and Ralph M. Richart, "The Use of Nurse-Midwives To Insert the Lippes Loop in Barbados, B.W.I.," Nov. 1966, which concludes that "the use of well-trained nurse-midwives to insert IUD's is not associated with a significant increase in pregnancy, expulsion, removal for medical reasons, or infection.") The Pakistan experience needs to be followed carefully, but at the moment it would appear that the problem of using paramedical personnel is more politico-professional, in the sense of acceptance by the medical community, than it is technical.

32. The average years of protection is estimated from W. Parker Mauldin et al., "Retention of IUDs: An International Comparison," *Studies in Family Planning*, No. 18, Apr. 1967, p. 7; and the figure for birth prevented is estimated from the middle estimate in the paper prepared by Robert G. Potter for this symposium, "Estimating Births Averted in a Family Planning Program."

33. There is some preliminary evidence to show that termination rates are low (1) where alternate methods of contraception are not readily available; (2) where medical consultation or service is not readily available, as in the case of mobile teams that do insertions and then leave the area or of women traveling some distance for the insertion; (3) where substantial numbers of women within a community or neighborhood have had insertions, so that social support is at hand, and especially (4) where the doctors have been thoroughly trained in providing full knowledge about possible side effects to the women and reassuring them in advance and at follow-up consultations.

34. I am indebted to my colleague Harry Levin for these estimates, as of May 1967. For later information, see Gavin W. Jones and W. Parker Mauldin, "Use of Oral Contraceptives," in *Studies in Family Planning*, No. 24, Dec. 1967.

35. The IUD data are from Mauldin et al., *op. cit.*, p. 3, and the sterilization data from P. S. G. Nair and K. S. Ayyappan, "Demographic Particulars of Sterilized Persons in Trichur District, 1964-1965," Paper No. 33, Demographic Research Centre, Bureau of Economics and Statistics, Trivandrum, 1966, p. 6. A similar correspondence in parity between IUD and vasectomy acceptors in India is presented for a district in Kerala in David A. May, "Strategy for Family Planning in India," unpublished manuscript.

36. Ronald Freedman, "Family Planning Programs Today," in Berelson et al., *op. cit.*, p. 819.

37. See S. B. Hong, *Induced Abortion in Seoul, Korea* (Dong-A Publishing Company, 1966), and Hernan Romero, "Chile," in Berelson et al., eds., *op. cit.*, p. 244. It is this same order of magnitude in several Eastern European countries that have legalized the practice, as reported in the articles by Mehlan and by Klinger, in Berelson et al., eds., *op. cit.*

38. And not just there, either. In this connection a noted public health worker has drawn a parallel with the mass treatment of tuberculosis. Before "the discovery of tuberculostatic drugs and the mass application of the BCG vaccine . . . it was considered that the control of tuberculosis was related to the prosperity of the country and that nothing substantial could be done if the standards of living were not improved." Nusret H. Fisek, "Problems in Starting a Program," in Berelson et al., op. cit., p. 304.

39. A specific example makes the same point. The oral contraceptive used today causes some degree of nausea in some women. How much is too much? Nausea is both socially defined and differentially tolerated depending on motivation. Can this deficiency in the method be best overcome by minimizing the nauseating agent or by persuading women to raise their motivation and hence heighten the cut-off point? Both should be tried, but the former will be more effective for mass purposes. And the same point can be made about technical, engineering-type improvements in both the material and the form of the IUD in order to promote retention.

40. Or, more completely, first perceived as acceptable by the appropriate medical community. Not only must a contraceptive method be screened and judged acceptable by the local doctors as a professional group. Beyond that, acceptability by the recommending doctor is often the key factor in securing acceptability by the woman. That is, the women accept what the trusted doctors recommend, so that a system of "free choice" is more often his than hers.

41. As in the case of Chulalongkorn Hospital in Bangkok, noted above, and in the well-documented case of Taichung, where see John A. Ross, "Cost Analysis of the Taichung Experiment," Studies in Family Planning, No. 10, Feb. 1966, p. 10

42. With this number, incidentally, the Pakistan family planning program is reported to be the third largest employer in that country, after the Army and the railroads.

43. Sources, in order, are: Studies in Family Planning, No. 13, p. 6-7; Studies in Family Planning, No. 13, p. 8; unpublished reports; Studies in Family Planning, No. 13, p. 5-6; Studies in Family Planning, No. 13, p. 1-3; Seoul National University, Sungdong Gu Action-Research Project in Family Planning: A Progress Report, Apr., 1966, p. 59; Studies in Family Planning, No. 8, p. 1-7; Studies in Family Planning, No. 22.

44. Information provided by Ronald Freedman; to be documented in forthcoming Freedman-Takeshita publication. Some relevant data appears in table on p. 372.

45. Hong Kong may be the exception, depending upon the definition of a national program (Hong Kong's effort is run by the private family planning association with some government support) and upon the starting point. A careful analysis indicates that during the period 1961-65, about 75 percent of the birth rate decline was due to changes in the age structure and 25 percent to a genuine decline in fertility, part of which may be due to the efforts of the Family Planning Association. More importantly, between 1965 and 1966 the birth rate fell by 3 points, and almost none of that decline was due to age structure. The genuine fertility decline occurring between 1965 and 1966 was probably due in large part to the FPA effort, since in the period from early 1964 to April 1966 a large number of IUD's were inserted. This appears to demonstrate that a substantial in-

crease in the service rate for a program can make a substantial difference in the birth rate in a very short time. (From unpublished material developed by Ronald Freedman in cooperation with the FPA of Hong Kong).

46. Ronald Freedman and L. P. Chow, "Taiwan: Births Averted by the IUD Program," *Studies in Family Planning*, No. 20, June 1967, p. 7. The effect on the birth rate is in process of analysis.

47. From unpublished data distributed by Ronald Freedman at the NIH conference on *Behavioral Sciences and Family Planning*, June 1967. The same result can be shown in different form for 204 rural townships (also provided by Dr. Freedman):

Acceptance rates, 1963-March 1965	Percentage changes in total fertility rates, all women	
	1961-1963	1963-1965
Under 3.0 (72 townships)	−1.4	− 6.2
3.0—5:9 (83)	−3.1	− 9.3
6.0 & above (49)	−2.8	−11.0

48. Mauldin *et al. op. cit.* p. 11. This is an extremely difficult type of analysis to carry out particularly in view of the substitution problem, but this seems to be the best that can be done at this time. The technical problems of measuring the effect of a family planning program on the birth rate have not been solved.

49. Even among sophisticated analysts in the United States, with full access to data, a similar question on the impact of the oral pill on the declining birth rate is hard to answer. See the article by Norman B. Ryder and Charles W. Westoff. "The United States: The Pill and the Birth Rate, 1960-1965," *Studies in Family Planning*, No. 20, June 1967, p. 1-3, which concludes, after several ingenious attempts at analysis: "The acceleration in fertility decline between 1964 and 1965 and the simultaneous acceleration in the adoption of oral contraception is unlikely to be merely a coincidence."

50. One of the key but largely unappreciated problems of interpretation in social research is what I like to call the *fully-only* problem: once the statistic is established, does one say *fully* X percent or *only* X percent? This is graphically illustrated recently in a highly sophisticated analysis of the IUD retention rates in Taichung concluding that the average first insertion protected for *only* "less than four years" (Robert G. Potter *et al.*, "IUD Effectiveness in the Taichung Medical Follow-up Study," *Studies in Family Planning*, No. 18, April 1967, p. 13-20), even though that figure was well above the protection provided by earlier methods used in mass programs.

51. For example, see "Variables for Comparative Fertility Surveys," *Studies in Family Planning*, No. 21, June 1967, p. 8-11; and the series of evaluation manuals now in preparation at the Population Council. This is perhaps a good place to stress again that in the absence of solid data of these kinds, the reviewer is forced to make the best estimates he can— which I have tried to do here. This is a double admonition: to the reader, to appreciate the statistical situation; and to the technicians, to improve the statistical situation. It is also a good place to observe that Korea and Taiwan receive substantial attention in this review partly because their programs are advanced and partly because their evaluation provides the data.

52. For a suggestion of the administrator's viewpoint, see pp. 806, 808, and 810 in Berelson *et al.*, eds., *op. cit.*

53. These correspond to the needs of professional practice as against academic discipline, and the two have important divergences, as I have tried to suggest in my article, "Sociology in Action: In Population and in General," in Arthur B. Shostak, *Sociology in Action*, Dorsey Press, 1966, p. 15-21; and in my unpublished memorandum, "Evaluation of Family Planning Programs: Propositions," Dec. 1965. On the general movement in the field, note that the proceedings of the major conferences in 1960 and 1965 were entitled, respectively, *"Research* in Family Planning" and "Family Planning and Population *Programs."*

54. By Lyle Saunders, in his "Research and Evaluation: Needs for the Future," in Berelson *et al.*, eds., *op. cit.*, p. 784.

55. Notably by Howard C. Taylor, Jr., M.D., "A Family Planning Program Related to Maternity Service," in Berelson *et al.*, eds., *op. cit.*, p. 433-41.

56. In an unpublished memorandum, "MCH Care and Family Planning" by Howard C. Taylor, Jr., M.D., and Bernard Berelson, June 1967.

57. See Sloan Wayland, "Family Planning and the School Curriculum," in Berelson *et al.*, eds., *op. cit.*, p. 353-62; and the materials prepared under his direction: "Critical Stages in Reproduction" by Lucile Spence, and "Teaching Population Dynamics" by Hazel W. Hertzberg, both issued by the Population Instructional Materials Project, International Studies Program, Teachers College, Columbia University, 1965 and 1966.

58. See the stimulating remarks by Michael Young, mentioned above, at the meeting on "Behavioral Sciences and Family Planning" at the National Institutes of Health, June 1967.

59. Ansley J. Coale and C. Y. Tye, "The Significance of Age-Patterns of Fertility in High Fertility Populations," *Milbank Memorial Fund Quarterly*, 39, 1961, p. 645.

60. My colleague Dorothy Nortman, Research Associate, Demographic Division of the Population Council, analyzed the effect upon births in India of a 2-year rise in the age of marriage. It appears that with no change in completed family size about 7 percent fewer births would occur in the 10-year period following the shift in age at marriage. Since the effect on the number of births changes over time the impact on the intrinsic rate of increase was also analyzed, and it was found that with no change in completed family size the decline was about 4 percent and about 15 percent if the births of the 2-year period of delay never occur. These are useful approximations and further work is needed on such questions; in addition, and perhaps even more, we need some way(s) to effect what most experts consider a desirable development, given the objective of lowering the birth rate.

61. See, for example, Stanford University, *Advanced System for Communications and Education in National Development,* June 1967.

62. One other possibility, deliberately omitted here on ethical grounds but slowly coming into consideration, is governmental compulsion to limit births, as in the Indian proposal noted above, now dead.

63. As quoted in John D. Rockefeller III, "Opening Remarks," in Berelson *et al.*, eds., *op. cit.*, p. 4.

RECENT TRENDS IN ATTITUDES TOWARD FERTILITY CONTROL AND IN THE PRACTICE OF CONTRACEPTION IN THE UNITED STATES

Charles F. Westoff
Princeton University
and
Norman B. Ryder
The University of Wisconsin

JUDGING FROM BOTH DISCUSSION in the popular press and increasing governmental action in the field of family planning, we are in the midst of a veritable revolution in attitudes toward a subject which until recent years was completely taboo. Has this change in attitudes toward fertility control and contraception in the public mind been paralleled by change in private attitudes? Have American married women in general radically altered their perception of the desirability of controlling the number and timing of children? Have the attitudes and contraceptive practices of Catholic women in particular been affected by the extensive publicity given to the possibility of modification of the official Church position on birth control? Have American women in fact changed their attitudes toward fertility control or their practice of contraception in recent years? And, if they have, have such changes been uniform throughout the population or have different age groups and socioeconomic strata changed more than others? Three studies of fertility and fertility planning in the United States conducted in 1955,[1] 1960[2] and 1965[3] offer a unique opportunity to assess such trends in both attitude and practice in recent years.

Attitudes Toward Fertility Control

Has the attitude of American women toward fertility control become more favorable in recent years? Strictly speaking, the data from the three surveys do not permit a precise answer because of differences in the phrasing of the respective questions and in the coding of responses; nevertheless, the procedures were sufficiently similar in the 1960 and 1965 studies to encourage comparisons.[4]

The questions asked in 1960 are:

Q. 61. "Many married couples do something to limit the number of pregnancies they have or to control the time when they get pregnant. In general, would you say you are *against* this, *for* it, or what?"

Those who replied "against"—20 percent—were then asked:

Q. 61 c. "Some married couples use only a natural method—rhythm or safe period—to keep from getting pregnant too frequently. Would you say you are *against* this, *for* it, or what?"

The questions asked in 1965 are:

Q. 63. "Many married couples do something to limit the number of pregnancies they will have. In general, would you say you are *for* this or *against* this?"

All respondents, regardless of their answers, were then asked:

Q. 64. "Some couples use a natural method—rhythm or safe period—to keep from having too many pregnancies. Would you say you are *for* this or *against* this?"

The main differences between the two sets of questions appear to be: (1) the primary question in 1960 includes the phrase "or to control the time when they get pregnant" while the 1965 version confines the question to the limitation of the number of pregnancies; (2) the 1965 questions reversed the ordering of the options *for* and *against*; (3) the word "only," used in the 1960 question on rhythm, was deleted in 1965. It is impossible to estimate how serious these differences are; it seems, however, that some counterbalancing is involved.

The responses of white women to these questions are presented for both samples in Table 1. In terms of response where method is unspecified, it appears that the answer to our initial question is yes: there has been an increase in the proportion of women who endorse the idea of fertility control. The increase is due primarily to a substantial change in the attitude of Catholic women. If we define a "favorable" attitude to include endorsement of the rhythm method only (the following tables include both measures) the change is less pronounced, and possibly even nonexistent for non-Catholic women. Among Catholics, there appears to have been some increase in favorability—from 85 percent in 1960 to 93 percent by 1965. In particular, there has been some shift among Catholics away from restricting endorsement to the rhythm method toward approval of fertility control in general.[5]

Protestant women, who by 1960 were already overwhelmingly

in favor of fertility control, reveal virtually the same pattern of response in 1965. Particular denomination seems to make little difference with the exception of members of fundamentalist sects who are slightly (5 percent) less favorable (tabular detail not presented).

As noted above, the question on rhythm was asked in 1960 only of women who replied "against" to the more general question, but was asked of all women in 1965. A substantial fraction of the latter (one-third of all white women and nearly one-quarter of Catholic women) say they are "against" the rhythm method but for fertility control in general. This interesting pattern may reflect a combination of anti-Catholicism for some non-Catholics and anti-traditionalism for some Catholics as well as for others an attitude shaped by negative experience with the method.

Cohort Analysis

Table 2 has been prepared to permit examination of the trend in attitude toward fertility control by birth cohort. The percentages on each upper diagonal are from the 1960 study; those on the lower diagonals are from the 1965 study.

Comparisons of the proportions favorable across cohorts for women at the same age reveal a distinct time trend in which all cohorts seem to have participated. The increase in proportion favorable —most of which we have seen occurs in the Catholic group—does not appear to be concentrated only among the more recent cohorts.

If we focus on age differences within cohorts, there seems to be some tendency for the increase in favorable attitude to have been larger among the younger women, who are probably more responsive to change.

Education

Analysis of the trend in attitude toward fertility control by wife's education (Table 3) reveals a pattern only for Catholic women, among whom the amount of change is directly associated with amount of education. This differential indicates a radical change in the position of the Catholic women who have attended college. In 1960, only 39 percent of college-educated Catholic women were favorable, less than that for any other educational category; five years later the proportion reached 67 percent. Comparison of the proportions including women only favorable to rhythm reveals that the explanation lies in a substantial shift of Catholic college-educated women away from an exclusive endorsement of rhythm toward a more general endorsement of fertility control.

The reasons for such a dramatic change over such a short period of time can only be conjectured. It seems plausible that educated women would have been exposed more to the publicity about the discussions on birth control within the councils of the Catholic Church and the attitudes of some have probably been affected by the atmosphere of uncertainty and doubt about the official position. However, even if this interpretation is correct, it does not explain why Catholic women who attended college were so little in favor of fertility control in 1960. The explanation seems to lie in the fact that more educated Catholic women tend to be more religious and attend Catholic educational institutions, in part because they are disproportionately Irish in origin, a circumstance which in turn implies more orthodox Catholicism.

Religion of the Couple

Thus far our observations about the influence of religion on attitude toward fertility control have been restricted to the affiliation of the wife irrespective of her husband's religion. Table 4 has been prepared to show the influence of the husband's religion, and also the trend in attitude among couples in terms of the religion of both spouses. It is quite clear from this tabulation that the attitude of the Catholic wife/ Protestant husband combination—formerly more like that of the Catholic couple than the Protestant wife/Catholic husband couple— has moved sharply toward the Protestant position. In the most general terms, the fact of being Catholic is becoming less significant as a factor in shaping attitudes toward fertility control and, as we shall see subsequently, in the practice of contraception itself.

Religiousness of Catholic Women and
Attitudes Toward Fertility Control

Past research on social factors influencing Catholic fertility and contraceptive practice has consistently disclosed strong associations with devoutness, as measured by religious practice; the two earlier studies both indicated similar relationships with attitudes toward fertility control. In Table 5 we have tabulated attitudes toward fertility control by the frequency with which Catholic women receive the sacraments. Several features of this analysis are noteworthy. If we include in the concept of "favorable" endorsement of rhythm specifically, Catholic women are now uniformly (and nearly unanimously) in favor of fertility control regardless of degree of devoutness. On the other hand, devoutness still strongly differentiates this attitude if those in favor of rhythm only are not included.

The largest change in the 5-year period seems to have occurred among Catholics who are more than nominally and less than extremely devout, that is, women who report receiving sacraments more than a few times a year but less than once a week or more. The category of the most devout women, however, has experienced some increase in overall favorability despite the absence of change in the proportion endorsing rhythm only.

Attitude and Practice

Much of our interest in the study of attitudes toward contraception resides in the assumption that attitudes relate to behavior. Ignoring the questions of the temporal sequence of attitude and practice, and of their interaction, the evidence in Table 6 clearly sustains this assumption. Among Catholic women (for whom there is sufficient variation in attitude to make the question interesting) there is a rather strong association between attitude and practice.[6]

Trend in Attitude Among Nonwhite Women

Comparison of the change in attitude among white and nonwhite women (Table 7) reveals a trend toward convergence; a difference of 12 percent in 1960 has diminished to 3 percent by 1965. Subdivision by region of residence and wife's education indicates that changes in the South and among the less educated nonwhites are responsible for this convergence, although small numbers of nonwhites require caution. The same pattern of change viewed from a different perspective is manifest in the sharp reduction among nonwhites in the amount of association between education and attitude over the five years compared with little change among whites. A substantial part of the explanation of convergence is the rapidly improving educational composition of the nonwhite population as reflected in successive samples of women 18-39 years of age.

Cohort analysis of the trend in attitude among nonwhites (Table 8) indicates that all cohorts (at each age) have participated in the rise in proportions favorable toward fertility control, and that the rise appears to be somewhat greater for the younger cohorts.

The Use of Contraception

Attention in the past few years has focused on the emergence of two radically new techniques of contraception—the pill and the intrauterine contraceptive device. Indeed, one of the main reasons for conducting the 1965 National Fertility Study was to estimate the use and demographic significance of the pill[7] (the IUD appeared much later) and it was discovered that by late 1965 the pill had "become the most popular method of contraception used by American couples."[8]

In the present report, we are concerned not with the specific methods of contraception used but rather with the trend in the use

of contraception in general, an analysis which assumes added significance in view of the recent decline of fertility in the U.S. In the first
part of this paper we reported a trend over the decade in the direction
of a more favorable *attitude* toward contraception; we turn now to
the question of whether a similar trend prevails in the *use* of contraception.

Comparability of Estimates

The questions used in the three interview surveys forming the basis
for our estimates of the trend in the use of contraception differ in some
details. Although the wording of the main question varied somewhat
in each study,[9] the major difference is that the 1955 and 1960 studies
both asked a question initially about whether the couple had *ever*
used any method, whereas the questions on use in the 1965 study were
located in the context of a pregnancy history beginning with use
before the first pregnancy; estimates for 1965 of the proportion of
women who ever used contraception were then derived by examining
successive intervals. The differences in the procedure followed in 1965
and that in the previous studies would appear to have opposite effects.
On the one hand, the use of repeated questions for successive intervals
to derive estimates of "ever use" possibly reduced underreporting; on
the other hand, the absence of follow-up questions probing possible
use of methods not listed on the card shown to the respondent probably resulted in some underreporting.

Other procedures were similar. In all three interview schedules
the attitudinal questions analyzed earlier preceded questions on use.
In all three studies, the rhythm method is included in the concept of
contraception. And, although details vary, a distinction has been
maintained consistently between what has been called use on an "action" and on a "motive" basis. The present report deals only with the
use of contraception for the explicit purpose of controlling the timing
and/or number of pregnancies.[10] The primary measure of contraceptive use is simply whether the woman reports that she and her
husband have *ever* used any method of fertility control. This crude
classification does not measure regularity, effectiveness, or length of
use, all of which will be analyzed in subsequent reports.

The Extent of Use of Contraception in the U.S.

As of 1965, 84 percent of married white women 18-39 years of age
report having used some method of contraception (Table 9). If we
add to this figure the number of women who say they expect to use a
method later (many being women married only a short time) the proportion reaches 90 percent. And finally, if we exclude women report-

ing problems of subfecundity, we find that the proportion of fecund women who have ever used or expect to use contraception is 97 percent. Clearly the norm of fertility control has become universal in contemporary America. This widespread use of contraception in the United States has not just developed in the past few years. In 1955, 70 percent reported having used contraception and by 1960 the figure had reached 81 percent. The increase to 84 percent by 1965 simply continues this trend. The same pattern of increase is also evident when the proportion expecting to use in the future is included. With practice approaching universality, the rate of increase must of course diminish with only little opportunity for further expansion.

Among the subfecund, the changes in the proportions who have used are in the same direction; this probably implies a growing tendency to use earlier in married life.

Duration and Parity

Data on duration and parity are useful to indicate the time pattern of adoption of use. In every study the proportions who have used are highest for duration 5-9 and for parity three. The decline for higher durations probably represents a combination of recall error, onset of subfecundity with age, and increased tendency to use (and use earlier) among successively more recent cohorts. The same explanations are relevant for the small declines with advancing parity with the additional important contributing cause that the women in higher parities are self-selected in ways that are relevant to use or nonuse. Accordingly it is of interest that in 1965 there is much less decline with advancing parity than there was in 1955 and 1960.

Cohort, Age, and Religion

Table 10 shows estimates of past or prospective use of contraception, by cohort, age, and religion. The data in the upper diagonal of each panel are from the 1955 study, those in the middle diagonal are from 1960, and those in the lower diagonal from 1965. Comparing successive cohorts at the same age (reading down each column), there have been monotonic increases over the entire sequence for both Protestant and Catholic subsamples alike; this observation applies to the percent who have used as well as the combined percent who have used or expect to use. Variations by age within each cohort (reading across each row) are likewise generally positive.

The bottom panels of Table 10 show the differences over time between Protestants and Catholics in the proportion who have used, and in the proportion who have used or expect to use. It is apparent from both of these tables that, for each cohort as age advances, and from cohort to cohort at each age, the difference is becoming attenuated. The convergence is particularly marked in the table which combines those who have used with those who expect to use. The inference from this observation is that young Catholics begin to use contraception later than young Protestants.

It is probable that there has been some intercohort increase in the likelihood of using contraception before the end of the childbearing period. This is particularly so among Catholics, in part because not much increase could be expected beyond the high values already recorded for Protestants, given the circumstances that accruing sterility problems obviate for many the necessity for use. Nevertheless, it is likely that the major changes, especially for the young, represent a decline in the age at which contraception is used rather than a rise in the likelihood of it ever being used.

Age and Education

In 1955 there was a strong differential by education in contraceptive practice (Table 11). This differential was sharply reduced between 1955 and 1960 and again between 1960 and 1965, except among women reporting having used contraception who have had only a grade school education. Essentially the same story is revealed once an age control is introduced, with the important qualification that the low proportion of grade school respondents reporting that they have used or expect to use is revealed as a consequence of the reports of women now past 30; among the 18-29 the proportion has approached equality with those for women with more education. Furthermore, the proportion of women 18-39 with a grade school education has declined from 14 percent in 1955 to 9 percent in 1965, and is less than 7 percent among the 18-29 in 1965. Thus in one way or another, the last component of never-users is being erased from the population. The remaining discrepancy is apparently the tendency for young women now past 30; among the 18-29 the proportion has approached because the differential remains substantial if attention is confined to those who have already used contraception.

Religion and Education

The estimates in Table 12 show that differentials by education in the two measures of contraceptive use prevail in each survey year within the Protestant and Catholic subsamples. The strongest difference by education, regardless of religion, is that between the proportion of those with grade school education, and the proportion for those at a higher educational level. However, a closer inspection of the table reveals that a previous pattern of use by education has vanished by 1965. In 1955, and to a somewhat lesser extent in 1960, the Catholic-Protestant difference was much greater at the college level than at the lower educational levels. This is no longer the case. The marked shift of behavior and attitude of college Catholics between 1960 and 1965 is one of the most striking findings of this analysis. The outstanding difference remaining between Protestant and Catholic use patterns, with educational level controlled, is at the grade school level. Since that differential is large only in the "have used" category, the implication is that it is a difference in timing of use. As noted above, there are reasons related to the distribution of the population by age and education to believe that this particular differential may grow smaller, and in any event become less significant as the proportion in the category declines.

Husband's Income and Occupation and Wife's Work History

The changing influence of other socioeconomic factors on contraceptive practice is shown in Table 13. Variations in the use of contraception are observable in each of the three time periods by husband's income estimated for the year preceding each survey: there is an irregularly direct but very weak relationship of use, and of use or expectation of use, to income. Through time the relationship appears to be weakening a little. Although it may be of interest that even a weak relationship persists, such analysis must proceed with caution because of changes in the meaning of the income categories through time. For example, the category $10,000 plus has shown an increase from 3 percent in 1955 to 11 percent in 1960 and to 19 percent in 1965, while the proportion in the under $3,000 category has declined from 21 percent to 14 percent to 6 percent in the same period.

The same observations are broadly applicable to differentials by husband's current occupational status. The differences are small, they are persistent through time, but they seem to be weakening a little as the groups with the lowest proportions increase somewhat more than those with the highest proportions. In detail it appears that the farm category has now replaced the lower blue-collar class as the occupational category with the lowest proportion; this observation must be tempered with the fact that the proportion in the farm category has shrunk from 9 percent in 1955 to 4 percent in 1965. As for the division of couples on the basis of whether the wife has or has not worked since marriage—an admittedly crude dichotomy—the absence of difference holds in 1965 as it did in 1955 and in 1960.

Race

The difference between the proportions of whites and nonwhites in 1960 who reported ever having used contraception was 22 percent for women 18-39; five years later the difference had diminished to 7 percent. An even more dramatic change is apparent in the proportions who have used or expect to use contraception where the race difference has all but disappeared.

As indicated in Table 14 which presents the cohort-age trends (the 1960 estimates are on the upper diagonal and the 1965 estimates are on the lower diagonal) these changes have been brought about mainly by the most recent cohort (1941-45) although increases are evident for all four intercohort comparisons. The greatest intracohort change is evident among women of the 1936-40 cohort across the age span 20-24 to 25-29. There is now a strong differential by age within the nonwhites, suggesting a definite trend toward greater use, and the possibility that this particular differential will disappear. This hypothesis is even more strongly suggested by the bottom tier of Table 15 which shows the pattern of rapidly declining differences between the two races.

The bulk of the nonwhite couples in both surveys were residents of the South where most of the dramatic increases in contraceptive practice appears to be concentrated (Table 15). The change in the fraction of nonwhites in the South ever using contraception has gone from half to three-quarters in the five-year period.

The increase in the use of contraception is particularly evident among nonwhites currently living on a Southern farm though they are only a small minority of this nonwhite population. The greater increase of use in this category has resulted in narrowing the difference between nonwhites on a Southern farm and all others.

A similar pattern exists when the differences between the races are examined in the light of wife's education and husband's income; although a positive association persists in 1965 it is not as strong as in 1960. In 1960 the relationship between contraceptive practice and education among nonwhites was stronger than among whites; in 1965 this is no longer true. In fact, with education or income controlled, there are only small differences in contraceptive practice between white and nonwhite couples.

Summary and Conclusions

On the basis of data collected from three national sample surveys in 1955, 1960, and 1965, trends in attitudes toward fertility control and in the use of contraception have been analyzed.

The major findings in connection with changes in attitudes since 1960 are: (1) American women have become increasingly favorable toward the principle of fertility control; (2) the greatest change has occurred among Catholic women, many of whom have moved away from exclusive endorsement of the rhythm method; (3) this change in Catholic attitude has been especially marked among the better educated Catholic women; and (4) the gap between white and nonwhite attitudes has narrowed considerably by 1965 because of the rapid change in nonwhite attitudes, due in part to increasing education.

Analysis of trends in the proportion of women who report ever having used contraception and those who expect to use leads to the following conclusion: (1) The upward trend evident between 1955 and 1960 has continued to 1965 though necessarily at a reduced rate; (2) couples appear to be adopting contraception earlier in marriage; (3) Protestant-Catholic differences in use are continuing to diminish; (4) use of contraception has increased most sharply among the more educated Catholic women; (5) education generally is becoming less important in differentiating use; and, (6) due to a substantial increase in use among nonwhite women, especially young women in the South, the white-nonwhite differences in proportions using contraception will probably disappear in the near future.

Table 1. Attitude of White Women Toward Fertility Control by Religion, 1960 and 1965

Attitude	Total[1]		Protestant		Catholic	
	1960	1965	1960	1965	1960	1965
For fertility control, method unspecified	80	85	91	92	52	70
For rhythm method only	13	10	5	4	33	23
Against fertility control	5	4	3	4	9	6
Not ascertained	2	1	1	—	5	1
Percent total	100	100	100	100	100	100
Number of women	2414	2918	1596	1907	668	846

[1]Includes women of other religions.

Source: The 1960 estimates are derived from Whelpton, Campbell, and Patterson, *op.cit.,* p. 178.

Table 2. Percent of White Women in Favor of Fertility Control by Religion, Cohort, and Age, 1960 and 1965[1]

Cohort	Percent Favorable, Method Unspecified					Total Percent Favorable, Including Rhythm Method Only					Number of Women				
	20-24	25-29	30-34	35-39	40-44	20-24	25-29	30-34	35-39	40-44	20-24	25-29	30-34	35-39	40-44
Total[2]															
1916-20					77					90					572
1921-25				80	82				92	95				677	821
1926-30			80	82				94	93				624	740	
1931-35		81	85				94	95				600	762		
1936-40	78	87				91	97				440	649			
1941-45	86					95					641				
Protestant															
1916-20					87					94					351
1921-25				90	89				97	96				425	534
1926-30			90	89				97	95				405	478	
1931-35		93	92				96	97				396	482		
1936-40	88	92				94	98				312	433			
1941-45	93					96					424				
Catholic															
1916-20					52					79					178
1921-25				54	62				82	92				192	241
1926-30			49	65				87	89				174	206	
1931-35		50	70				87	93				176	242		
1936-40	53	74				87	97				112	176			
1941-45	69					93					189				

[1]Estimates for 1960 and 1965 appear on the upper and lower diagonals respectively.

[2]Includes women of other religions.

Source: The 1960 estimates are derived both from Whelpton, Campbell, and Patterson, op. cit., p. 181, and from the original data.

Table 3. Percent of White Women in Favor of Fertility Control by Religion and Education, 1960 and 1965

Education	Total[1]		Protestant		Catholic	
	1960	1965	1960	1965	1960	1965
	Percent Favorable					
	Method Unspecified					
College	86	89	96	97	39	67
High school 4	83	87	93	93	55	73
High school 1-3	80	85	88	89	58	72
Grade school	68	69	79	79	46	52
	Total Percent Favorable					
	Including Rhythm Method Only					
College	97	98	99	98	88	96
High school 4	95	97	98	97	88	96
High school 1-3	93	94	95	95	87	90
Grade school	82	82	87	89	74	75
	Number of Women					
College	427	585	284	400	79	136
High school 4	1153	1422	752	910	341	439
High school 1-3	579	644	392	437	168	177
Grade school	255	267	168	160	80	94

[1]Includes women of other religions.

Source: The 1960 estimates are derived from Whelpton, Campbell, and Patterson, *op. cit.,* p. 177.

Table 4. Percent of White Women in Favor of Fertility Control by Religion of Wife and Husband, 1960 and 1965

Religion		Method Unspecified		Rhythm Only		Total Favorable		Number	
Wife	Husband	1960	1965	1960	1965	1960	1965	1960	1965
Prot.	Prot.	91	92	5	4	96	96	1454	1701
Prot.	Cath.	78	90	10	6	88	96	106	127
Cath.	Prot.	59	83	28	11	87	94	114	133
Cath.	Cath.	52	67	34	25	86	92	525	691

Source: The 1960 estimates are derived from Whelpton, Campbell, and Patterson, *op. cit.,* p. 180.

Table 5. Percent of White Catholic Women in Favor of Fertility Control by Frequency of Receiving Sacraments,[1] 1960 and 1965

Frequency Receive Sacraments	Method Unspecified		Rhythm Only		Total Favorable		Number	
	1960	1965	1960	1965	1960	1965	1960	1965
Never	72	83	19	7	91	90	84	145
Once a year or less	78	85	15	10	93	95	61	92
Few times a year	59	72	29	21	88	93	160	169
Once a month	48	70	35	23	83	93	191	177
Two or three times a month	35	65	49	29	84	94	78	107
Once a week or more	33	47	47	46	80	93	94	153

[1] In 1960, the question referred to receiving Sacraments and in 1965 to receiving Communion.

Source: The 1960 estimates are derived from Whelpton, Campbell, and Patterson, op. cit., p. 179.

Table 6. Attitude of White Catholic Women Toward Fertility Control by Type of Contraception Used, 1965

Attitude Toward Fertility Control	Never Used Any Method	Have Used Only Rhythm	Have Used Any Other Method	Percent Total	Number of Women
For fertility control, method unspecified	15	19	66	100	588
For rhythm method only	33	47	20	100	196
Against fertility control	64	9	27	100	56
All Catholic women[1]	22	25	53	100	846

[1] Includes six women whose responses to both questions do not permit classification.

Table 7. Percent of Nonwhite and White Women in Favor of Fertility Control by Region of Residence and Education of Wife, 1960 and 1965

Characteristic	Percent Favorable Method Unspecified				Total Percent Favorable Including Rhythm Method Only				Number of Nonwhites	
	Nonwhite		White		Nonwhite		White			
	1960	1965	1960	1965	1960	1965	1960	1965	1960	1965
Total	68	82	80	85	81	91	93	95	270	837
Region:										
Northeast	76	88	74	82	90	95	90	95	41	158
North Central	77	77	76	83	87	90	92	94	74	131
West	*	95	83	91	*	98	*	97	19	46
South	60	79	86	87	74	89	95	94	136	502
Education:										
College	89	85	86	89	97	94	97	97	37	106
High School 4	85	87	83	87	90	94	95	97	73	285
High School 1-3	64	80	80	85	78	90	92	94	86	290
Grade School	47	72	68	69	67	84	81	82	74	156

*Too few cases.

Source: The 1960 estimates are derived from the original data.

Table 8. Percent of Nonwhite and White Women in Favor of Fertility Control by Cohort and Age, 1960 and 1965[1]

Cohort	Percent Favorable, Method Unspecified 20-24	25-29	30-34	35-39	Total Percent Favorable Including Rhythm Method Only 20-24	25-29	30-34	35-39	Number of Women 20-24	25-29	30-34	35-39
Nonwhite												
1921-25				61				73				66
1926-30			70	77			83	87			79	182
1931-35		74	81			82	90			65	202	
1936-40	68	82			84	93			50	200		
1941-45	87				92				214			
White												
1921-25				80				92				677
1926-30			80	82			94	93			624	740
1931-35		81	85			94	95			600	762	
1936-40	78	87			91	97			440	649		
1941-45	86				95				641			

[1] Estimates for 1960 and 1965 appear on the upper and lower diagonals respectively.

Source: The 1960 estimates are derived from the original data.

Table 9. Percent of Couples Who Have Used or Expect to Use Contraception by Fecundity, Duration of Marriage, and Parity: 1955, 1960, and 1965

	Percent Have Used			Percent Have Used or Expect to Use			Number of Couples		
	1955	1960	1965	1955	1960	1965	1955	1960	1965
Total	70	81	84	79	87	90	2713	2414	2912
Fecundity									
Fecund	83	89	93	91	96	97	1794	1674	2030
Subfecund	45	62	63	55	68	72	919	740	882
Duration of Marriage									
Under 5	65	75	82	81	91	93	649	544	661
5-9	75	86	87	83	91	93	869	649	755
10-14	73	82	86	79	86	89	686	702	719
15 or more	65	78	82	68	80	84	509	519	778
Parity									
0	42	55	56	59	72	75	419	301	358
1	71	74	81	82	85	90	603	463	491
2	78	89	89	84	93	92	843	682	758
3	81	89	91	87	92	93	468	499	613
4	73	87	90	78	90	94	190	263	372
5	67	80	90	74	84	93	104	119	161
6 or more	57	76	81	65	78	84	86	87	160

Source: The 1955 and 1960 estimates are from Whelpton, Campbell, and Patterson, *op. cit.*, p. 214.

Table 10. Percent of White Couples Who Used or Expect to Use Contraception, by Cohort, Age at Interview and Religion: 1955, 1960, and 1965[1]

Cohort	Percent Have Used					Percent Have Used or Expect to Use					Number of Couples				
	20-24	25-29	30-34	35-39	40-44	20-24	25-29	30-34	35-39	40-44	20-24	25-29	30-34	35-39	40-44
Total[2]															
1916-20				65	76				69	77				695	572
1921-25			73	77	78			79	80	79			748	677	821
1926-30		73	83	81			83	88	84			714	624	740	
1931-35	71	84	84			85	91	88			464	600	762		
1936-40	79	86				92	93				440	649			
1941-45	85					94					641				
Protestant															
1916-20				70	79				74	80				457	351
1921-25			76	81	80			82	84	82			505	425	534
1926-30		80	85	82			89	89	85			461	405	478	
1931-35	76	89	87			90	93	89			320	396	482		
1936-40	83	90				93	94				312	433			
1941-45	88					95					424				
Catholic															
1916-20				55	66				58	67				209	178
1921-25			63	67	71			72	69	71			212	192	241
1926-30		59	75	77			70	80	81			220	174	206	

[1]Estimates for 1955, 1960, and 1965 appear on the upper, middle, and lower diagonals respectively.

[2]Includes women who are neither Catholic nor Protestant.

Table 10.—Cont.

	Percent Have Used					Percent Have Used or Expect to Use					Number of Couples				
	20-24	25-29	30-34	35-39	40-44	20-24	25-29	30-34	35-39	40-44	20-24	25-29	30-34	35-39	40-44
Catholic															
1931-35	58	71	79			73	85	86			128	176	242		
1936-40	65	78				87	89				112	176			
1941-45	79					91					189				
Protestant Minus Catholic															
1916-20				15	13				16	13					
1921-25			13	14	9			10	15	11					
1926-30		21	10	5			19	9	4						
1931-35	18	18	8			17	8	3							
1936-40	18	12				6	5								
1941-45	9					4									

Source: Estimates for the 1916-30 cohorts in 1955 from Freedman, Whelpton, and Campbell, *op.cit.,* p. 106. The 1931-35 cohort statistics for 1955 are derived from the original data. Estimates for the 1916-35 cohorts in 1960 are from Whelpton, Campbell, and Patterson, *op.cit.,* pp. 207, 218. The 1936-40 and 1916-20 cohort statistics by religion for 1960 are derived from the original data.

Table 11. Percent of White Couples Who Have Used or Expect to Use Contraception by Wife's Age and Education: 1955, 1960, and 1965

	Percent Have Used					Percent Have Used or Expect to Use					Number of Couples				
	Total	18-24	25-29	30-34	35-39	Total	18-24	25-29	30-34	35-39	Total	18-24	25-29	30-34	35-39
Wife's Education															
Total															
1955	70	68	73	73	65	79	84	83	79	69	2713	556	714	748	695
1960	81	78	84	83	77	87	92	91	88	80	2414	513	600	624	677
1965	84	84	86	84	81	90	94	93	88	84	2912	762	649	762	740
College															
1955	85	86	85	88	80	88	89	90	92	82	417	76	115	112	114
1960	88	83	88	92	87	93	95	95	94	90	427	59	121	121	126
1965	88	87	88	89	87	94	97	94	93	91	585	124	158	166	137
High school 4															
1955	74	70	78	77	69	83	88	87	83	72	1236	271	347	348	270
1960	83	78	89	84	80	90	93	94	90	81	1153	278	286	290	299
1965	86	85	88	89	83	92	94	93	93	86	1420	375	309	375	361
High school 1-															
1955	66	62	69	71	62	76	80	82	78	65	681	166	174	176	165
1960	78	78	75	82	76	85	92	85	86	77	579	145	137	138	159
1965	83	84	83	78	84	88	95	89	81	86	641	209	144	140	148
Grade school															
1955	49	51	46	46	51	59	67	61	54	58	377	43	76	112	146
1960	66	74	71	67	59	72	81	82	71	65	255	31	56	75	93
1965	65	0	77	59	61	75	89	95	68	65	267	54	39	80	94

Source: The 1955 and 1960 estimates are from Whelpton, Campbell, and Patterson, *op. cit.,* p. 217.

Table 12. Percent of White Couples Who Have Used or Expect to Use Contraception, By Wife's Education and Religion: 1955, 1960, and 1965

Education	Total[1]			Protestant			Catholic		
	1955	1960	1965	1955	1960	1965	1955	1960	1965
Percent Have Used									
Total	70	81	84	75	84	87	57	70	78
College	85	88	88	90	93	90	62	67	81
High school 4	74	83	86	80	86	88	61	73	82
High school 1-3	66	78	83	70	80	86	59	73	75
Grade school	49	66	65	53	73	72	41	54	55
Percent Have Used or Expect to Use									
Total	79	87	90	83	90	91	67	80	87
College	88	93	94	92	96	95	71	82	89
High school 4	83	90	92	88	92	92	71	83	90
High school 1-3	76	85	88	79	87	90	68	80	85
Grade school	59	72	75	63	77	79	49	64	72
Number of Couples									
Total	2713	2414	2912	1817	1596	1902	787	668	845
College	417	427	584	306	284	399	73	79	136
High school 4	1236	1153	1420	794	752	909	396	341	438
High school 1-3	681	579	641	457	392	434	208	168	177
Grade school	377	255	267	260	168	159	110	80	94

[1]Includes women who are neither Catholic nor Protestant.

Source: The 1955 estimates are partly from Freedman, Whelpton, and Campbell, *op. cit.,* p. 109 and partly from tabulations of the original data. The 1960 data are from Whelpton, Campbell, and Patterson, *op. cit.,* p. 201.

Table 13. Percent of Couples Who Have Used or Expect to Use Contraception by Husband's Income and Occupation and By Whether the Wife Worked Since Marriage: 1955, 1960, and 1965

Characteristic	Percent Have Used			Percent Have Used or Expect to Use			Number of Couples		
	1955	1960	1965	1955	1960	1965	1955	1960	1965
Total	70	81	84	79	87	90	2713	2414	2912
Husband's Income									
$10,000 or more	76	89	89	81	91	92	88	261	540
$7000-$9999	81	84	88	84	89	90	156	405	730
$6000-$6999	80	85	86	84	89	89	186	312	421
$5000-$5999	77	80	82	85	88	88	393	423	486
$4000-$4999	73	81	78	81	88	87	583	380	301
$3000-$3999	69	77	81	78	85	86	619	306	185
Under $3000	59	70	70	71	82	80	581	327	168
Husband's Occupation									
Upper white-collar	81	86	88	85	90	93	620	725	804
Lower white-collar	76	84	87	82	89	91	286	312	390
Upper blue-collar	69	79	83	77	86	88	644	465	708
Lower blue-collar	62	76	81	74	84	88	765	670	765
Farm	63	81	78	74	84	85	242	154	130
Wife Worked Since Marriage									
Never worked	67	80	82	77	87	90	819	683	725
Worked	71	81	85	79	87	90	1866	1713	2193

Source: Estimates for the income categories above $6000 in 1955 derived from the original data. All other estimates are mainly from Whelpton, Campbell, and Patterson, *op. cit.,* pp. 185 and 216.

Table 14. Percent of Couples Who Have Used or Expect to Use Contraception, by Cohort, Age at Interview, and Race, 1960 and 1965.[1]

Cohort	Percent Have Used				Percent Have Used or Expect to Use				Number of Couples			
	20-24	25-29	30-34	35-39	20-24	25-29	30-34	35-39	20-24	25-29	30-34	35-39
Nonwhite												
1921-25				53				58				66
1926-30			66	65			77	71			79	182
1931-35		65	74			85	84			65	202	
1936-40	50	82			80	90			50	200		
1941-45	84				96				214			
White												
1921-25				77				80				677
1926-30			83	81			88	84			624	740
1931-35		84	84			91	88			600	762	
1936-40	79	86			92	93			440	649		
1941-45	85				94				641			
White Minus Nonwhite												
1921-25				24				22				
1926-30			17	16			11	13				
1931-35		19	10			6	4					
1936-40	29	4			12	3						
1941-45	1				−2							

[1]Estimates for 1960 and 1965 appear on the upper and lower diagonals respectively.

Source: The 1960 estimates are from Whelpton, Campbell, and Patterson, *op. cit.*, pp. 207, 359 and the original data.

Table 15. Percent of Nonwhite and White Couples Who Have Used or Expect to Use Contraception, By Region of Residence, Southern Farm Residence, Education of Wife, and Income of Husband, 1960 and 1965

Characteristic Age:	Percent Have Used Nonwhite		Percent Have Used White		Percent Have Used or Expect to Use Nonwhite		Percent Have Used or Expect to Use White		Number of Nonwhites	
	1960	1965	1960	1965	1960	1965	1960	1965	1960	1965
Total	59	77	81	84	76	86	87	90	270	837
Region:										
Northeast	76	84	77	84	95	91	85	89	41	158
Northcentral	59	74	82	84	76	79	88	91	74	131
West	*	83	80	83	*	93	89	92	19	46
South	51	75	83	87	68	85	88	88	136	502
Southern Farm Residence:										
On farm now	36	63	86	76	52	80	87	82	33	67
All other	62	78	81	84	79	86	87	90	237	770
Wife's Education:										
College	86	85	88	88	95	88	93	94	37	106
High school 4	67	83	83	86	81	91	90	92	73	285
High school 1-3	56	79	78	83	79	87	85	88	86	290
Grade school	42	58	66	65	57	71	72	75	74	156
Husband's Income:										
$6000 or more	76	82	86	88	88	90	89	90	25	183
5000-5999	63	81	80	82	81	89	88	88	32	162
4000-4999	59	79	81	78	73	85	88	87	51	172
3000-3999	56	75	77	81	80	82	85	86	45	156
Under $3000	56	68	70	70	71	81	82	80	117	155

*Too few cases.

Source: The 1960 estimates for nonwhites are from Whelpton, Campbell, and Patterson, *op. cit.*, pp. 358-59 and from the original data.

Notes

1. Ronald Freedman, Pascal K. Whelpton, and Arthur A. Campbell, *Family Planning, Sterility and Population Growth* (New York: McGraw-Hill, 1959).

2. Pascal K. Whelpton, Arthur A. Campbell, and John E. Patterson, *Fertility and Family Planning in the United States* (Princeton, N. J.: Princeton University Press, 1966).

3. The 1965 data were collected in the National Fertility Study under a contract between Princeton University and the National Institute of Child Health and Human Development. The authors would like to acknowledge

the able assistance of Shirrell Buhler and Susan Hyland of the Office of Population Research, Princeton University, who were responsible for the data processing. We would also like to express our appreciation to Larry Bumpass for preparing several special tabulations of the 1955 and 1960 data.

4. The 1955 data are not included because the question did not make any allowance for women who approved of the rhythm method but objected to other methods of birth control. In addition, the question was open-ended and thus required coding. In both 1960 and 1965 separate questions were asked about the rhythm method and they were mainly pre-coded.

5. Although the shift could be simply the result of a more permissive style of response among Catholics—the reduction from 5 to 1 percent in the "not ascertained" category may be pertinent here—other data on methods of contraception actually used by Catholics support the hypothesis of a real change in attitude. See Westoff and Ryder, "United States: Methods of Fertility Control, 1955, 1960 and 1965," in William T. Liu, ed., *Family and Fertility*, University of Notre Dame Press, 1967, pp. 157-69. (Reprinted in *Studies in Family Planning*, February 1967.)

6. The association is diluted, of course, by such factors as sterility and young women recently married who have not begun to use contraception.

7. Norman B. Ryder and Charles F. Westoff, "Use of Oral Contraception in the United States, 1965," in *Science*, 153, September 9, 1966, pp. 1199-1205. Also see Norman B. Ryder and Charles F. Westoff, "Oral Contraception and American Birth Rates" in William T. Liu, ed., *Family and Fertility, op. cit.,* pp. 171-84 (reprinted as "The United States: The Pill and the Birth Rate" in *Studies in Family Planning*, No. 20, June 1967, pp. 1-3.)

8. Westoff and Ryder, "United States: Methods of Fertility Control, 1955, 1960 and 1965," *Family and Fertility, op. cit.,* pp. 164-65.

9. The main questions in the three studies were: *1955*—Q. 43. "Now in your own case, have you or your husband ever done anything to limit the number of your children or to keep from having them at certain times?"

1960—Q. 65. "Here is a card with the names of methods some married couples use to keep from getting pregnant. Have you or your husband ever used any of them?"

If the wife said "yes" she was asked which methods had been used. If she said "no" she was asked:

Q. 65b. "Have you ever used any methods not shown on this card?"

1965—Q. 100. "Here is a card with the names of methods couples use to delay or prevent having a baby. During this time, which method or methods, if any, did you or your husband use?"

This question was repeated for each interpregnancy interval.

10. This excludes the use of douching for cleanliness only, as well as the use of the "pill" for non-contraceptive reasons. The latter is estimated in Ryder and Westoff, "Use of Oral Contraception in the United States," *Science, op. cit.,* p. 1200.

ESTIMATING BIRTHS AVERTED IN A FAMILY PLANNING PROGRAM

Robert G. Potter, Jr.

Brown University

MODERN CONTRACEPTIVES, notably oral pills and intrauterine devices (IUD), are characterized by high acceptability, low pregnancy rates, but often rather high discontinuation rates. The effectiveness of these contraceptives may be addressed from two fundamental viewpoints. First, one may ask what the contraceptive is doing for the acceptors themselves in terms of periods of protection conferred. How long do "segments" of successful use from adoption of a method to its discontinuation last and what are the causes of discontinuation? Second, from the standpoint of the population of which the acceptors are a part, one may ask how many births are being averted and what is the manner in which the time flow of births is being modified. The terms "use effectiveness" and "clinical effectiveness" have been applied synonymously to the former viewpoint and "demographic effectiveness" to the latter.[1]

Through use of life table techniques, the measurement of use effectiveness has recently been strengthened.[2] Given data from an adequate follow-up study, one can, by means of a life table analysis, derive the proportions of acceptors successfully using or discontinuing the contraceptive for specified reasons as a function of time elapsed from adoption of the method. That is, within the period of follow-up, one can obtain for each duration both the proportion of couples retaining as well as rates of discontinuation for classified causes.

The demographic effectiveness of a contraceptive in a given population depends on the number of acceptances, but just as importantly on the lengths of successful retention and fertility foregone during retention. To date there has been little work done on the problem of combining life table statistics on retention with additional information relating to potential fertility in the absence of the particular contraceptive in order to estimate births averted. The one impressive

413

previous attempt is that of Lee and Isbister relating to births averted by IUD's in the family planning program of South Korea.[3] However, as discussed in the next section, there are at least three assumptions carried by their argument which it is desirable to modify.

The utility of credible estimates of births averted per acceptance of a contraceptive hardly needs emphasis. To know whether more births are being averted in one stratum than another is of great value in setting priorities in a family planning program. For instance, is more accomplished by inserting IUD's into younger women who tend to have higher potential fertility or a like number of older women who tend to wear the device longer? To assist planning one might want to evaluate the reduction in birth rate to be expected from given annual numbers and age-schedules of insertions; or conversely for a given age schedule of IUD insertion one might want to assess the annual numbers of insertions needed to achieve a specified reduction in birth rate. As Lee and Isbister have demonstrated, one can profitably tackle these problems through component projection, but before one can adjust age-specific birth rates to register the effects of stipulated regimes of IUD, one must make assumptions about the number of births being averted per segment of IUD each consecutive year after insertion.

The purpose of this paper is to present a revision of Lee and Isbister's procedure as it pertains specifically to estimating births averted per segment of IUD. To illustrate the procedure, application is made to data from Taichung, Taiwan with a specific objective of testing certain conclusions reached by Lee and Isbister and by Chow[4] concerning the relative impact of IUD among different age classes. Like the scheme of Lee and Isbister, the procedure described below is general enough so that, in situations affording enough information, it could be adapted to other types of contraception. However, it will simplify exposition to deal in the present report solely with births averted per first segment of IUD.

The present analysis was developed in connection with the writer's participation in a collaborative project of the Taiwan Population Studies Center and the University of Michigan Population Studies Center. Acknowledgement is owed to Drs. L. P. Chow and C. H. Lee for use of their data, to A. K. Jain and C. Ludvigh for preparing a number of special tabulations, and to Dr. R. Freedman for coordinating the project and contributing many valuable ideas and comments. Financial support for the larger project has come from the Ford Foundation and the Population Council. The writer has undertaken the present analysis under support from the Ford Foundation.

Lee Isbister model

Lee and Isbister set themselves the task of deriving a set of formulas that would enable them to estimate:

(1) "the effect of a given birth control program on the fertility of a particular future year,"

(2) "the total effect that IUD's will have during all the years they remain in use," and

(3 "the scale of the IUD program required to achieve specified objectives."

These objectives are tackled within the framework of component projection. As a result, the task requiring methodological innovation is narrowed to that of estimating the effects upon age-specific fertility of posited schedules of IUD acceptance. Broadly speaking, these effects depend on the lengths of time devices are retained and the fertility foregone during these periods of protection.

Lee and Isbister present as their basic formula:

$$f_{i,t} = \frac{F_{i,t} \cdot f_{i,0} - Q_{i,t} \cdot g_i}{F_{i,t}} \quad ,$$

where $f_{i,t}$ birth rate of the ith age group, in year t,

      $F_{i,t}$ total women belonging to the ith age group in year t (derived by procedures of component projection),

      $f_{i,0}$ birth rate of the ith age group, in base year before IUD program is begun (derived from census and vital registration data or from a sample survey),

      g_i "potential" birth rate which acceptors of IUD of the ith age group would have experienced had they not adopted IUD,

      $Q_{i,t}$ number of women of the ith age group, in year t, who were practicing totally effective contraception, on the basis of IUD, in year t-1,

      and the subscript i = 1, 2, . . ., 7 refers to age— classes 15-19, 20-24, . . ., 45-49 years.

With respect to $Q_{i,t}$ it is assumed that effective contraception practiced during year t-1 by preventing conceptions during that year is averting births during the next year t. To estimate $Q_{i,t}$, it is necessary to know the number of women accepting IUD each previous year t-1, t-2, . . . and to know as well the fraction of these women who are still deriving protection from the device during year t-1.

Three features of Lee and Isbister's treatment call for improvement. First is their method for deriving the potential birth rates g_i of acceptors. Because the acceptors of IUD would have had higher fertility in the absence of IUD than their whole age class, it is not permissible simply to equate g_i with $f_{i,0}$, the birth rate of the ith age group in the base year. Instead, Lee and Isbister postulate that "without the program, acceptors' age-specific fertility rates would have been 20 percent above the marital fertility rates in the general population during the base year." Yet evidence from Ross[5], as well as data to be reviewed below, indicates that this difference in birth rates is not a constant proportion but a variable one increasing with advancing age. It is preferable then to have more empirical estimates of g_i-value based if possible on the previous performance of the acceptors themselves.

A second limitation is the lack of any provision for accidental pregnancy through failures of IUD. Lee and Isbister's basic formula forces them to assume that IUD is 100 percent effective so long as it is retained.

A third limitation is their unrealistic assumptions about the length of time that devices are retained. Lacking information available now, Lee and Isbister adopted a rather schematic set of assumptions reflecting the belief current then that the minority of the devices would come out quickly but the rest remain in place for long periods. These assumptions now appear to exaggerate length of retention and to distort the contrast among age classes. It is plainly desirable to replace these schematized assumptions with more empirical ones.

The procedure to be described below is designed to remove the three limitations just enumerated. Lee and Isbister's convention respecting lengths of retention is replaced by a formula that makes it possible to incorporate life table results pertaining both to duration-specific proportions retaining and rates of accidental pregnancy. In addition, alternative estimates of potential fertility are derived from prior fertility data collected from the acceptors themselves.

To be tested with the revised procedure is a main conclusion of Lee and Isbister, namely, that: "A family planning program is made much more effective by securing younger participants."[6] Applying their scheme to the family planning program of South Korea, and using an empirical distribution of ages at insertion averaging 33 years, Lee and Isbister calculated that 1.5 births are averted on average per first segment of IUD. When they substituted a hypothetical age distribution averaging 29.5 years, their estimate was increased to 1.9 births averted per first segment of IUD.

Also worth testing is a much quoted rule of thumb derived by L. P. Chow for Taiwan. According to the rule, five insertions of IUD avert one birth per year for at least 5 years. Chow's reasoning, as interpreted by Ross[7], is:

(1) "Of 5 IUD's inserted this year, two will come out before they

have time to do much good. The others will stay in at least 5 years.

(2) The marital fertility rate among acceptors would be about 333 in the absence of a program. Consequently:

(3) Five IUD's inserted this year will prevent one birth next year and another birth each year for at least four more years. Thus, each IUD inserted this year prevents one birth within 5 years, on the average."

Rationale

Two assumptions guide much of the development below. First of all, it is assumed that acceptors of IUD are doubly selected, having higher fecundity than average for their age class and partly for that reason also higher than average interest and initiative with respect to family planning. The intensities of these two selectivities may be expected to vary from population to population and within a population from age class to age class. As a consequence, it is too much to hope for a fixed relationship between the potential fertility of acceptors and marital fertility of the general populace. It appears necessary to draw estimates of ɩotential fertility from the experience of the acceptors themselves. A second basic assumption is that estimates of retention span are best obtained through life table analyses of use effectiveness, with the results then subjected to a series of corrections lest they exaggerate the periods of protection being conferred.

At any time during her reproductive period, a married woman who is still fertile may be thought of as being in one of three states: pregnant, amenorrheic, or fecundable. If in the fecundable state and not practicing contraception, the woman has a certain monthly chance of conceiving, termed her "natural fecundability."[8] Contraception reduces fertility by lowering natural fecundability and thereby tending to prolong stays in the fecundable state. Such a prolongation by interrupting the cycle of pregnancy-delivery-amenorrhea-fecundability-pregnancy is suspending the childbearing process for a time. Depending on the length of this interruption and upon the woman's potential rate of childbearing during this period of suspension, a certain number of births are being averted, at least in the short run.

Thus a contraceptive averts births by delaying the next conception when the woman is in her fecundable state. Nothing is accomplished if a sterile couple practice contraception or if a nonsterile couple practice contraception when the female partner is amenorrheic or already pregnant. For an estimate of births averted per segment of IUD, two kinds of statistics are needed. The first are estimates of the prolongations of stay in the fecundable state resulting from retention of the device. Second, to convert these prolongations into births averted, it is necessary to divide them by a constant representing the average marriage duration per birth that might have been required by the couples had they not adopted IUD.

Retention of IUD as estimated by a simple life table analysis such as used in the measurement of use effectiveness overstates the extent to which IUD is prolonging stays in the fecundable state. A corrected estimate of the latter would allow for: (1) the proportions of couples whose union is disrupted by death or divorce while still using the contraceptive; (2) the proportions of acceptors who were already sterile or who became sterile during retention of the device; (3) the amount of overlap between amenorrhea and practice of the contraceptive; and (4) the accidental pregnancies that occur despite presence of the device.

It is convenient to summarize these matters by two equations applicable to any contraceptive but defined below in terms of IUD.

(1) $I = F(R - A - PW)$, where all durations are in months and

$I =$ average duration that childbearing is interrupted—i.e., mean prolongation of stay in the fecundable state,

$F =$ proportion of couples fertile at time IUD is inserted,

$R =$ mean time device is retained among couples at fertile time of insertion,

$A =$ allowance for amenorrhea,

$P =$ proportion becoming accidentally pregnant, i.e., pregnant with device in situ or position undetermined,

$W =$ penalty per accidental pregnancy;

(2) $B = I/D$, where I is defined above and

$B =$ births averted per first segment of IUD, and

$D =$ average duration per birth that might have been required had IUD not been adopted.[9]

Since the wearing of a device by couples sterile at time of insertion accomplishes nothing, equation (1) properly focuses on that fraction F of couples who are fertile at time of insertion. R refers to the mean interval from insertion to death of a spouse, divorce, onset of secondary sterility, or loss of the device through pregnancy, expulsion, or removal, whichever occurs soonest. A convenient shorthand for pregnancy, expulsion, or removal is "PER." R is best estimated from a life table analysis in which mortality (together with separation and divorce, if need be), sterility, and PER are treated as three competing risks. The estimates A and P relate to women belonging to unions fertile at time of insertion. A denotes the overlap between amenorrhea and use of IUD, which overlap is shortened when death, sterility, or PER intervenes before end of amenorrhea. P designates the proportion of acceptors belonging to unions fertile at insertion for whom accidental pregnancy is the cause of ending useful retention of IUD rather than mortality, divorce, sterility, expulsion, or removal. It will be convenient to use "EUROD" as an abbreviation for "end of useful retention of IUD."

If an accidental pregnancy occurs despite the device, then it is proper to impose a "penalty" by subtracting "W," the remaining term in equation (1), from R for each such pregnancy. W signifies the mean fecundable period that would have been required for pregnancy among still fertile acceptors if they had not had a chance to elect IUD. IUD is not prolonging stays in the fecundable state unless it is extending the mean fecundable period per pregnancy over what it otherwise would have been. If IUD were substituting for a contraceptive superior to it in effectiveness, with the consequence that IUD's were actually shortening stays in the fecundable state, then it would be appropriate for the estimate of childbearing interruption I to be negative, a result obtained when the term PW exceeds R − A. Thus the magnitude of W depends closely on the extent and effectiveness of family planning activity for which IUD is substituting. A low potential fertility by implying lengthy stays in the fecundable state determines a large W-value. At the other extreme, if not introducing IUD would have meant no birth control, then W would take its minimal value.

A given interruption of childbearing (I) averts more births, the less effective is the contraception (or the less frequent its practice) for which IUD is substituting. In equation (2), a less effective regime of potential family limitation is expressed by a shorter duration D per potential birth. However, it must be kept in mind that not only D, but also W, one of the variables appearing in the expression for I, is affected by the assumed effectiveness of the contraception for which IUD is substituting. Hence there exists a dependence between I and D and it is not meaningful to think of the two values as varying independently of each other.

To estimate births averted per segment of IUD during each successive year following insertion, one analyzes the total interruption of childbearing into additive annual subtotals $I_1, I_2, \ldots$ and divides each by the common appropriate D-value. Following Lee and Isbister, it is assumed that no births are averted the first year so that I_1/D represents births averted during the second year, I_2/D births averted during the third year, and so on. Strictly speaking, one should think of the duration D per potential birth as continuously changing as a function of the woman's age and motivation to practice family limitation and accordingly I_1, for example, would be divided by a slightly different value of D than I_2. However, except possibly near the end of the reproductive period, the changes of D are not so rapid as to make such a refinement seem worth attempting and as a first approximation one may be satisfied with dividing the several annual subtotals of useful retention by a common D-value specific to the 5-year age class and appropriate to the other assumptions being adopted at the time.

As a last general point, before turning to procedure and results, note should be taken of another form of substitution ignored by Lee and Isbister and to be ignored in the analysis below. Let us say that among n acceptors, the interruption of childbearing averages x months per segment of IUD, while in the absence of IUD, y months would have been required on average to produce a birth. Therefore x/y births are being averted per segment of IUD in the short run. Whether these births are averted in the long run in the sense of representing subtractions from completed family size depends on whether the women are limiting or merely postponing. In the latter case, current postponements of births may mean later postponement of family limitation practices and hence at that later period more childbearing than otherwise would have been the case. Accordingly some of the presently averted births are cancelled by later births that otherwise would not have been allowed. To this extent, the cohort's childbearing has merely been spread out in time rather than reduced in volume.

This second aspect to substitution will be ignored in the analysis below. According to a series of monthly reports, about 85 percent of the Taichung acceptors are using IUD's for limitation rather than spacing purposes.[10] However, in the youngest age class to be considered, 20-24 years, the proportion of spacers is appreciable and the estimates of births averted are to be interpreted only as births averted in the short run.

Interruption of childbearing
Estimates of I, the interruption of childbearing, involve a rather long list of parameters, with each derivation requiring several steps. A full description of procedure is contained in an unpublished technical appendix.[11]

The analysis is carried out separately for four age classes: 20-24, 25-29, 30-34, and 35-39 years. Acceptors of the present sample are distributed among these age groups in proportions of .13, .32, .32, and .23. Results for the total sample are derived as weighted averages of age-specific results. This approach offers two advantages. First, assumptions that acceptors are homogeneous with respect to monthly risks and that these risks are constant in time are less damaging simplifications when taken over an age span of 5 years rather than over an entire reproductive span. Secondly, it becomes possible to assign different sets of weights to the four age classes and in this manner to treat the acceptors' age distribution as a variable for study.

That the various estimates used in the derivation of I are subject to error follows not only from limitations of the available data but from deliberate simplifications of concept aimed at making computation and estimation easier. However, as far as possible the expedient of assuming independence where there is appreciable dependence has been resisted. For example, W, the penalty for an accidental pregnancy, is defined in specific relation to the effectiveness of family planning which it is assumed that IUD is replacing. When two or more factors shortening retention of IUD are competing with each other, that competition is operationalized through a life table or other type of analysis. For example, in the derivation of mean retention span R, mortality, sterility, and PER are treated as competing risks; in evaluating P, the proportion experiencing accidental pregnancy, the risk of pregnancy is treated as being in competition with risks of expulsion and removal as well as mortality and secondary sterility. Even in the development of A, account is taken that EUROD may antedate end of amenorrhea and to that degree abbreviate the overlap of amenorrhea with useful retention of IUD.

However, to achieve the above refinements and still keep estimation and computation (on a desk calculator)[12] within practicable limits, free use has been made of such expedients as substituting expected values for distributions, assuming homogeneity of risk within 5-year age groups, and treating age-specific risks as constants unvarying with time elapsed from insertion. These expedients make it possible to take repeated advantage of the very convenient properties of the exponential density, formulas for which are reviewed in the first section of the aforementioned technical appendix. Perhaps the most serious simplification is the composite assumption that among women fertile at insertion, a proportion x lose their device "immediately" whereas the remaining $(1 - x)$ are exposed continuously to three constant, competing risks, namely, of mortality m, of secondary sterility s, and of PER p. While justification will be adduced later for assuming the constancy of p, and while the level of mortality in the present application is low enough at all relevant ages to render it unimportant, it must be admitted that the risk of secondary sterility s is not realistically treated as a constant, especially in the oldest age class where its level is high enough to make it an important factor and where that level is changing rapidly as a function of age. In a later version of the present analysis, it is hoped to remove this restriction.

Regarding secondary sterility, measured by the parameters F and s, the basic assumption adopted is that any acceptor is fertile at the time of her last birth prior to insertion, but then becomes subject to the risk of secondary sterility characteristic of her age class. The magnitude of this risk is taken from the work of Henry on the brash premise that involuntary sterility operates in contemporary Taiwan as Henry estimates it to have operated in a congeries of historical European populations.[13] Use is made of data from the Taichung respondents concerning the average interval (in each 5-year age class) between last preceding birth and first insertion of a device.

Respecting m, the age-specific monthly risk of a marriage being disrupted by death of one of the partners, it is assumed, on the authority of Chow, Hsu, and Hsu,[14] that U. N. Model Life Table No. 80 (e_0 of 60.4 years)[15] best typifies current mortality in Taiwan. Although it is one of the causes of EUROD, divorce is considered infrequent enough in the present population so that it may be ignored without fear of serious distortion.

Other things equal, the overlap A between useful retention of a device and amenorrhea is greater when either postpartum amenorrhea is longer or else the interval from last birth to insertion is shorter. Average length of postpartum amenorrhea is estimated at 8 months, based on Mohopatra's intensive analysis of birth intervals of the Taichung women.[16] The detailed data on duration from preceding birth to insertion are again exploited.

Another necessary estimate is P, the proportion among women fertile at insertion who become accidentally pregnant with the device. For the first two years following insertion, a direct estimate is available from the Taichung IUCD Medical Follow-up Study.[17] For the subsequent period an extrapolation based on these same data is made consistent with assumptions concerning the course of the combined risk p of accidental pregnancy, expulsion, and removal. W, the age-specific penalty per accidental pregnancy, requires detailed assumptions about fecundity including risks of spontaneous wastage and lengths of gestation and amenorrhea conditional upon outcome of pregnancy. The reason for stipulating a mean of 8 months for postpartum amenorrhea has already been mentioned. The remaining stipulations have to rest on the premise that level and age changes of Taiwan fecundity broadly correspond to those found in other populations.[18] More specifically, it is assumed that the ratio of pregnancies (including spontaneous abortions and stillbirths) to live births is roughly 1.2 in the youngest age class, rising to 1.33 in the oldest.

The estimate of R is dominated by the value assumed for p, the constant monthly risk of PER. Available from the Taichung IUCD Medical Follow-up Study is an estimate of the proportion who, exposed solely to PER risks, still retain their device at the end of 24 months, designated as U(24), for each age class. From the same analysis,[19] a graph of the monthly risk of losing the device if retaining it up to the start of the month shows appreciable decline during the first three months but very little decline thereafter. Following the lead of Mauldin and Stephan,[20] a monthly rate of device loss is estimated on the basis of months 6 through 24 and this constant rate is assumed to prevail at all durations after insertion. To allow for the relatively high rates of the initial 2 or 3 months, a proportion of "immediate" device losses is postulated, namely, that proportion which together with the estimated constant rate of device loss p will yield the proportion U(24) estimated from the original life table analysis of data from the Taichung Medical Follow-up Study. The resulting estimates of proportions of women retaining the device for specified intervals will prove conservatively low if it turns out in the long run that there is a gradual decline in the monthly risk of device loss to PER. It is also to be kept in mind that these proportions of retention relate to first segments of IUD with no provision made for reinsertions and ensuing segments of IUD.

Illustrative results are given in Tables 1-3. Table 1 carries a comparison of parameters U and R, the former being an uncorrected estimate of mean retention span and the latter an estimate of the same quantity corrected for mortality and secondary sterility. Both U and R increase rapidly with advancing age of wife. While differences between U and R are negligible for age classes 20-24 and 25-29 years, the two estimates diverge rapidly across the next two age intervals.

Table 2 indicates that of the three causes of EUROD—mortality, secondary sterility, and PER—PER dominates in all age classes. It accounts for over 70 percent of EUROD even in age class 35 years and over and for greater proportions in the younger age classes. In no age class is mortality of much significance. Only in the oldest age class is sterility of more than secondary importance and of minor, though not trivial importance, in age class 30-34 years.

In Table 3 are assembled the values entering into an estimate of

Table 1. Mean Span of Useful Retention of IUD, Allowing for Mortality and Sterility,[1] in Comparison with an Uncorrected Estimate, by Age Class of Wife

Age class	Monthly rates of attrition[2]			Three causes com- bined	Propor- tion losing device at once	Mean span of re- tention (months)		Differ- ence
	PER	Mortality	Sterility			Cor- rected	Uncor- rected	
	p	m	s	u^3	x	$R = \dfrac{(1-x)}{u}$	$U = \dfrac{(1-x)}{p}$	U-R
20-24	.0561	.000562	.000715	.0574	.069	16.2	16.5	0.3
25-29	.0355	.000589	.001138	.0372	.075	24.9	26.0	1.1
30-34	.0218	.000667	.002093	.0246	.064	37.9	43.0	5.1
35-39	.0151	.000793	.005475	.0214	.072	43.3	61.4	18.1
All ages[4]	—	—	—	—	.070	32.1	38.2	6.1

[1]Among women fertile at time of insertion.

[2]Among the proportion $(1-x)$ who do not lose the device immediately.

[3]$u = p + m + s$

[4]Estimates derived as weighted averages of age-specific results.

Table 2. Proportions of Women Ending Useful Retention of IUD Because of Mortality, Secondary Sterility, and PER (Pregnancy, Expulsion, or Removal), by Age Class of Wife

Age class	Percent of EUROD† attributable to:			Total
	PER	Mortality	Sterility	
20-24	97.9	0.9	1.1	99.9
25-29	95.7	1.5	2.9	100.1
30-34	89.4	2.5	8.0	99.9
35-39	72.7	3.4	23.8	99.9
All ages*	88.7	2.2	9.0	99.9

*Estimates derived as weighted averages of age-specific results.

†Ending of useful retention of an intrauterine device.

I, given "medium" assumptions about potential fertility. The proportions of acceptors fertile at insertion are too close to unity for the parameter F to have much bearing on the results. The allowance A for overlap with amenorrhea also proves of secondary moment. The proportions P experiencing accidental pregnancy are low enough to

Table 3. Interruption of Childbearing by IUD, Given the Medium Assumption about Effectiveness of Family Planning in the Absence of IUD, by Age Class of Wife

Age class	Proportion of women fertile at insertion	Span of useful retention	Mean overlap with amenorrhea	Proportion becoming accidentally pregnant	Penalty per accidental pregnancy	Allowance for accidental pregnancy	Interruption of childbearing	Difference
	F	R	A	P	W	PW	I = F(R-A-PW)	U-I
20-24	.9945	16.2	2.1	.11	5.9	0.6	13.4	3.1
25-29	.9910	24.9	1.7	.18	11.0	2.0	21.0	5.0
30-34	.9816	37.9	1.5	.23	21.2	4.9	30.9	12.1
35-39	.9520	43.3	1.6	.12	36.1	4.0	35.9	25.5
All ages*	.9796	32.1	1.7	.15	19.3	3.2	26.5	11.7

*Estimates derived as weighted averages of age-specific results.

keep the PW correction at modest levels. The most critical term in deciding the relative lengths of childbearing interruption amongst the four age classes is R, which, except for the oldest age class, is determined largely by p, the monthly risk of device loss from PER.

If it is posited that IUD is substituting for no family planning activity, then the value of W is reduced to its minimum of 6 to 12 months, the value within this range depending on age, and the correction PW is correspondingly reduced. On the other hand, if a conservative assumption in the sense of belittling potential fertility is adopted, then W and hence PW may be increased by a factor of 2 or 3 over values observed in Table 3.

Time distribution
The allocation of useful retention of IUD to successive years following insertion is the next topic for consideration. In the aforementioned technical appendix, an argument is advanced for expecting these annual subtotals, $I_1, I_2, \ldots$ when expressed as proportions of I to conform approximately to the proportionate distribution of corresponding subareas under a decay curve with parameter $u = m + s + p$, where m, s, and p are defined as in Table 1. The argument rests on the assumptions that u is constant within 5-year age classes and that frequency of accidental pregnancy is proportional to the number of fertile women still wearing the device. The chief deviation from this hypothesis is caused by the fact that the entire overlap A between

amenorrhea and retention of IUD has to be subtracted from the I_1 of the first year.

To test L. P. Chow's generalization alleging a uniform impact over the first 5 years, it is of interest to estimate subtotals of child-bearing interruption during each of the first 5 years and for the sub-sequent period. These subtotals are given as proportions in Table 4, again for the case of "medium" potential fertility—to be defined in the next section. Actually, altering the assumption about potential fertility produces only second order effects upon the proportions contained in Table 4. As one would expect from the argument cited above, amongst the youngest women whose risk of device loss u is high, the annual impact of IUD diminishes rapidly. Over 40 percent of total useful retention is expended in the first year and over two-thirds in the first two years. In sharp contrast, among the oldest women with a much lower monthly risk of EUROD, only about one-fifth of the useful retention of IUD is concentrated in the first year, with the subsequent decline in retention slow enough so that about 30 percent of the total impact is felt after 5 years. Of course, if impact is defined in terms of births averted rather than conceptions post-poned, the proportionate effects documented by Table 4 are displaced roughly one year to the right, with zero impact assigned to the first year.

Potential fertility

Attention now turns to potential fertility, to be measured in terms of duration D per potential birth. As remarked earlier, the double selectivity of acceptors with respect both to fecundity and family planning initiative banishes hope for a simple relationship between

Table 4. Useful Retention of IUD during Successive Years following Insertion, by Age Class of Wife

| Age Class | Proportionate distribution of useful retention of IUD | | | | | | |
	First year	Second year	Third year	Fourth year	Fifth year	Sixth year or later	Total
20-24	.42	.29	.15	.07	.04	.03	1.00
25-29	.31	.25	.16	.10	.07	.12	1.01
30-34	.22	.20	.15	.11	.08	.24	1.00
35-39	.19	.18	.14	.11	.08	.29	.99
All ages*	.27	.22	.15	.10	.07	.18	.99

*Estimates derived as weighted averages of age-specific results.

the potential fertility of acceptors and the marital fertility of all women. It is necessary, therefore, to look to the acceptors' own experience as a basis for estimation. This task is made practical by an analysis of Freedman and Takeshita relating to a probability sample of Taichung women first interviewed in late 1962.[21] Information about these 2132 couples includes: (1) a birth rate for the 3-year period directly preceding first interview[22]; (2) use or nonuse of birth control prior to the interview; (3) sterilization or not before a second interview approximately one year after the first; and (4) acceptance or not of IUD before July, 1965, approximately 2½ years after the initial interview. Sterilizations are not uncommon in this sample. Of the respondents aged 36 years or over, 17 percent report sterilizing operations to themselves or their husbands. With regard to the majority who report no sterilizing operations, the selectivity of acceptors is affirmed by their having consistently higher fertility than nonacceptors with the differential increasing at older ages. Moreover, this increasing differential persists within categories of use or nonuse of family planning prior to first interview.

Among the acceptors themselves, the fertility of those reporting no birth control before IUD declines only gradually with advancing age. This finding supports the premise that not only did virtually all the women believe themselves fecund at time of insertion—or why should they accept a device—but the great majority actually were still fertile at time of insertion. In contrast, the acceptors who reported previous practice of birth control show a more rapid decline in pre-insertion fertility with advancing age, indicative of an improving practice of family limitation.

From these findings it is plain that in the absence of IUD, the acceptors as a total group would have been lowering their fertility during the interval between the 3-year base period just prior to interview and the R-year period coinciding with IUD use. Presumably this decline would have reflected less a fecundity decline than an increased practice of family limitation. Now eventually there will be information both about the birth rates of acceptors after discontinuing IUD as well as before its initiation. Interpolations between these "before" and "after" sets of data will yield relatively firm estimates of potential fertility during retention of IUD.

For the present, however, only information respecting pre-insertion fertility is available. To gauge the potential fertility of acceptors aged 30-34 at first interview, for example, it is necessary to estimate by interpolation the base period birth rate of acceptors aged $30 + c$ to $34 + c$ years at time of interview, where c is chosen to represent the average interval between midpoint of the 3-year base period and midpoint of the period coinciding with IUD use. In addition, the calculation of potential fertility must allow for the possibility that in the absence of IUD a minority of the acceptors would have accepted sterilization during the R-year period coinciding with IUD retention.

Three sets of age-specific D-values have been derived on the basis of data from the analysis of Freedman and Takeshita. In the first set, the pre-insertion birth rates of acceptors reporting no previous practice of birth control are utilized to represent potential fertility in the absence of family planning. Provision is made for the slight declines in birth rates between base period and R-year period coinciding with IUD use. As with the estimates of childbearing interruption, a number of simplifications are allowed, mainly replacing distributions with expected values and working from these. The procedural details are not necessary here, but are described in the technical appendix mentioned earlier. It should be remarked that the estimates of potential fertility for the younger three age classes are based on interpolation and for that reason are firmer, though certainly not free from error, than the estimate for the oldest age class, which is based on an extrapolation.

A medium set of birth rates are derived from the pre-insertion birth rates of all acceptors. It is assumed that these birth rates reflect the frequency and effectiveness of indigenous birth control and that if IUD had not been introduced, the age-specific fertility of the acceptors would have persisted unchanged for a few more years at least. Adjustment is made for the interval between base period and period of IUD use. The provision for sterilization operations emerges as a surprisingly minor correction. A rate of 17 percent reporting sterilizing operations near the end of the reproductive period sounds impressive, but is still low enough so that it implies a rather low rate of new sterilizations per year. Only modest proportions of acceptors could be expected to resort to sterilization during the comparatively short periods coinciding with IUD use.

A third, deliberately conservative set of estimates is derived from the pre-insertion birth rates of acceptors reporting previous practice of family planning. The objective here is to assess the potential fertility that might have resulted if nearly every acceptor had tried some other method of birth control in the absence of IUD. The adjustment for fertility decline between base period and retention period is again incorporated into the estimates as well as the provision for sterilizing operations.

The three sets of durations per potential birth are compared in Table 5. One must keep in mind the greater uncertainty attaching to estimates relating to the oldest age group. The increase in D with advancing age from 25 months to 35 months, when no family planning is postulated, is not unreasonable in the light of available data on natural fertility.[23] The substituting of IUD for pre-existing birth control occurs more frequently among the older women. As is clear from Table 5, passage from a situation of no substitution to one of medium substitution and finally to one of nearly universal substitution hardly affects the potential fertility of the youngest women, but markedly reduces the potential fertility of the oldest women and to a lesser degree that of the intermediate age classes.

Births averted

Estimates of births averted per first segment of IUD are obtained from the simple ratio I/D. The principal results are grouped in Table 6.

The top row of figures relates to the hypothetical case where IUD is replacing an absence of family limitation. Accordingly, potential fertility is at its maximum. Even so, the estimated number of births averted per segment of IUD does not quite reach 1.0. In this special situation of no substitution, the older women over 30 years of age are estimated to avert slightly more births than their younger neighbors.

Table 5. Estimates of Duration D per Potential Birth in the Absence of IUD, by Age Class of Wife

Estimate	*Rationale*	*Wife's age at interview*				
		20-24	*25-29*	*30-34*	*35-39*	*All ages**
No family planning	Experience of acceptors when not practicing family planning	25	27	30	35	29.5
Medium	Experience of all acceptors with provision for sterilizing operations	25	31	43	67	42.2
Conservative (D-estimate too high)	Experience of acceptors when practicing family planning with provision for sterilizing operations	28	39	60	125	63.7

*Estimates derived as weighted averages of age-specific results.

Table 6. Births Averted per First Segment of IUD, by Age Class of Wife: Comparison of an Uncorrected Estimate with Three Corrected Estimates under Contrasting Assumptions about Effectiveness of Family Planning in the Absence of IUD

		Births averted per first segment of IUD				
Estimate of childbearing interruption	*Estimate of duration D per potential birth**	Age class				*All agest*
		20-24	*25-29*	*30-34*	*35-39*	
Corrected	Minimal D-estimate (no family planning)	.54	.80	1.12	1.10	.94
	Medium	.54	.68	.72	.54	.64
	Conservative (D-estimate too high)	.47	.51	.46	.24	.43
Uncorrected	Medium	.66	.84	1.00	.92	.88

*D-estimates are taken from Table 1.

†Estimates derived as weighted averages of age-specific results.

Their much longer retention spans are outweighing their lower potential fertility.

However, when proper recognition is given to the substituting of IUD for other forms of birth control, the picture changes drastically, as might be anticipated from Table 5. Under the medium assumption of potential fertility, the average number of births averted decreases by roughly a third. Furthermore, because substitution operates so much more strongly in the older age classes, the largest impacts are now recorded in age classes 25-29 and 30-34 years.

Moving to the conservative definition of potential fertility, predicated on nearly universal substitution, the average number of births averted declines still further and the greatest point of impact is now centered in age group 25-29 years. Obviously the strength of the substitution factor—as illustrated by the three different definitions of potential fertility in Table 6—exerts a tremendous influence both on the general level of IUD impact and the differentiation of that impact amongst age classes.

The last row of figures in Table 6 represents estimates of births averted based on the medium standard of potential fertility combined with the uncorrected estimate of mean retention span U. Estimating interruption of childbearing I entails a good deal of labor and it is fair to ask whether U might not serve as a reasonable stopgap, especially since it is a pure function of p, the monthly risk of device loss to PER, which has been shown to predominate in the determination of R. Unfortunately a comparison of the second and fourth rows of Table 6 indicates that the short-cut not only exaggerates births averted by a factor of over one-third, but seriously distorts age differentials as well.

Discussion

Before addressing the significance of the above results, it is worth emphasizing once more that the values contained in Tables 1-6 are subject to considerable error, especially those pertaining to the oldest age class, and have meaning chiefly as orders of magnitude and indicators of trend, rather than as point estimates. Four conclusions are now briefly discussed:

1. Obviously the present analysis has produced lower estimates of births averted per segment of IUD than did the analyses of either Lee and Isbister or Chow. According to present results, the one birth averted per segment of IUD promised by Chow is approached only when substitution effects are ruled out. When these effects are given recognition, the resultant number of births averted falls well short of 1.0 and of course even farther short of the 1.5 projected by Lee and Isbister. Much of the difference lies in the contrasting stipulations about retention length. Admittedly too, in the present case, only first segments are dealt with. However even if segments had been extended to encompass reinsertions, it is still doubtful that under the medium assumption of potential fertility, estimates of births averted among the Taichung women would have reached 1.0.

2. Present results also qualify Lee and Isbister's generalization that more is accomplished by securing younger participants in an IUD program. In Taichung, devices are retained so much longer by older women than younger that the most favorable balance between useful retention of IUD and potential fertility is found to coincide with the two intermediate age classes. Actually this outcome is a highly favorable one since it means, for Taichung at least, that IUD has its greatest impact in precisely those age classes which are furnishing the most acceptors. It is to be recalled that the proportions of Taichung acceptors aged 20-24, 25-29, 30-34, and 35-39 years are .13, .32, .32, and .23 respectively. Materials assembled by Mauldin[24] indicate that in some other populations besides Taiwan, but not in all, acceptors concentrate in the age range 25-34 years.

3. Third, exception may be taken to Chow's allegation that impact from IUD will be fairly uniform over the 5 years following insertion. Rather, after the initial year, the number of births averted

may be expected to decline and this decline will be the more rapid the shorter is the average span of retention. The situation he forecasts would be approached only if retention spans—apart from the very short spans due to early device loss—were consistently long.

4. Particular stress is placed on a fourth and final point. It would appear that several of the parameters entering into the calculations above, such as the parameters relating to secondary sterility, mortality, and amenorrhea, are often of secondary importance or at least may be expected to operate in a fairly uniform manner from one population to another. Then too, IUD and oral contraception typically vouchsafe low levels of accidental pregnancy. However, there are two factors—first, the degree to which the contraceptive under study is substituting for other methods of birth control and, second, the typical length of its use—which may be expected to vary greatly from one population to another and within a population from age class to age class.

This variation with respect to retention length has already been documented by Mauldin[25] and an important variation with respect to potential fertility is presumably in the process of emerging among nations having large-scale family planning programs. Given the paramount importance of potential fertility and typical lengths of usage of a contraceptive together with their widely varying combinations of value, one can only anticipate that the new contraceptives like IUD and the pills will exhibit widely varying levels of average impact and age differentiation from one family planning program to another. Hence, it is very unlikely that any universal rule of thumb—such as one birth averted per first segment of IUD—will find empirical support. For a serious evaluation of the demographic effectiveness of a specified contraceptive in a given population, there is no choice but to work for suitable information concerning the two most critical aspects. For this purpose we need, first, follow-up data on the acceptors to ascertain lengths of successful usage and to verify that low rates of accidental pregnancy obtain, and second, data regarding the acceptors' potential fertility and the selectivity of that fertility relative to the rest of the population.

Notes

1. C. Tietze, "The Clinical Effectiveness of Contraceptive Methods," *American Journal of Obstetrics and Gynecology*, 78 (1959), pp. 650-51. A third aspect of effectiveness distinguished by Tietze is "physiologic effec-

tiveness," use effectiveness under ideal conditions, i.e., when the method is used consistently and according to instructions.

2. R. G. Potter, "Application of Life Table Techniques to Measurement of Contraceptive Effectiveness," *Demography*, 3, No. 2 (1966), pp. 297-304; and C. Tietze, "Intra-uterine Contraception: Recommended Procedures for Data Analysis," *Studies in Family Planning*, 18 (Supplement), (Apr., 1967), pp. 1-6.

3. B. M. Lee and J. Isbister, "The Impact of Birth Control Programs on Fertility," in B. Berelson, *et al.* (eds.), *Family Planning and Population* (Chicago: University of Chicago Press, 1966), pp. 744-47.

4. J. A. Ross, "Cost of Family Planning Programs," in B. Berelson, *et al.* (eds.), *Family Planning and Population* (Chicago: University of Chicago Press, 1966), pp. 761-62.

5. J. A. Ross, *op. cit.*, pp. 762-64.

6. B. M. Lee and J. Isbister, *op. cit.*, p. 746.

7. John A. Ross, "Cost of Family Planning Programs," *op. cit.*, pp. 761-62.

8. J. C. Ridley and M. C. Sheps, "An Analytic Simulation Model of Human Reproduction with Demographic and Biological Components," *Population Studies*, 19 (March, 1966), 301-2. See also R. G. Potter, "Birth Intervals: Structure and Change," *Population Studies*, 17 (Nov., 1963), 164-65; and M. C. Sheps and E. B. Perrin, "Changes in Birth Rates as a Function of Contraceptive Effectiveness: Some Applications of a Stochastic Model," *American Journal of Public Health*, 53 (July, 1963), 1031-44.

9. Following Lee and Isbister, we could have let g designate the potential birth rate (per woman per year) and then, noting that $g = 12/D$, expressed equation (2) as $B = 12Ig$. Parameter D is used instead of g because D clarifies and enters into the calculation of W, the penalty per accidental pregnancy which is discussed below.

10. For example, Table 7 of the *Joint Monthly Report—December 1966*, published jointly by the Taiwan Provincial Department of Health, the Maternal and Child Health Association, and the Taiwan Population Studies Center.

11. Titled "A Technical Appendix on Procedures Used in Manuscript 'Estimating Births Averted in a Family Planning Program,'" this appendix is available on request from the Population Studies Center, University of Michigan, 1225 South University Ave., Ann Arbor, Mich. 48104.

12. It is proposed to program the analysis for an electronic computer in order to be able to relax some of the simplifying assumptions as well as to be able to undertake a wider set of calculations for purposes of studying the generality of some of the findings to be reported below.

13. Louis Henry, *Fécondité des Mariages*, Institut national d'études démographiques, Travaux et Documents, Cahier No. 16 (Presses Universitaires de France, 1953), p. 103. See also his, "Some Data on Natural Fertility," *Eugenics Quarterly*, 8 (June, 1961), 85.

14. L. P. Chow, S. C. Hsu, and T. C. Hsu, "The Future Population of Taiwan Projected by Three Fertility Assumptions," *J. of the Formosan Medical Association*, 64 (Sept. 1965), 565.

15. From United Nations, *Methods for Population Projections by Sex and Age*, Population Studies No. 25, ST/SOA/Series A, 1956, p. 73.

16. Partha S. Mohopatra, *The Effect of Age at Marriage and Birth Control Practices on Fertility Differentials in Taiwan* (unpublished Ph.D. dissertation, The University of Michigan, 1966), p. 126.

17. R. G. Potter, L. P. Chow, A. K. Jain, and C. H. Lee, *Expanded Report on Social and Demographic Correlates of IUCD Effectiveness: The Taichung IUCD Medical Follow-up Study* (University of Michigan Population Studies Center, Feb., 1967), unpublished paper, pp. 8-11.

18. L. Henry, "La Fécondité Naturelle: Observation—Théories— Résultats," *Population*, 16 (Oct.-Dec.), pp. 625-36, and his "Some Data on Natural Fertility," *Eugenics Quarterly*, 8 (June, 1961), pp. 81-91.

19. R. G. Potter, L. P. Chow, A. K. Jain, and C. H. Lee, *op. cit.*, pp. 11-16.

20. W. P. Mauldin, "Retention of IUDs: An International Comparison," *Studies in Family Planning*, No. 18 (Apr. 1967), p. 7.

21. R. Freedman and J. Takeshita, "Recent Fertility of Taichung Couples in Relation to Acceptance Status and Prior Use of Family Limitation" (University of Michigan Population Studies Center, Sept., 1966), unpublished paper.

22. Birth rates may also be computed for the 5-year period preceding first interview and these birth rates yield results virtually duplicating those for the 3-year period, to be used in the analysis below.

23. R. G. Potter, "Birth Intervals: Structure and Change," *Population Studies*, 17 (Nov., 1963), 159-62; and R. G. Potter *et al.*, "A Case Study of Birth Interval Dynamics," *Population Studies*, 19 (July, 1965), 89-92.

24. P. W. Mauldin, *op. cit.*, p. 3.

25. P. W. Mauldin, *op. cit*, p. 4.

GOVERNMENTAL RESPONSIBILITY FOR FAMILY PLANNING IN THE UNITED STATES

Leona Baumgartner
Harvard Medical School

THE ROLE OF GOVERNMENT in human affairs varies from one culture, one government, to another, may vary in different areas in the same country, and changes from one era to another. In health affairs in the United States the history of governmental involvement in family planning must be viewed in the light of the pioneer past of this country, in which the individual assumed responsibility for whatever personal health service his family needed and did not look to the government to help him, and in the light of our Puritanical and Victorian heritages, which frowned on discussion of matters related to sex. Family planning has not been a matter of governmental concern for most of our history for many reasons.

It was left for reformers like Margaret Sanger, Robert Latou Dickinson, the Stones, and the organizations they founded, for the students of population growth like Raymond Pearl, Frank Notestein, and for the foundations which supported a wide variety of demographic, medical, and social studies to lay the basis for programs of family planning. But until there was wide public discussion of the problem itself, government in this democratic, pluralist society of the United States did not act. This, too, is a common, though not universal, pattern here. Private groups pioneer in new areas; then the government follows.

Existing Legislative Authority Not Widely Used

There was no lack of authority, however, for federal, state, and local governments to support family planning. Local and state laws usually gave the right to protect the health of the citizens to some health official, who then initiated and sought support for specific programs. In some states there were restrictive laws regarding contraception.

435

At the federal level of the "general welfare" clause of the Constitution gives the Congress the right to legislate in this field and no constitutional objection exists unless any specific activity is prohibited by the Bill of Rights. In 1965, the U.S. Supreme Court struck down the 1879 Connecticut anti-birth control law which, in effect, prohibited the use of contraceptives, their distribution, and information about them.

Several pieces of legislation might have been interpreted as giving the federal government the power to support family planning programs had the climate of the times not discouraged discussion and activity in this field. They are:[1]

(1) The Basic Act of 1912, establishing the right of the newly formed Children's Bureau to investigate and report on all aspects of child life.

(2) The Social Security Act of 1935, which authorized grants to state health departments for the promotion of the health of mothers and children (Title V, part 1).[2]

(3) The Public Health Service Act (Sections 315 and 314c) which gives broad authority to the Surgeon General to disseminate information relating to the health of the public and to make grants to the states for public health programs.

(4) The various Foreign Assistance Acts passed after World War II, which have provided broad authorities under which family planning programs might have been financed, as have the Food Assistance Acts (P.L. 489, etc.).

(5) The recent office of Economic Opportunity legislation, which is now financing health and family planning services in poverty areas.

Despite the legislative authority, there was little action in the public sector except in the southern states and Puerto Rico. There, after 1935, available grant monies were used to establish public clinics but the activity was disguised at all levels. Supplies were called "gynecological" supplies; states were asked by federal representatives to delete any reference to birth control and support such activities as "maternal health" projects. Local and state governments were usually quiet about their activities in this field. Demographic activities and maternal and child health services were openly financed by foreign assistance funds and there is also some evidence that birth control activities were indirectly assisted. In many countries, of course, the basic demographic data and development of health services were essential before family planning could be supported. But the same taboos existed in the Department of State as in the Public Health Service and Children's Bureau.

The Years of Change

The past decade has seen remarkable changes in the attitudes and activities of government and the public in the United States in relation to understanding and assisting attempts to modify the effects of rapid increases in population growth rates of other countries as well as to provide governmental help for those who wish to limit the size of their families in this country. There has been developed what the nuclear physicist calls a "critical mass" of public opinion in favor of governmental activity. This has created a chain reaction of response.

The people have been ahead of their leaders. In the years when the topic of birth control was seldom mentioned publicly or even privately in this country, a substantial proportion of families of all faiths limited the size of their families. In recent years, public opinion polls have shown increasingly higher percentages of people (Catholic and non-Catholics) favoring governmental action. By 1956, for example, when many governmental leaders were loathe to enter any discussion of the problem, 65 percent of the U.S. population and 59 percent of Catholics of childbearing age favored governmental action.

By the early 1960's the picture was changing. In religious and other groups there was more discussion of responsible parenthood. The Rockefeller and Ford Foundations increased their interest and support. The Population Council expanded. Private groups of all kinds took up the fight so long led by advocates of birth control. There were marked shifts in the attitudes of newspapers and other mass media; business, religious, and educational leaders; and professional groups. The rapid change in 1963 in the mass media, including television, was of particular importance.

It must also be remembered that after World War II, the U.S. obviously became increasingly involved in what was going on in the rest of the world. The walls of rigid isolation crumbled. Air travel, business expansion, cultural exchange, and a host of activities led to a feeling on the part of an ever-increasing proportion of U.S. citizens that what happened elsewhere in the world was a matter of practical concern to *them,* and not just to diplomats, missionaries, individual businessmen, and scholars. Universities opened centers for the study of various, non-European areas; private groups devoted themselves to a variety of activities related to the developing countries; business leaders sought new business partners abroad; young people turned as eagerly to Africa or Asia as their forefathers had to the unknown West or Europe. In one way or another, the problems associated with rapid population growth in some of these areas were brought home to the American public. After 1962, the "population explosion" became an acceptable topic for discussion in many fields of public and private life in this country. The way for dialogue, for action, was open. It began in the reorganized Agency for International Development[3] which was responsible for assisting the developing countries with their social and economic development.

Specific Factors Leading to Change in Federal Policy
The attitude of the federal government toward population problems underwent radical change after 1960, when President Kennedy took office. President Eisenhower had specifically called the problem one of private, not public concern. The change is related, of course, to the changes in public opinion noted above, but is related as well to at least seven other important factors.

First, there is much greater knowledge of the extent of population changes themselves. Before 1947, demographic facts in many parts of the world were scanty. Since then, largely under the leadership of the United Nations, many countries have developed the people and the machinery necessary to enable them to know the size of their population and its changing dimensions. The value of having figures cannot be overemphasized. India, the first country to establish a governmental family planning program, has been well-known for many years for the relative excellence of the demographic material coming out of its decennial censuses. Since 1947, an increasing number of the countries of Asia and Latin America have acquired their own professionally competent trained demographers. Many countries have taken their first regular censuses only recently. The various foreign-aid programs of the U.S. government from the 1940's on have helped with such fact-gathering. In Asian and Latin American countries, reliable population figures are becoming increasingly available. In Africa, the situation is still less clear.

Second, national recognition of a country's population problem is seen as one of achieving a favorable balance of people and resources, the number of people the resources must support, and the abilities of the people to use these resources. In other words, the interrelatedness of economic and social growth and development with *rapid* increases of population is now recognized by policy-makers in many countries. In some countries, more people may wish to achieve a satisfactory balance, but effective population control programs are seen increasingly as critically important to the achievement of desired rates of savings and economic and social development in most of the non-industrialized, developing countries. Where growth rates are accelerating the pressure for food, schools, teachers, health services, jobs, and houses, they are resulting in reappraisals and concern for the long-term aspects of rapid population growth. The need for increased food production and slowing down of population growth are seen as essentials in some countries.

Third, the importance of switching from short-term to long-term planning for economic and social development programs to meet the needs of aid-receiving countries is a critical factor leading to change in the federal government's policy on population. It was of major importance, for it turned attention to looking farther ahead than many economic advisers had been accustomed to looking.

Fourth, many families in the developing countries are now more concerned with the kind of life they can achieve for themselves and their children. They are moving from their traditional societies where the status quo is accepted as a way of life to a modern society which believes it can, at least in part, determine its own future. As infant mortality decreases and their children survive, many see that they do not have to have as many children to carry on the work the family must do and the traditions it must support. In some countries, particularly in Latin America, families, church, medical, and governmental leaders have become increasingly concerned with the high incidence of child abandonment and abortion, and with the health, fiscal, and moral implications of these practices. In this country the pressures for schools, houses, recreation space, etc., have made our people see the problems associated with population growth more clearly.

Fifth, more is known about the physiology of human reproduction. There have been technical advances in methods of regulation of pregnancy, which have made family planning programs of wide scope more possible and have given new hope that these countries will be able to do more about the rapid increases in population. The behavioral sciences have shown that it is possible to determine the knowledge, the attitudes, and the practices of family planning in given populations. There is a growing research and development approach to the whole field even though it is poorly organized, inadequately supported, and still lacking much knowledge.

Sixth, the importance of population problems has been increasingly recognized in the United Nations system. This has stimulated interest in all countries. The pressures from the developing countries themselves, particularly those in Asia, are forcing action on the United Nations and the specialized agencies, and on western leaders. It was the pressure originating in the Asian Population Conference in 1963, for example, that forced the question of supporting technical assistance on the agenda at the United Nations in 1965. Its approval led as well to changes in the position of the World Health Organization.

Seventh, the increasing rate of illegitimacy among the poor in this country also began to concern those with responsibilities for them in this country. There was a growing interest in poverty and a realization that the poor had, for all practical purposes, little access to family planning services and thus were discriminated against. In a period of renewed emphasis on the importance of equality of opportunity for each individual, it seemed clear that family planning should no longer be the quiet privilege of the rich and the middle class but should become a common right enjoyed by all.

Policies Which Guided U.S. Government Activities
In Changing Its Policy On Family Planning
The following points of view have been of critical importance throughout the recent development of U.S. governmental policy. Each of them was finally adopted for specific reasons. These have proved sound, particularly from the political point of view vis-à-vis the developing countries and potential opposition in this country as well.

First, what the U.S. government does and says is founded on its concern for human beings. The quality of life is a matter of importance to us. Economic and social progress, laudable as they are, are not ends in themselves. Neither is slowing down, increasing, or stabilizing population growth. They are one means whereby countries as well as families enhance the development of healthy, self-reliant human beings.

Second, it is U.S. policy to support the building of a great world society of independent nations where every family can find a life free of crippling poverty, hunger, and disease—a life offering a sense of personal dignity and a chance for jobs; and where each country can have the opportunity to develop its own resources and to sustain its own economic and social development. We recognize that the world's political, social, and spiritual leaders, as well as public opinion, are increasingly recognizing the necessity of facing the many social, economic, and political problems associated with rapid population growth. The U.S. recognizes that there is no one solution to such problems and so supports a variety of activities which will raise the level of economic, social, and family life. At the same time, it considers that action in fertility control is indicated in certain areas, for we recognize that rapid growth of population threatens the development these countries hope to achieve.

Third, the increased availability of new methods of fertility control and their potential acceptability to a broad spectrum of religious, cultural, social, and economic groups now makes possible more effective family planning programs. Birth rates have been reduced in certain very limited areas where such methods are intensely used, but there are still many problems to be solved if birth rates are to be reduced in many countries.

Fourth, the U.S. is concerned about various problems associated with population growth in its own country and is attempting amelioration through a variety of actions. The government at all levels is increasingly supporting domestic programs of fertility control. It believes that in its own pluralistic democratic society full freedom should, in tax-supported institutions, be extended in the selection and use of such methods of regulating family size as are consistent with the creed and mores of the individual concerned.

Fifth, the government believes that in working in other countries it is important to point out that population problems are not solved in the U.S. This point assumes greater significance as one recognizes the sensitivity of other nations, particularly Asia and Africa, to any indication that the wealthier predominantly white nations want them to curtail their non-white populations. A similar point of view is becoming important in this country. The position of communist countries is also recognized.

It is also helpful for the U.S. to recognize the continuing pressures for action in the developing countries themselves and the leadership coming from them. Many of them want help to get on with the job themselves. They often resent inferences that we are ahead of them or wish to show them how to solve their problems in family planning.

Sixth, population policies, plans, and programs in other countries are to be made by the individual country concerned and by its families, in accord with their own needs and values. AID has nevertheless believed that fertility control should, when practical, be made available through health services to families and that it is an essential part of maternal and child health and social welfare activities. In view of the evidence that limiting family size usually follows a decline in the infant mortality rate, further specific efforts to achieve the latter are important.

Seventh, the U.S. government is firmly committed to cooperating with the United Nations, with other countries, and with private organizations in assisting the developing countries which request assistance with their population problems. There is increasing emphasis on channeling U.S. aid whenever possible through multilateral or private institutions, instead of via the direct bilateral route.

Eighth, there is great need to stimulate and support research in the many fields which may contribute to solving the problems of fertility control. United States research and development capabilities can make unique contributions. Research is interpreted by each group concerned in its own terms. The demographer thinks of demographic research, the biologist or physician of biomedical research, the economist of the relation of population growth to economic development, the behavioral scientist of the attitudes, knowledge, and practices of the people. More knowledge in all fields is necessary. The quest for better methods of fertility control must be maintained. The successful implementation of family planning programs needs systems and operational research. The U.S. government is committed to all these research efforts at home and abroad.

Ninth, AID has taken the position that it is interested in action and not words. There is enough of a consensus that what is important now is to get on with the jobs to be done.

Tenth, in other countries the U.S. government will support research, training, and technical assistance in the family planning field as well as in the demographic and related fields. It will also encourage and support population and demographic analyses on the macro-economic level of GNP growth rates, import requirements, and at the sectoral level, e.g. employment, education, and housing. The one element excluded from AID support when the new policy was adopted in late 1964 was the provision of already manufactured contraceptives or machinery to manufacture them. There were marked differences of opinion at the time. Some saw inclusions as raising so many questions and so much opposition in the Congress, particularly from members who were Catholics, that AID appropriations would be threatened. Others were not as concerned with appropriations but felt the move to include these materials would prove to be politically embarrassing to the President. Others saw clearly that with the rapid changes in public opinion and growth of family planning programs in the developing countries this restrictive policy would have to be reversed in the near future. They felt, too, that it would be wiser to avoid the inevitable question, "Do you really want to help us?" and the appearance of inconsistency on the part of the U.S. At that time, however, a clear case could not be made for the lack of contraceptives being a stumbling block in the AID-assisted countries in which the government was backing an active program, so the support of contraceptives was not included. This policy was reversed in early 1967. By then, the need for help was much more clear.

A second question discussed was the possibility of considering family planning efforts as a "self-help" measure in those countries where population growth was seriously threatening economic development. This has not been felt to be consistent with the stated beliefs of, nor in the best interests of, the United States, which supports the concept that each country should have the freedom and responsibility to choose what it feels is best for its own people.

How Was Governmental Policy Developed?

To look back historically and determine exactly the steps, the people, and the circumstances which have influenced the development of U.S. governmental policy in this controversial field of birth control is problematic. Each historian will probably see the process in a slightly different way. Some may overlook the importance of the climate at one particular time, another the influence of one or another specific event. Indeed, in so complicated a development it is difficult to reconstruct the impact of one factor on all others. Much was done behind the scenes. Headlines usually meant less than unrecorded conversations and contacts.

It seems clear, however, that in the 3-year period from 1962 through 1964 the major decisions which allowed the U.S. government to take an active role in supporting birth control services with tax funds were being shaped. Action occurred first in relation to foreign aid programs—not domestic ones. Once the policy was set for work abroad it became policy at home, too.

There was no overall directive to move ahead. Individuals in the White House, Department of State, AID, and in the Congress quietly took the initiative. Many active in the Executive branch were newcomers. Much was acomplished through speeches made by governmental officials, often cleared by the White House before delivery. Public reaction could thus be assayed. If no great difficulty was encountered, another step could be taken.

Persons were quietly recruited to work full-time on family planning, and many others spent a major portion of their time working on the problems. Conversations with leaders in other countries, universities and research institutions, and experts from the private groups long active in the field were carried on over many months. Research and action programs were planned and some financed using existing legislative authority. Economists studied the situation in different countries. On the basis of available data from certain countries projections were made of probable changes in per capita income under different assumptions of population growth rates. It seems fair to state that developmental economists in general had been little interested in the subject of family planning because they doubted that much could be done to lower birth rates anyway. They were suspicious of the emotional pleas being made by many of the prophets of doom who talked of the population "explosion." They were intellectually sure that long-term predictions in the economic field were unsound. The turn-around of top economists in government on the value of supporting family planning was important in the change in federal policy.

Two policies were of strategic importance at home and abroad. Supporting full freedom of choice in the democratic, pluralistic society of this country in the selection and use of such methods for the regulation of family size as are consistent with the creed and mores of the individual concerned was of key importance in the domestic political scene. This was publicly announced in a speech at an International Conference on Population at the Johns Hopkins University on May 28, 1964.[4] The recognition that the U.S. believed the population and practices of any country should be determined by that country was of key importance in foreign policy. This was stated on December 10, 1962, in a speech at the U.N. with an offer to help other countries, on request, to find potential sources of information and assistance on ways of dealing with population problems.[5]

By the summer of 1964 major policy lines were laid down and had White House approval. It was decided that in addition to information already sent AID missions, a firm policy statement could and should be sent out—though there were still those who feared too open action. The foreign aid program was already in enough trouble with Congress. In the meantime work was going on. Foundations, universities, private groups, and government officials from some countries were discussing programs to be financed by U.S. funds with governmental representatives of this country.

With the death of President Kennedy, there was some uncertainty about the attitude of the new President. The work in AID continued as if the previous approvals for moving ahead had been restated.

By December, 1964, a position paper on the issues presented by population growth trends in the less developed countries was completed. It had been prepared by the AID's population and economic experts in consultation with regional, desk, and mission representatives, representatives of the Departments of State, Commerce and Health, Education and Welfare, the United Nations, and related agencies, several U.S. universities and foundations, and private groups. It was discussed at an executive staff meeting on December 1, 1964, with staff from AID, the Bureau of the Budget, the President's office, and the Department of State present. The position and policy related above was agreed upon.

One additional question was widely discussed in the closing months of 1964. What should be said or done by the newly-elected President, Lyndon Johnson? All kinds of pressures were put on his office by citizens who had long fought for governmental action to have him deliver a major address on the subject, call a White House Conference, or name a Commission. Some, who favored governmental action, feared reactions if anything was done. So the arguments continued. In the meantime, AID officials, who had long been consulted by staff of the President's Science Advisor on population matters, discussed the question with them. Statements by various governmental officials were reviewed. It was decided that a short statement in the State of the Union message would be helpful. The President's Science Advisor took one to the Texas White House just after Christmas. The President accepted the idea and stated on January 4, 1965, "I will seek new ways to use our knowledge to help deal with the explosion in world population and growing scarcity in world resources." Federal policy was thus finally announced at the top.

In concluding this brief story of the development of U.S. government policy up to 1965, it should be noted that although some complained that progress was too slow and others that it was too rapid, a complete change of policy was made between 1959 and 1965. It was made with a minimum of friction, one step at a time. It now seems firmly established. The agencies could implement whatever programs of action seemed desirable. This was only the first step— but one which was essential to all future action, so essential that the change in policy almost appeared as the end itself. At last the government was free to act openly.

Implementation

But implementation of policy creates its own set of problems, for action does not necessarily flow neatly or automatically out of policy statements. It takes time to adapt a general statement of policy to specific problems. Old bureaucratic attitudes must be changed, money must be appropriated, an organization set up, personnel recruited and trained, logistics and tactics determined. A two-year lag may well ensue before a federal agency is ready to act with even moderate effectiveness after policy is set. Before federal funds are spent in local areas here and abroad more time may elapse. Though many of the dedicated persons who worked so long to move governments in the United States to participate openly and actively in family planning efforts have thought progress far too slow, much has happened. By January of 1966 the new Secretary of Health, Education, and Welfare had issued a policy statement for that department. Both it and the State Department appointed population officers. In 1967 AID brought together its War on Hunger program with its Family Planning and greatly increased family planning staff in Washington and in missions abroad. The National Institute of Child Health and

Human Development increased its activities after 1965. The Office of Economic Opportunity entered the field to help serve the poor. The Armed Forces liberalized their existing policies. The Department of the Interior approved services for population groups that they serve.

The Congress held extensive hearings on population problems and family planning. It also made several amendments to the Foreign Assistance and the Social Security Acts, which strengthen the positions of the Department of Health, Education, and Welfare and AID to support family planning efforts at home and abroad. Comparison of various departmental directives based on these legislative acts indicates a continuing liberalization of previous positions. Of particular interest is the policy of requiring state welfare departments in the United States to offer birth control to assistance recipients, who had, as noted above, largely been denied access to service. The principle of freedom of choice is also written into the federal legislation. The prohibition of coercion, feared by many religious leaders, was spelled out.

Since that advent of Title XIX (Medicaid) of the Social Security Act, private physicians have been paid to prescribe birth control and materials in the same manner as for other medical services. The Children's Bureau was enabled to expand services. In 1967 there were some 54 projects to develop comprehensive medical and social services for selected mothers in low-income areas, primarily in cities. They contribute in varying amounts to family planning. In the southern part of the United States, where public health departments had long supported birth control service in clinics, the new federal dollars seem to have gone primarily to support additional service in clinics. In the north, where fewer tax-supported clinics existed, Title XIX Medicaid funds appear to have been more widely used. The Office of Education has done little to support educational efforts which would be useful.

To document accurately the actual growth in tax dollars spent or patients served in this country or abroad is impossible. Figures are incomplete, but better reporting schemes are being set up. Federal government figures overlook the services supported by state, local, or private funds. Reports from state health departments show a rise from 1963 to 1965 of 591 to 843 local health departments giving family planning service. This is exclusive of organized clinics privately financed and of the thousands of women who get service from their own doctors or take pills on their own. The situation varies widely. Some areas finance all service from local or state funds. Others operate on federal funds, still others on combinations.

More recently, the tendency of the federal government seems to have been to overestimate the amount it spends on family planning. This is in sharp contrast with the pre-1962 policy of hiding any expenditures. It may be a reaction to continuing criticism that Washington talks but fails to act aggressively. The best current estimates of federal expenditures for all family planning activities by the Department of Health, Education, and Welfare and the Office of Economic Opportunity show a rise from about $23.8 million for 1967 to $48 million for 1970.[6]

Expenditures for family planning activities abroad are similarly difficult to document, but there is evidence that they have risen from less than $3 million in 1964-65 to almost $9 million projected for 1966-67. Monies have been used in many ways: for public education, personnel training, conferences, purchasing transport, medical supplies (including contraceptives) and audiovisual aids, development of evaluation methods, finance of travel to learn elsewhere, advisors, finance of administrative structures, support services to individuals, and research. They have been spent directly, through grants to other governments groups, or through contracts of one sort or another with different domestic university organizations. Funds have also been given to international groups.

The accelerated movement in the population field throughout the world has been assisted in many ways, but certainly the expansion of governmental responsibility in the United States has been and promises to be more and more helpful. There is now some danger of pushing too hard and too fast without adequate knowledge of what to do and how to do it. Raising expectations too high has caused setbacks in many health efforts. Pushing other countries faster than they are ready to go can backfire.

But progress in family planning has never been easy, nor does it promise to be so now. The ways in which, and the reasons why, people do or do not respond to bring about declining birth rates must constantly be explored and evaluated. The obstacles are not all known or understood. The day-to-day decisions of millions of individual people, changing economic forces, and social and political ideals are all involved. There are obstacles in the bureaucratic procedures of public and private agencies at home and abroad. Flexibility of approach, the ability to move quickly, and continuing evaluation of results are essential. Tools for evaluation need polishing and development. The developing countries and local communities in this country often lack the dynamic administrators, the machinery, and the personnel to absorb effectively the help offered. They know far too little about the readiness of their own people to limit the size of their families or about how to reach them.

The need for continuing research and evaluation, dynamic

leadership, effective administration, innovations, and better training programs are all too evident. The responsibilities of governments everywhere, but particularly in this more affluent society, are clear. A greater commitment is obviously important at a time when the world population is increasing at a rate, which, if continued, will double in the next 35 years.

Notes

1. Authority to support research is not discussed since service programs are the focus of this chapter.

2. In 1963, amendments to the same title (part 4) specifying that grants for comprehensive maternity care for mothers, especially those living in poverty ghettos, as well as certain other sections, notably, Title XIX, gave specific support for current activities.

3. To be called AID in this chapter.

4. Baumgartner, Leona. "Population and Public Health Policy." In: *Population Dynamics*, Muramatsu, Menora, and Harper, Paul. The Johns Hopkins Press, 1965, viii, 248 pp.

5. Gardner, Richard. Delivered U.N. General Assembly, December 1962.

6. Harkay, Oscar; Wishik, Samuel M.; Jaffe, Frederick. "Implementing DHEW Policy on Family Planning and Population." A Consultant's Report. Mimeographed. Washington, D.C. Sept. 1967, 36 pp. plus 3 attachments.

V. FERTILITY PLANNING IN THE DEVELOPING WORLD DURING THE NEXT DECADE

Editors' Note

The plan of the Conference included a final session to which leaders in eight of the major family planning programs in the world were invited to contribute papers anticipating important problems for their programs during the next decade. Promising alternative means of preventing or solving these problems were then to be sought from a panel of experts at the Conference.

Because of the growing intensity of program demands at home for immediate attention to immediate problems during 1967, two of these leaders felt unable to accept the invitation and three who did accept were unable to complete their papers or to attend the Conference. The three papers that were prepared and discussed at the Conference, therefore, do not provide as wide a range of programs and problems as orginally intended but do present some important aspects of "Fertility Planning in the Developing World" from the viewpoints of three widely separated nations with three different settings, programs, and problems. We are particularly grateful to Drs. Chow and Hsu of China, Dr. Fisek of Turkey, and Dr. Requena of Chile for these three papers.

A CHINESE VIEW OF FAMILY PLANNING IN THE DEVELOPING WORLD*

L. P. Chow
and
S. C. Hsu

Taiwan Population Studies Center, Taichung
Joint Commission on Rural Reconstruction, Taipei
Taiwan

Introduction

For the first time in history high fertility rates in various parts of the world have become a universal concern. The concern is justifiable, particularly in the "developing" world where governments have been striving for the betterment of the life of their people. Toward this end, a number of them have adopted policies to promote fertility control programs.

The present paper will discuss the following questions:

(1) What is the current status of fertility control programs?
(2) What are their current problems?
(3) What changes are anticipated during the next decade?
(4) How can the desired changes be brought about?

The phrase "developing world" used in the present paper indicates countries in Asia, Africa, Latin America, and other parts of the world where fertility is high and control of fertility is an urgent need.

Some data will be quoted from program experiences in Taiwan, the Republic of China, to illustrate the problems and to support the arguments. It is hoped that these data will be interpreted in the context of actual conditions in various countries in the "developing world."

Current Population and its Future Growth

In 1963, the estimated population in Africa, Latin America, and Asia totalled 2273 million consisting of 72 percent of the world total of

*Thanks are due to Mr. George P. Cernada of the Population Council for his assistance in editing this manuscript. He also contributed a number of valuable ideas to this paper.

3160 million. According to the median assumption of the United Nations, the total population in these three continents will increase to 2816 million, an increase of 24 percent, consisting of 74 percent of the world total of 3828 million in 1975.[1]

The birth rates in these areas are still rather high. The death rates also have been rather high, braking the rate of population growth. It is most likely, however, that the death rates in these areas will sharply decline after introduction of modern technical changes and application of inexpensive public health methods. The rate of natural increase in these areas during the next decade will increase rather than decrease, unless fertility control programs are implemented promptly and successfully.

Generally speaking, the current gross reproduction rates in the developing world are in the vicinity of 2.5 to 3.0, and the expectancies of life at birth range somewhere between 40 to 60 years. On the assumption that these conditions will continue, vital rates have been estimated by the United Nations (Table 1).

Current Status of Fertility Control

Most of the governments in the "developing world" have been concerned with improving the standard of living of their people by implementing long- or short-term plans to accelerate economic development. One inevitable consequence has been the realization of the impact of rapid population growth, which minimizes the net results of their efforts. Assumption of responsibility by governments for family planning is but a logical step toward achievement of their ultimate goals.

Table 1. Vital Rates in Selected Stable Populations when the Specified Conditions are Maintained Constantly

GRR	$e^0{}_0$	Births per 1000 per year	Deaths per 1000 per year	Natural increase per 1000 per year
	40	46.0	23.3	22.7
3	50	44.9	15.8	29.1
	60.4	48.8	9.6	34.2
	38.3	39.5	24.9	14.6
2.5	50.8	38.3	15.5	22.8
	64.1	37.4	8.4	29.0

GRR = Gross Reproduction Rate

$e^0{}_0$ = Life Expectancy at Birth

The degree of governmental commitment for fertility control, however, varies from those countries which have positive policies to those which have never had any organized effort. In between are countries which are still in the "pilot study" stage. Some countries do not have population policies favoring family planning but do realize the problem and support morally, technically, or financially family planning programs carried out by voluntary organizations.

The goals of the programs
The goals of the family planning programs in most of these countries are in general expressed in terms of reduction of birth rates or growth rates. The crude birth rates in these countries lie between 30 and 50 per 1000, and most of the programs aim to reduce the rates by about 30 percent in about 10 years (Table 2).

Methods for attaining the goals
Most of the programs have emphasized the Lippes' loop. In some countries such as India and Korea, sterilization, vasectomy in particular, has also been emphasized, although the degree of emphasis varies.

Because of the rather high termination rate of the loop and the reduction in cost of oral contraceptives, the latter gradually have been included in some of the national family planning programs. The Taiwan program has started to offer the pills to women who discontinued the use of the loop or to those who cannot wear the loop. Conventional contraceptives are distributed but their program significance appears less.

Induced abortion is "illegal" in most of these countries unless it complies with rather rigid "medical" justifications. The enforcement of related regulations, however, seems to be rather loose generally. The prevalence of "illegal" induced abortion is probably much higher than the statistics or survey results show.

Table 2. Goal of Family Planning Programs in Selected Countries[2] (Percent reduction in birth rates)

Country	From:	To:
Ceylon	3.6% at present	2.4% in 10 years
China (Taiwan)	3.6% in 1963	2.4% by 1973
India	4.0% at present	2.5% over 10 years
Singapore	3.0%	2.0% in 5 years
Korea	2.9% in 1962*	2.0% by 1971*
Pakistan	5.0%	4.0% during 1965-70

*Natural Increase Rate

Administrative set-up

The administrative set-up to carry out the program activities varies from country to country also. In a few countries, such as India and Pakistan, family planning has been given a much higher political and administrative status in the government. In Malaysia, an autonomous board administers the family planning program. In the Republic of Korea the MCH Section of the Ministry of Health and Social Welfare is responsible for implementation.

Current Problems and Future Perspectives in Fertility Control

The accomplishment of man in controlling death has been most successful. He has not yet shown the ability, however, to control birth in a sufficiently large population through a deliberate effort. The next decade will give him an opportunity to demonstrate his ability to do so.

The goals of the national fertility control programs are set rather high in most countries, calling for most painstaking efforts, including intelligent planning and dynamic implementation to achieve them.

The following discussion will point out some of the major problems encountered or predicted in carrying out these programs in the developing world during the next decade.

Administrative

(1) Official policy

Some governments are still rather reluctant to be involved in the controversial issue of "population control." During the next decade, it is almost certain that more governments will realize the need of, and will take more positive steps for, family planning.

An official policy for family planning is not a "must" but will greatly facilitate its progress. It also facilitates securing international aid for the program.

Those countries with a policy ought to strive to convince others, through their membership in such international organizations as the United Nations Children's Fund, the World Health Organization, and the United Nations Economic Commission for Asia and the Far East. It has been said that when it comes to family planning the UN itself is only a "backward" country. Organizations whose central personnel are headquartered in one part of the world and largely influenced by agencies within a few hundred miles of their office must try harder to think in terms of needs thousands of miles way.

A positive government attitude toward family planning may include the amendment of related laws and regulations in favor of dissemination of knowledge about and supplies for fertility control. A more liberal attitude toward sterilization and induced abortion may be expected once an official policy is established.

(2) Administrative set-up

Because of the acuteness of the problem and the goals to be attained within a rather short period of time, the administrative set-up of organizations responsible for carrying out family planning should have maximum authority and autonomy, no matter where the unit is placed.

The often-heard notion that family planning units should be "integrated" as a part of the Maternal and Child Health (MCH) Section of the Ministry of Health is excellent in theory only, at least within the next decade[3]. Although provision of family planning services through MCH services seems to be the most satisfactory arrangement in the "developed" areas, it seems advisable to create an independent autonomous organization within public health to push the program vigorously in those developing areas where the MCH unit is weak or virtually nonexistent.

(3) Role of voluntary organizations

Voluntary family planning organizations in most countries have played important roles in "pioneering" related activities. They still assume major responsibility in many countries in promoting family planning programs. When programs are expanded to the national level with active government participation, some voluntary organizations may find difficulties in justifying their existence.

Others will take on roles in training and public information that the government is unable to handle. All voluntary agencies ought to be developing plans to find a definite helpful role in areas where the government is soon going to take on the responsibility for family planning. Solution of this problem will be another challenge to the related administrators in the next decade.

(4) Allocation of resources

It is understood that the family planning program is to accelerate the nation's economic development. On the other hand, the program cannot be fully successful unless some degree of social and economic development has been achieved. The policy-makers should seriously study the interrelationship of various factors to ensure the "optimum" allocation of resources, which are limited.

(5) Personnel

Many questions remain to be answered regarding the type, qualification, number, recruitment, and training of workers in family planning programs, and regarding the status, authority, and autonomy of executive staff and incentives for workers, allied professional personnel, and community leaders to work for the program.

The problems of population are multi-dimensional and require well trained personnel of various disciplines who are in short supply in the developing world.

(6) Method of approach

The "planned parenthood" approach to family planning in the United States and elsewhere has been criticized as having a "medical" bias,[4] one of its most serious disadvantages being emphasis on "individual" rather than "community." This involves mainly the private physician providing services to the individual patient on consultation basis in the clinics.

It is apparent that the program goals can never be attained through the "clinical" approach. The need is to expand to deal with the "community" as a whole. Family planning programs must evolve from "clinical medicine" to "public health" orientations in the next few years.

(7) International organizations

A more active role in family planning is expected for various international organizations not only because the program is related directly to the welfare of the people that they aim for, but also because the success of their past efforts, e.g., in health, have helped make the population problem more acute.

(8) Integration into the general health and welfare services

Although an independent autonomous unit to execute the program is desirable now, when the "acute" phase of the program is over, the related activities should be gradually "integrated" into the existing administrative organizations of the health or welfare services.

Technical problems

The Lippes' loop and oral contraceptives have brought about a "breakthrough" in the technology of contraception. Nevertheless, both fall short of expectation because of some weaknesses. It is likely that other technical "breakthroughs" in methods of fertility control will come during the next decade. However, the immediate concern is to discover a better "strategy" in the use of various presently available contraceptives.

(1) Intrauterine Device (IUD)

The most serious problem of the IUD is that retention rates appear discouragingly low. A carefully designed follow-up interview[5] conducted on samples of IUD acceptors in Taiwan revealed that the retention rate was 61 percent at the end of 12 months, and 51 percent at the end of 18. Surveys conducted in other countries tend to confirm this finding.

Retention rates are closely associated with such characteristics of acceptors as age, parity, education, place of residence, experience of induced abortion, prior use of contraceptives, etc. Age and parity are the two most important variables (Table 3). "Medical removal" has been the most important cause of device loss. The future problem is not only to get more IUD cases, but also to keep the loops in the uterus longer.

Other problems of program importance are (a) "exhaustion" of higher parity women and (b) bad "word-of-mouth" circulation about the loops. When the program reaches the stage, such as in Taiwan, where the acceptance rate exceeds 19 percent of the total married women of childbearing age, a "plateau" of acceptance may occur. If this happens greater attention must be given to finding methods to recruit the "less motivated" women.

Similarly, the "word-of-mouth" communication helped accelerate IUD use initially may gradually operate in the opposite direction, if more dissatisfaction with IUD's develops.

(2) Oral contraceptives

The importance of pills in fertility control programs is ever increasing. In Taiwan, pills have recently been offered at reduced cost of NT$10 (U.S. 25 cents) to women who discontinued the use of IUD because of medical or other reasons, and for whom the IUD is not indicated.

The pills seem to fall short of expectation because of a higher termination rate than that of the IUD. In a pilot study in Taiwan,

Table 3. Cumulative Net Termination Rates of the Lippes' Loop at End of 12 Months per 100 Initial Insertions Under Field Conditions by Age Group and Parity of Women Results of 1965 Taiwan Island-wide IUD Follow-up Interview[5]

	Type of Termination			
	Pregnancy	Expulsion	Removal	Total Termination
Age of wife				
17-24	11.3	22.5	42.9	60.7
25-29	7.3	13.4	31.8	45.2
30-34	7.8	10.0	23.9	36.8
35+	4.6	4.2	19.5	26.4
No. of live births				
2 or less	8.8	19.0	44.3	58.9
3	8.7	16.2	31.7	47.8
4	6.2	9.0	25.4	36.4
5 or more	6.5	6.8	21.2	31.4
All samples	5.6	9.0	24.6	39.1

offering the pills at reduced cost through mail order, 42 percent of acceptors continued to use them at the end of 12 months. Side effects, sustaining motivation needed, and suppression of lactation are important weaknesses of the pills. The recent development of using low dosage progesterone may partly solve the problem in the future.

(3) Sterilization

Sheps et al.[6] have demonstrated by a stochastic model that a fertility control method of higher efficacy accepted by less people brings the birth rate down faster than less effective methods accepted by more people. Sterilization programs, therefore, may need further emphasis in the next decade.

Sterilization is fairly acceptable to people in the Orient. In Taiwan, the 1965 Province-wide sample survey[7] showed that of 23.5 percent of the respondents who were currently practicing fertility control, 23 percent had been sterilized. The ratio of male to female sterilization was about 1 to 10, consistent with the male dominant cultural pattern. A survey[8] in Taiwan of 3043 former traditional contraceptive practicers indicated that 29 percent "would accept either tubal ligation or vasectomy" if the service were offered "free of charge."

(4) Induced abortion

In Korea, a 1966 national fertility survey[9] indicated that 13.5 percent of respondents had experienced at least one induced abortion. The percentage is 9.7 percent in the 1965 Province-wide survey in Taiwan. The statistics in most of the countries grossly underestimated the actual prevalence of induced abortion.

Medical opinion seems gradually to have been shifting to favor a more liberal attitude toward induced abortion. In fact, a few countries have started to study carefully the desirability and consequences of liberalizing induced abortion.

The demographic impact of induced abortion, however, must be carefully assessed. Japan's success in halving the birth rate within a decade is not simply because of liberalization of induced abortion per se but rather that it is accepted as a method to "correct" contraceptive failure.

(5) Social class differentials

Higher fertility among lower socioeconomic status women is a universal phenomenon. In Taiwan, the 1965 fertility survey revealed that a woman without formal education had an average of 4.02 living children compared to an average of 2.92 for a woman of senior high school or above education.

The desire to have a smaller family is always stronger for the higher educated, suggesting that the fertility differentials by socioeconomic status may be broadened further. The acceptance rate for

IUD's in Taiwan up to the end of 1966 was 13 percent for women without formal education but more than 21 percent for those with junior high and above education.

What impact the fertility differentials will have on the quality of population is an important issue. Children of less fortunate parents may not be inferior in their hereditary qualities. Nevertheless, considering the less favorable environment in which they will grow up and the lesser opportunities they may expect in the future, fertility differentials by social class deserve some concern from the viewpoint of population quality.

(6) Demographic impact of various fertility control methods

An important question that is often asked and for which an answer still is not available is "How many births will be prevented by an IUD insert?" A rather crude estimate made by L. P. Chow[10] was that 5 IUD's inserted probably could prevent 1 live birth per year for 5 years. This, however, was a guess based on limited evidence. Recently Robert Potter, Jr.[11] has made a more realistic estimate based on the Taiwan program experience. According to his findings, the number of births averted per IUD insertion falls short of 1.0; ranging from 0.43 to 0.94. Data on the demographic impacts of sterilization, induced abortion, and pills under actual conditions in various countries are also needed for better program planning.

Knowledge, attitudes, and practice

(1) Knowledge

A major barrier to the promotion of the program in the developing world is people's lack of knowledge about family planning. In the 1965 fertility survey in Taiwan 53 percent of respondents had never heard about loops, although the island-wide IUD program had been in operation for nearly two years. Pills were known of by less than one-third of respondents (31 percent). Although 78 percent knew at least one contraceptive method, only 54 percent of them cited the Japanese Ota ring, 46 percent sterilization, and 48 percent the Lippe's loop. New ways of bringing information to all must be developed and old ones improved.

(2) Attitudes

The agrarian economic setting and higher child mortality in the past have favored a larger family in the developing world. Numerous children not only add more working hands on the farm, but also are a prime source of security when one gets old. In Taiwan in 1965 78 percent of respondents indicated that they expect to live with their children or grandchildren when they are old even though they have sufficient means to live by themselves.

Despite the idea that the traditional family concept seems to be resistant to substantial change, the desire to have less children has been spreading. Surveys in a number of countries indicate that most women now wish to have less than 4 children although they would have 5 to 6 if the current fertility persists. An overwhelming majority of 92 percent of respondents in Taiwan approve of family planning.

The average age at first marriage of girls has direct association with their subsequent fertility. In 1965 in Taiwan women of ages 40-44 had 2.91 living children if they had married at the ages 30-34, compared to 5.94 children if they had married at an age less than 20.

The strong sex preference for male children in most oriental cultures motivates some couples to have additional children in the hope of having a male baby thereby increasing fertility.

Inasmuch as the acceptance of family planning is closely related to the status of women in the community and within the household, the program should actively seek a change in community attitudes toward women and endeavor to raise the wife's status in the family and in community organizations.

(3) Practice

In 1965 a survey in Taiwan showed that 23.5 percent of respondents were currently practicing fertility control methods; of whom 22 percent were loop users, 27 percent wore the Ota ring, 23 percent had been sterilized, 25 percent were using traditional contraceptives, and less than 3 percent were pill users.

Fertility control methods are used mainly for stopping rather than spacing birth. In Taiwan 66 percent of contraceptive users started to practice after having had more than 3 living children and 84 percent of those accepting the loop wanted no more children.[12]

If the program goals of various countries are to be achieved, a high proportion of married women of childbearing age need to accept loops or practice other methods which are as effective as loops. In Taiwan, although the acceptance of loops has exceeded 19 percent of married women, 20 percent more will have to be recruited during the next few years. The need for better motivational techniques in the future is apparent.

Education and motivation

Although the need for family limitation is growing, most of the people, those less educated in the rural areas in particular, in the developing areas do not know how to regulate effectively their family size. Better communication and motivation are needed. Following are some major issues on this subject.

(1) "Why" *vs.* "how" to control fertility

A study in Taiwan indicated that women are currently more in-terested in "how" than in "why" to control fertility. After an educa-tional campaign teaching both "why" and "how" in one township, samples of women were interviewed six months later.[13] About 97 percent of them were able to recall the "how" materials compared to 35 percent who recalled the "why". The former also circulated more among women who did not attend the educational meeting.

Although programs in developing countries have been bringing information on "how" to many people, attempting to convince people "why" they should practice birth control is difficult. The acuteness of the problem has led to implementation of "crash" programs. This often means stressing contraceptive methods rather than the reasons for using them. What effect hasty efforts to reach goals by a "crash" type of approach will have in the long run needs to be carefully studied during the following decade.

(2) Mass media *vs.* face-to-face motivation

The "crash" program approach usually requires intensive and extensive use of mass education media. Some people think that mass media are "singularly ineffective"[14] because "family planning deals entirely with the intimate and deeply personal area of life for which mass media are rarely persuasive." A contrary view was expressed by Professor Donald Bogue[15] of the University of Chicago, who believes that "family planning in Asia won't really get off the ground until mass communication methods are used."

(3) Emphasis on "individual welfare" *vs.* "collective interest"

Prof. Bogue has said that the often-heard notion that the popula-tion problem must always be presented to the public in terms of its own self-interest, not the collective national interest, may be a false dichotomy. Others are opposed to this viewpoint. What is the best theme for family planning communications?

(4) "Passivity" *vs.* "individual commitment"

Most of the national family planning programs seem to stress overly the need for "free" service brought to the door of each house. This over-encouragement of "passivity" in the program may not be a gain in the long run. Family planning practice demands personal involvement and commitment.

Another factor of significance in terms of "saturation" levels in field work is that face-to-face motivation is effective but if conducted too long or repeated too often, it may soon invite resistance rather than cooperation.

(5) Health advantages *vs.* economic incentives

The planned parenthood approach emphasizes the health advantage of family planning. Studies in various areas tend to show that economic motives are the major reasons for accepting fertility control methods.

Intelligent use of monetary incentives to encourage the public and the workers to promote a family planning program deserves special consideration. This may mean a kind of bonus system for field workers as in Taiwan or an overall "no-birth" bonus for women. The latter, however, must be weighed against the dangers of "passivity" mentioned previously. Perhaps the best approach is gearing educational materials to stress the economic advantages of family planning.

(6) Stopping *vs.* spacing birth

Emphasis on the health advantages of family planning tends to stress the values of spacing, yet women in the developing world are more interested in stopping births altogether than in spacing.

(7) School curriculum

The advantages of smaller families should be tactfully emphasized through basic school education. Teaching in fertility control methods should be an integral part of medical education. Roles of universities in the national fertility control programs should be carefully defined.

(8) Post-partum education

Women are generally thought most receptive to family planning during the post-partum period. This may have to be somewhat qualified in the devevloping world where prolonged lactation is the usual practice; women generally believe themselves to be sterile during lactation and show less interest in family planning.

Evaluation and research

Should fertility in the developing world decline as planned during the next decade, it will be a significant historical event. Careful evaluation and record-keeping of the process of change, therefore, is a historical undertaking.[16]

Evaluation and record-keeping are also important for better program planning. Unfortunately, in most of the countries in the developing world the basic statistical system is still not well developed. Lack of baseline data on population and vital events make evaluation of program achievement difficult.

More exchange of information needs to take place among the developing countries. Centers could be located in developing countries which have more advanced statistical systems and used as model demonstration areas for training of staff of other countries. Major efforts needed should also include:

(1) Instituting or improving the basic statistical system for col-

lection of population, natality, mortality, and other demographic data. As statistical systems improve, recorded fertility rates will probably rise because of more complete registration.

(2) Conducting good surveys to estimate the population and vital rates; and

(3) Conducting regular surveys of good quality to provide benchmark data as well as to evaluate the effect of the fertility control program.

Other major research needs include:

(4) Acceptability studies on various fertility control methods;

(5) Development of methodology for evaluating family planning;

(6) Education and communication techniques for dissemination of knowledge about fertility control and for motivation of people to accept family planning;

(7) Studies on the health advantages of birth control and child spacing;

(8) Undertaking operations research or field experiments to discover more efficient and effective methods to implement programs.

Another urgent need is to find better contraceptive methods acceptable to a majority of people in the developing world. They must be inexpensive, effective, and free from untoward side effects.

General socioeconomic development

Professor Ronald Freedman[17] said that fertility will decline first and most rapidly when significant social development has already occurred.

In most of the countries in the developing world, the per capita annual income is less than US$200. While a few countries have literacy rates as high as 70 percent, most have rates as low as 20 percent. More than half the people are agricultural, living in rural villages. Their natural resources are limited and food production barely meets local demands. Under-employment is prevalent.

These conditions are barriers to the success of fertility control programs. Concerned efforts to accelerate socioeconomic development must not only be continued but should be intensified to create the "felt-need" of people for fertility control.

Conclusion and Summary

The potentiality of population growth during the next decade in the "developing world" is still great. With the introduction of modern technology and extensive application of inexpensive public health measures, mortality will fall sharply, resulting in a higher natural rate of growth.

Most of the governments in the developing world have been concerned with implementing long or short-term economic development plans to uplift the standard of living of their people. They have come to the realization that population growth offsets their net results. Adoption of policies to control fertility is a logical step to their ulimate goals. During the next decade, it appears that most of the other countries will take more active steps to regulate fertility.

The problem of population growth in the developing world is extremely acute. Most of the countries, therefore, have set goals which are rather high and achievement of which calls for tremendous efforts. Best ways to achieve the goals include adoption of official policies, effective administrative organization to carry out the programs, and optional strategy in using various fertility control methods.

Intrauterine contraceptive devices and oral contraceptives are technical "breakthroughs" in the methodology of fertility control. Unfortunately they fall short of expectations, mainly because of the high termination rates. Sterilization, vasectomy, in particular, is another effective method which should be promoted more in the next decade.

Induced abortion, which is illegal in most of the countries, has played an undeniable role in fertility control. Statistics have always underestimated its prevalence. Medical and social opinion has been shifting to favor a liberal attitude toward it. However, it should be resorted to as a method to correct contraceptive failures, rather than as a fertility control method itself.

A major barrier to spread of fertility control practice in the developing areas is lack of knowledge among the people. Although surveys in various parts of the world clearly indicate the growing desire for family planning, a majority of the people still do not know how to plan and limit their families.

Better motivation and communication techniques are also needed when the program reaches a "plateau" by skimming off the higher parity and strongly motivated ones. Higher fertility among the lower socioeconomic class of people is a universal phenomenon. The socioeconomic differentials of fertility deserve further concern.

Opinions vary as to emphasizing "why" or "how" to plan family size, a "crash" program or a long-range one, mass media or individual contact, and stress on individual or collective interest in motivating people to practice fertility control. Family planning should not overencourage the "passivity" of people, should make the best use of economic incentives, and should stress stopping as well as spacing births. The post-partum program in the developing world, where prolonged lactation is the usual practice, needs some modification.

The effort which is being made in the developing world to demonstrate man's ability to control fertility through organized programs requires adequate evaluation and record-keeping to record the process of change properly. In most countries improvement of the statistics systems is an urgent need. Surveys of good quality should be undertaken to provide the benchmark data for evaluation.

Fertility control programs in the developing world should strive for "variety" during the next decade. Highly imaginative and dynamic leadership is needed for the programs. Efforts of the governments in accelerating economic development should be strengthened further because fertility control programs flourish best upon the ground of general social development.

Before concluding, let us add that for the first time in man's history, the rate of population growth has become a universal concern. Whether it can be brought down significantly during the next decade through planned efforts, is a real challenge to man's ability. People in the developing world have been provided with a unique opportunity to write a most significant chapter in the history of mankind. In what way this will be written rests entirely upon the intelligence and determination of those who are directly or indirectly involved in these programs.

Notes

1. United Nations, *The Future Growth of World Population*, UN ST/SOA/ Series A/28, 1958.

2. UN Economic Commission for Asia and the Far East, *Report of the Working Group on Administrative Aspects of Family Planning Programmes*, March 1966, Bangkok, Thailand.

3. Chow, L. P., "Some Aspects of the Integration of MCH and Family Planning Activities in the General Health Services" (mimeographed paper prepared for the Technical Discussions of the 1967 Western Pacific Regional Conference of the World Health Organization).

4. Kiser, C. V. (ed.), *Research in Family Planning*, pp. 477-502 (Princeton: Princeton University Press, 1962).

5. Chow, L. P., R. Freedman, R. G. Potter, Jr., and A. Jain, "Correlates of IUD Termination in a Large-Scale, Mass Family Planning Program: The First Taiwan IUD Follow-up Survey," (mimeographed draft), 1967.

6. Sheps, M. C. and E. B. Perrin, "Changes in Birth Rates as a Function of Contraceptive Effectiveness: Some Applications of a Stochastic Model," *American Journal of Public Health*, July 1963, pp. 1031-44.

7. Taiwan Population Studies Center, *Joint Monthly Report*, Feb. 1966.

8. Taiwan Population Studies Center, "Follow-up Interview of Conventional Contraceptive Users in Nantou County" (under preparation).

9. Ministry of Health and Social Affairs, Republic of Korea, *The Findings of the National Survey on Family Planning, 1966,* Dec. 1966.

10. Chow, L. P., Unpublished data.

11. Potter Jr., R. G., "Estimating Births Averted in a Family Planning Program" (draft paper prepared for the Sesquicentennial Celebration of The University of Michigan). Published in Part IV of this volume.

12. Taiwan Population Studies Center, *Joint Monthly Report,* Dec. 1966.

13. Lu, Laura, "Group Meeting as a Method of Community Health Education for the Family Planning Health Program," *Proceedings of the IPPE Regional Conference—Western Pacific Region, May 1965,* Seoul, Korea.

14. DuiBois Cora, *et al.,* "A Strategy for Population Control," *Harvard Public Health Alumni Bulletin,* Vol. 22, No. 1, Jan. 1965.

15. Population Council, *Studies in Family Planning,* No. 3, Apr. 1964.

16. Chow, L. P. "Evaluation Procedures for a Family Planning Program," *Family Planning and Population Programs,* (Chicago: University of Chicago Press), pp. 675-89.

17. Freedman, R., "The Transition from High to Low Fertility: Challenge to Demographers," *Population Index,* Vol. 31, No. 4, Oct. 1965.

PROSPECTS FOR FERTILITY PLANNING IN TURKEY

Nusret H. Fisek
Hacettepe Institute of Population Studies,
Hacettepe University, Ankara

Introduction

UNTIL 1965 THE TURKISH GOVERNMENT prohibited not only the sale and use of contraceptives but also the dissemination of knowledge pertaining to birth control under authority of specific articles in the Turkish Penal Code. Prior to 1965 extensive official measures were taken to promote a rapid growth of the population to increase the diplomatic prestige and military strength of the country. Five years (1960-1965) of effort and enormous strife were required before the Parliament passed legislation which allows the sale and use of contraceptives and places population control among the responsibilities of the government (1,2). Although this new policy was accepted, the government has been facing great difficulties in getting the programs underway. Among the major problems have been an active opposition from some intelligentsia, a relatively low level of education, and the inadequacy of rural health services (3). In 1965, the population of Turkey reached 31.9 million and the population growth rate was 2.49 percent (4).

One of the most crucial factors that determines either the success or failure of a birth control program is, of course, the attitude of the public. In Turkey a national sample survey of public knowledge, attitudes, and practice of birth control, conducted in 1963, showed that a sizable majority of the population favored having small families and government-sponsored programs for family planning (5). Currently, Turkey's Second Five-Year Development Plan is up for discussion in the Parliament. This document reflects that the present government, in a manner similar to its predecessors, maintains interest in population control (6). Thus the *sociocultural and political climate for family planning appear favorable*. Two years of past experience, however, in the implementation of the program have shown beyond doubt that the desire for action, the availability of resources, and the existence of knowledge about contraception are not dependable guarantees of success.

In this paper, I wish to present a number of factors, other than public opinion and governmental interest, which will substantially affect future developments in Turkey's family planning program.

Major Social Factors Affecting Fertility
Some of the major factors contributing to the decrease of fertility in Europe over the past 150 years can be listed as industrialization, urbanization, and education. During the coming decades, the same factors will certainly affect fertility in all developing countries. It is not, however, readily possible to make safe predictions without considering basic factors.

Education   An inverse correlation is widely found between the level of education and the rate of fertility; e.g., family size tends to decrease as the level of education goes up. In general, education promotes and facilitates the acceptance of new and progressive ideas and practices.

In Turkey within the next decade the cohort of females of reproductive age (15-44) which now has a low literacy rate (Table 1) will be replaced by another having a relatively higher literacy rate.

Table 1. Literacy Rates in Turkey (1965) (7)

	Male			Female		
		Literate			Literate	
Age Groups	Population (1000's)	No. (1000's)	Rate (percent)	Population (1000's)	No. (1000's)	Rate (percent)
10-14	2043	1605	78.6	1805	1021	56.6
15-19	1549	1245	80.4	1370	704	51.4
20-24	1210	979	80.9	1155	470	40.8
25-29	1069	813	76.1	1170	390	33.3
30-34	1132	790	69.8	1139	306	26.9
35-39	995	656	65.9	935	228	24.4
40-44	684	429	62.7	669	142	21.2
45-49	444	243	54.7	430	77	17.9
49+	2050	741	36.1	2256	183	8.1
Total	11176	7501	67.1	10929	3521	32.2

This undoubtedly constitutes a very favorable factor for the future of family planning programs in Turkey.

Religion   Ninety-eight percent of the Turkish population adheres to Islam. Unlike some of the other major religions, Islam has no religious provisions directly curtailing fertility control practices. One could be tempted to conclude prematurely that religion poses no hindrance whatsoever to the implementation of fertility control programs. However, in considering this point, it should be remembered that an organized religious clergy does not exist in Islam. Every imam (parochial leader) or even every faithful has the right and the privilege to interpret and practice his faith as he understands it. Since interpretations vary from person to person, this variance has a direct effect on the implementation of fertility control programs. A great contribution to the success of fertility control programs would certainly be made in Moslem countries, if, for example, imams were to propogate the desirability of, and the necessity for, small families. Whether or not Islam encourages large families is highly controversial. The prophet Mohammed had said: "Marry and reproduce so that I may be proud of you before God." On the basis of this statement and in the absence of any direct reference to it in the Koran, some argue "the prophet encourages large families," while others contend that the case is quite to the contrary in this "Mohammed had actually emphasized pride rather than mere numbers, and, families should bear no more children than they can amply support." Therefore, proper education, especially among the imams, can provide fertility control programs with the accelerating and stimulating effect of religious sanction.

Industrialization and Urbanization   The phenomena of industrialization and urbanization are among the most important variables influencing fertility patterns in the world. Compared to agrarian areas, the lower age limit of the economically active population is higher in urbanized and industrialized communities where joining the labor force requires learning certain specialized skills and legislation prohibits child labor. In a predominantly agricultural society, where technological development is at a minimum and labor-intensive methods of production are employed (a common characteristic of all underdeveloped countries) children as young as 5 to 9 years take part in the livelihood of the family.

Recent studies conducted in Turkey confirm the effect of industrialization on family size there. A survey carried out in Eregli, one of Turkey's major steel production centers, shows that whereas the extended family was predominant prior to the advent of industrialization, the average number of children per family is now 2.24(8).

The Turkish Demographic Survey has found that the average birth rate in three metropolitan centers is 29.7 per thousand persons per year. In cities and towns of Central Anatolia and the Black Sea regions, the birth rate is 35.0 per thousand, whereas this rate increases to 48.7 per thousand in the rural parts of the same regions (9).

Urbanization and industrialization are rapidly taking place in Turkey. The percentage of urban population rose from 18.5 to 29.9 percent during the last fifteen years (Table 2); and may reach 60 percent in 1985. Both the industrialized population and the share of industry in the GNP grew considerably during recent years. Industrial employment has amounted to 7.8 percent during the last 5 years. The share of industrial product in GNP rose from 4.84 percent in 1962 to 15.88 percent in 1966. It is expected that this share will go up to 20.52 percent by 1972 (6,7,11). This trend of industrialization and urbanization can be expected to lower the high fertility rate of Turkey in the coming decade.

Early Marriage The age of marriage is relatively high in Turkey (Table 3) and is steadily going towards higher age groups. In 1965, only 22 percent of all women under 19 years of age were married, taking both the rural and the urban areas together. This rate was 33 percent in 1960. The same trend is also observable for the male population (7).

Health Services and Fertility Control The success or failure of any program of fertility control is greatly dependent on, and closely interrelated to, the health infrastructure of the country. The inadequacy of the health services not only hinders the development of the program directly but also discourages families from practicing effective birth control indirectly because of high infant and child mortality.

Table 2. Percentage of Urban Population in Turkey

Year	Total Population (1000's)	Urban Population* (1000's)	Percent Urban
1940	17,821	3172	17.8
1945	18,790	3439	18.3
1950	20,947	3875	18.5
1955	24,065	5078	21.1
1960	27,755	6828	24.6
1965	31,391	9395	29.9

*Communities with population over 10,000.

Table 3. Unmarried Population in Turkey (1965)

Age Group	Male Population (1000's)	Single (1000's)	Percent	Female Population (1000's)	Single (1000's)	Percent
14-19	1907	1757	92.1	1711	1339	78.3
20-29	2279	877	38.5	2326	241	10.4
30-39	2127	97	4.6	2074	44	2.1
40+	3180	61	1.9	3355	54	1.6
Unknown	14	5	35.7	15	7	46.7
Total	9507	2797	29.4	9481	1685	17.8

Many babies must be born to assure survival of the needed number of children.

Organization of Health Services   The Ministry of Health and Social Assistance is the main organization providing medical care and public health services in Turkey. Presently Turkey's health organization follows two distinctly different patterns. The old health organization pattern consists of hospitals and district medical offices. These two organizations are independent and cooperate little in their work.

Turkey is divided into 67 provinces and 637 administrative districts (counties). The rural population in these districts varies from a minimum of 2149 to a maximum of 142,199. The districts in turn are subdivided into villages, of which there are 35,441 with a median population of about 300. There are one or sometimes even more medical officers stationed in the district medical office. They may, in addition to their official work, have private practice. The district medical officers come under the control of the district governor. The male public health nurses and rural midwives employed in the district are attached to the medical officer. The number of paramedical workers needed falls well below the present demand. Such a health infrastructure is highly inadequate for successful implementation of family planning programs in the rural areas.

The total number of hospital beds in Turkey is 75,900 (1967) or 22 beds per 100,000 population. Of these hospital beds, 94 percent belong to the public sector. It can be assumed, that if appropriate administrative measures were taken, the hospitals and private doctors located in the urban areas could meet the needs of the public for family planning clinical services.

In 1961, the Turkish government decided to change the existing system for health services by introducing a National Health Service Plan. The health units of this service constitute the mainstead of the organizational pattern. A health unit is staffed with one medical officer, two nurses and two or three midwives. One health unit serves an average of 7000 inhabitants. The health personnel in these units, medical doctors included, cannot have private practice. Within their responsibilities are ambulatory and home care, all preventive work, and active participation in community development. The work in the health unit is supported and/or supplemented by hospitals and public health specialists under the direct supervision of the provincial health director. 16.9 percent of the present population of Turkey is covered now by the National Health Service. An additional 7.3 percent is planned to be covered in the very near future. According to national plans, by 1977, the former health organization pattern will be entirely replaced by the National Health Service. This nationalization of health services will provide the organizational set-up for a more successful implementation of the family planning programs. In fact, preliminary data obtained by Serinken, (12) who is studying the potentialities of using health units for carrying out family planning programs in rural areas, show that one gynecologist or trained general practitioner and two educators in addition to local health unit personnel can provide in 4 months, intrauterine contraception for 12 percent of all married women under 50 years of age served by 7 health units (60,000 total population).

Health Manpower Turkey has 1 medical doctor per 3150 population. About 500 new M.D.s graduate every year. This figure is expected to rise to 750 by 1975. The major problem of physician manpower arises not from the availability of an adequate number of M.D.s, but from inequality of their geographical distribution. The National Health Service has contributed appreciably to leveling off these disparities by the extension of medical services by doctors residing in rural health units.

A most critical question that gives rise to severe problems is the shortage of para-medical personnel (male and female public health nurses and midwives). The ratio of para-medical workers to total population is 1:2065. The First Five-Year Development Plan had assigned high priority to the training of para-medical personnel. The results are inspiring, for the number of graduates in various para-medical fields has increased from 325 in 1963 to 1742 in 1967. According to plan targets, this figure will be doubled during the coming 5 years.

The Medical Profession and Fertility Planning
Inadequacy of interest shown by the medical profession towards fertility control is a worldwide problem. Guttmacher (*13*) lists ethical drawbacks, fear of unpopularity, avoidance of "playing God," and political worries as the basic factors contributing to the observed attitude of the medical doctors. Going one step further, the following may be added: The lack of proper and comprehensive perspectives in tackling the social aspects of medicine, and the obviously old-fashioned attitude or value orientation that a doctor's work starts and ends in his surgery or in the hospital. These attitudes can be attributed, as a whole, to the inadequate scope of medical education that generally aims at teaching patient care and training research workers, without due emphasis on the study of environmental factors affecting health.

No systematic study has been conducted on the attitude of Turkish medical doctors towards fertility control. It seems that a great majority are not opposed but it remains doubtful whether they are conscious of the magnitude of the problem. There are reasons to believe that this generalization may hold true for many doctors working in the local health services, as well as those having responsible positions in the government. Some doctors oppose fertility control and spare no effort in supporting the anti-planning undercurrents.

The National Population Planning Program
The population planning policy and program in Turkey were introduced for the first time in the First Five-Year Development Plan. During the First Five-Year Plan period, the government amended existing legislation, made intrauterine contraception devices (IUD's) and oral contraceptives available to the public, established 215 family planning clinics, and 3 mobile rural teams, and trained 425 gynecologists and general practitioners for inserting IUD's. By May, 1967, the number of IUD's inserted was over 50,000 and the estimated number of women using oral contraceptives around 60,000 (*14*). These are very modest figures if compared to the fertile married female population which totals 4.6 million.

The Second Five-Year Development Plan provides that 5 percent of the female population in the fertile age group should be reached every year and that two million women should be practicing some measure of birth control by 1972. In order to achieve these targets, the government will add 0.50 Turkish lira (9TL = 1 $US) per capita to the state budget in addition to the usual health expenditure allocations. Provincial family planning directorates will start utilizing mobile teams; emphasis will be given to adult education; mass media techniques will be used; and similar educational programs will be carried out in the schools and in the units of the Armed Forces.

Hacettepe Institute of Population Studies
The Hacettepe University, in response to the world wide implications of fertility control and the difficulties encountered in the implementation of the National Population Policy, has established an Institute of Population Studies (15). The purposes of this Institute are to:
"1. Set up an Information-Documentation Center and collect data systematically concerning population and population planning in Turkey and other countries, to distribute these data to official and private organizations for their use.
2. Establish a Public Education unit; improve public education methods and materials, do research, convey the results to official and private organizations.
3. Train technical and administrative personnel in population planning and do research in this field."
The Institute is organizing an Information-Documentation Center, is supporting an educational program in population dynamics at the master's level in cooperation with the Hacettepe Graduate School, and has started a rural adult education pilot program.

Additional Considerations
Adult Education
The population planning program which officially started in 1965 has not developed as rapidly as was expected. One of the major reasons for the slow progress is the shortage of manpower in public education, especially those who can organize and implement the adult education programs linked to family planning. The medical doctors in charge of the action programs in family planning do not assume responsibility for adult education. For the reasons listed above, the intelligentsia have to be oriented so that they will give high priority to family planning programs; the medical doctors need to be urged to step up adult education efforts; the public has to be enlightened on the various aspects of family planning and above all the public has to be so motivated that they will put pressure on the government and politicians for a quick realization of their wishes. Furthermore, it is of utmost importance that all educational media in the country be influenced and even conditioned so as to be permissive to the purposes and policies of fertility control.

The attitudes of medical doctors are conditioned to a great extent by the present educational system. Doctors are trained as specialists of certain fields, with complete disregard of paramedical and social disciplines. This education undoubtedly results in the doctors' shallow understanding of health as a whole. Future medical doctors have to be so educated that they will grasp the holistic view of phenomena encountered. They will have to appreciate that man is not an independent being, but he is a part of and a product of his environment. His attitude and ability for medical team work as well as his aptitude for cooperation with other professionals need be furthered.

Operational Research

Administration today is a substantially different discipline than the common sense practices of the past. Present-day administrators have to base their policies and decisions more on scientific findings and channel their efforts to purposes partly pinpointed by science. Operational research has to be conducted in a variety of fields, including family planning. Research of this nature has to be encouraged, results evaluated, and strategy planned accordingly.

Rural Health Services

Any government considering the implementation of family planning programs has to provide a service network which can reach even the remotest villages. In the regions of Turkey, where health services are being nationalized, this will not pose an important problem. In villages where proper health services have not been established, the use of mobile health teams will bring temporary relief. The permanent or temporary employment of medical doctors in rural areas is a crucial problem faced by a great majority of the developing countries. To break through these barriers, countries will have to start from the beginning—improving medical education and conceiving a workable overall plan for better mobilizing all resources and manpower.

Contraceptive Methods

Contraceptive methods are an important factor affecting the outcome of fertility control programs. Only 10 years ago, those voicing the necessity for a decline in fertility had little to offer but a wish for a change in sociocultural factors. The use of oral pills and IUD's has greatly changed this somewhat resigned point of view. The discovery of more modern techniques and devices which will cause less side reactions, give better protection, and be more easily used will pave the way to a successful action program.

Summary

In summary the success of a fertility control program is substantially dependent on such factors as adult education, the extension of health services to rural areas, and the utilization of scientific methods in administration. Family planning, like all social action, is not an independent variable. The successes recorded in one area will determine the destiny of others. For these reasons, no effort should be spared in accelerating such phenomena as industrialization, urbanization, and the transition from a traditional to a progressive society.

The level of education in present-day Turkey is rising slowly but steadily. Turkey is industrializing and consequently urbanizing. The age of marriage is being prolonged. Prospects of using religious sanction in promoting family planning programs are good. The traits characteristic of traditional societies are gradually disappearing. For the next decade or so, a well organized national fertility control program superimposed upon a progressive sociocultural environment, described above, will provide sufficient protection from the danger of a population explosion.

REFERENCES

1. Fisek, N. H. "Responsibilities of the State in Family Planning," p. 197 *in Sex and Human Relations,* International Congress Series no. 102, Excerpta Medica Foundation, Amsterdam, 1965.

2. "Family Planning in Turkey and Its Development," U.N. Economic and Social Council E/ICEF/CRP/66-13, United Nations, New York, 1966.

3. Fisek, N. H. "Problems Starting a Program," *in* Berelson, B. *et al.,* eds., *Family Planning and Population Programs* (Chicago: University of Chicago Press), 1966.

4. *Nufus Haberleri Bulteni* (in Turkish), No. 1, Hacettepe Institute of Population Studies, Ankara, 1965.

5. Berelson, B. "Turkey: National Survey on Population," *Studies in Family Planning,* No. 5. New York: The Population Council, 1964.

6. The Second Five-Year Development Plan (1968-1972), The Turkish Republic, Prime Ministry, State Planning Organization, 1967.

7. *Population Census of Turkey* (Oct. 24, 1965), Publication No. 508, State Institute of Statistics, Ankara, 1966.

8. Kiray, M. B. "Eregli: Agir Sanayiden Once Bir Sahil Kasliasi" (in Turkish), State Planning Organization, Ankara, 1964.

9. Bulletin of the Turkish Demographic Survey No. 1, School of Public Health, Ankara, 1967.

10. "Urbanization Problems" (in Turkish), State Planning Organization, Ankara, 1966.

11. Census of Population (Oct. 23, 1960), Publication No. 452, State Institute of Statistics, Ankara.

12. Serinken, H. Unpublished data, Hacettepe Institute of Population Studies, Ankara.

13. Guttmacher, A. F. "The Responsibility of the Public Health and Medical Profession" *in Proceedings of the Eighth International Conference of IPPF,* Chile, Apr. 9-15, 1967, International Planned Parenthood Federation, London, 1967.

14. Metiner, T. "Recent Development in Family Planning in Turkey," paper presented at International Conference organized by Ankara Gynecological Society, June 8-10, 1967.

15. Fisek, N. H. "A New Institute of Hacettepe Science Center: Hacettepe Institute of Population Studies," *Turkish J. Ped.,* 8:237, 1966.

CHILEAN PROGRAM OF ABORTION CONTROL AND FERTILITY PLANNING: PRESENT SITUATION AND FORECAST FOR THE NEXT DECADE

Mariano Requena B.
Latin American Demographic Center

THE OBJECTIVE OF THIS PAPER is to make a forecast for the next decade about the Chilean Program of Abortion Control and Fertility Planning (P.A.C.F.P.). This is a complex and dangerous task. A forecast in science—and I am referring to a forecast based on the knowledge of factors of change and not to the simple projection of trends—is always a hard enterprise. Difficulties increase as we move away from the physical sciences and approach the social sciences, not only because of the complexity and variety of the determinant factors but because of the singularity that concrete situations present.

For whoever ventures to make a forecast about P.A.C.F.P., it is indispensable to comply with two conditions. On the one hand, it is necessary to have a hypothesis that explains the complex of variables which determine the consecutive changes of a programmed action. On the other hand, it is necessary to know the present situation, its background, and the factors that have determined it.

Present State and Analysis of the Program
Chile is a country with an estimated population (*1*) in 1966 of 8,962,000 to 9,007,000 inhabitants, with an age distribution in which youngsters under 15 are 37.4 percent and with a crude birth rate, during the last 30 years, of 36 to 37 births per 1000 inhabitants per year. The crude death rate is 12 per 1000 inhabitants and the population growth rate is 2.2 percent per annum.

Since 1963, the year in which the first somewhat systematic public actions were initiated, the Chilean program has had a rapid growth (see Table 1). The number of women who, through the National Health Service (N.H.S.), initiated use of contraceptives in 1963 was

478

only 3200, all of them in Santiago. In 1966, three years later, this number had grown to 59,691, of which 17,010 (28.5 percent) were from outside Santiago.

Table 1. Women Initiating Use of Contraceptives Through National Health Service, Chile, 1963 to 1966

Area	1963*		1964		1965		1966	
	No.	%	No.	%	No.	%	No.	%
Santiago	3,200	100.0	12,878	99.5	27,834	86.1	42,681	71.5
Provinces	—	—	70	0.5	4,479	13.7	17,010	28.5
Total	3,200	100.0	12,948	100.0	32,313	100.0	59,691	100.0

*Data in 1963 were registered in only one out-patient clinic.
Source: Requena M. and T. Monreal[2]

The type of contraceptives used, which for the first year consisted of intrauterine devices only, has expanded to include oral contraceptives (39 percent usage in 1966). (2) Given this important growth in the use of contraceptives, our next step is to analyze the factors that have influenced it. We will look first at the factors that have determined program growth and then at the importance of the role that the community has played.

Program Factors
The first characteristic of the Chilean program is the decisive role that physicians and health professionals and personnel have played in initiating the actions that have been developed. Although it is true that there has been some participation from others in our national activities, they have never taken any executive initiatives. Their participation has been limited to giving advice and support about the problems on which they considered it only too natural that physicians should act.

In 1962, a group of physicians, all of them professors of obstetrics, gynecology, and preventive medicine, gathered in order to create the Chilean Committee for Family Protection. In the beginning their task was carried out in silence and was mainly to stimulate themselves in their isolated research efforts, started independently by each of them. Two years later, in 1964, the group became an autonomous organization, changing its name to Chilean Association for Family Planning, and it continues to act through the N.H.S. The actions that this group carried out had important characteristics which explain its subsequent evolution. In the first place, its main objective was not birth control, but prevention of the high incidence and high case fatality rate of induced abortion. Data from hospital discharges revealed an increase in the proportion between abortions and live births. Clinical experience and the epidemiological studies carried out (3) had demonstrated that at least one out of three pregnancies was interrupted by abortion. Induced abortion was obviously a new problem of high priority among the public health problems of the country. The members of the committee had another characteristic: besides being university professors, they were also Service Chiefs of the N.H.S., which permitted them to carry out activities within the service even though these actions were not officially recognized. The ability to act through the N.H.S. represents evident advantages. It makes it possible to reach the remotest places of the country, since the N.H.S. has at its disposal a very acceptable network of basic resources: buildings, equipment, and personnel. This situation not only facilitates supplying contraceptives to those who want them but also diffusing knowledge about contraception to women at moments of their lives when they are highly motivated to control their pregnancies. The multiparous woman who gives birth in a maternity ward, the woman who is in a hospital for complications of a recently induced abortion or the one who requests the pediatrician's care, are women in situations which make them more receptive and motivated to the use of contraceptives.

This has been empirically confirmed in recent years by the program started in 1964 in the western health district of Santiago.* In the beginning, it was carried out exclusively through the district outpatient clinics with educational action primarily through lectures given to women who were waiting for the pediatrician's care (4). Since the second half of 1966 contraceptives have been offered in the maternity wards to women who had just had an abortion or a live-born child delivery. In the case of women with a live-born child delivery there has been a rapid growth in the percentage of those who have accepted contraceptives, from 2.3 percent to 32.9 percent in one year (5). In the case of women who had undergone an induced abortion, the growth has been even more rapid. In other words, the experience of this program reveals an adequate acceptance by the most susceptible groups. This situation would not be possible if it was not carried out by the N.H.S.

In 1965, the authorities of the N.H.S., realizing that a program of

* For medical care purposes, the city of Santiago is divided into five health districts (northern, southern, eastern, western, and central). The western district has more than 500,000 inhabitants and it initiated its program of abortion control in May, 1964.

abortion control and use of contraceptives was being intensively carried out through it without its recognition and direction, decided to take its leadership in their hands. During the VIII World Conference of the International Planned Parenthood Federation held in Santiago, Chile in 1967, the Ministry of Health proclaimed publicly the basic principles of the P.A.C.F.P. (6), which may be summarized as follows:

1. Although at a determined moment in the economic development of a country, the level of population increase may become an important factor in economic and social development, it never becomes a necessary condition.
2. From the public health point of view, induced abortion is a problem. The respective authorities must act in order to control it and offer to susceptible groups a more rational method of birth control.
3. The human, free and responsible couples concerned should decide on the limitation and spacing of children.
4. All action taken for this purpose must be founded on adequate education concerning all existing efficient methods so that the choice may be as wide as possible.

These basic principles led to ambitious aims and objectives for 1967, which are summarized in Table 2.

Table 2. Birth Control Program of Santiago and Provinces N.H.S., Chile, 1967

	Population of fertile women under N.H.S.'s medical care	Program Objectives for 1967			
		100 percent of women discharged for abortion	40 percent of women discharged for delivery	10 percent of women not attended by abortion or delivery	Total
Santiago					
Number	446,140	25,567	28,250	34,993	88,839
Percentage		28.8	31.8	39.4	100.0
Provinces					
Number	836,690	29,053	45,682	69,141	143,878
Percentage		20.2	31.7	48.1	100.0
Total					
Number	1,280,830	45,620	73,932	104,134	232,747
Percentage		23.5	31.8	44.7	100.0

Source: "Programa de regulación de la natalidad según zonas de salud, provincias y áreas hospitalarias." Servicio Nacional de Salud, Dirección General, Fomento de la Salud, Chile, 1967.

One serious problem remains: the physicians and midwives,* who are the direct agents of the program, have not yet given to it their total support. This is one of the most important handicaps of the P.A.C.F.P. at present, since physicians and midwives do not easily change their opinions and attitudes concerning these matters. In an inquiry made this year to a random sample of 280 women who were discharged from the maternity ward of the western health district of Santiago, it was shown that only 151 (53.9 percent) had been informed about family planning (82 percent of those informed accepted the use of contraceptives).

The Community

Another aspect of the program which it is necessary to examine is the community's reaction and the acceptance achieved. These aspects are important not only in themselves but also in the influence they exert on the subsequent decisions of various authorities. Our impression is that, in Chile, while a few leaders opened the door to the possibility of rational fertility control, it was the community which, later on, demanded that these isolated services become generally available. In 1962 (the year during which programs began to be intensified), women were much more motivated than was supposed and the task of the leaders was to give them the resources which would permit them to put this motivation into practice.

Information gathered about practices, opinions, and attitudes regarding family formation (7) and the epidemiological characteristics of induced abortion (3) lead us to state that the Chilean community was motivated at the moment of the initiation of the programatic actions. The most important argument is found in the induced abortion practices themselves. The woman who undergoes induced abortion, whatever the causes may be, reveals an intense motivation, since its practice is never pleasant and there is always the possibility of meeting danger, of which the woman is generally aware. At the same time, the epidemiological studies (3) contradict the previous belief that abortion was largely a means to solve the problem of pregnancies resulting from illicit relations and indicate that it was used as a birth control means. These studies show that the frequency of its use is the same for married women, concubines, or single women; and higher for the multiparous woman and when there is unemployment.

Abortion had continued to increase up to the time that the program began. The ratio of 3.1 induced abortions per 100 pregnancies discharged from hospitals in 1931 grew to 22 per 100 pregnancies in

* Midwives in Chile are university professionals who have graduated from the School of Obstetrics.

1960. If we accept the limitations of hospital discharge data,* induced abortion has increased since the initiation of the program in 1963 among all women of fertile age (see Table 3).

Table 3. Hospitalized Inducted Abortion Rate Per 1000 Women 15 to 49 Years Old and Percent Change in Chile, Santiago, and Provinces, 1961 to 1965

	Santiago		Provinces		Chile	
Year	Induced abortions per 1000 women, 15-49 years old	Percent change	Induced abortions per 1000 women, 15-49 years old	Percent change	Induced abortions per 1000 women, 15-49 years old	Percent change
1962	35.57	—	22.89	—	27.44	—
1963	30.67	−13.78	24.17	5.59	26.55	−3.24
1964	40.43	31.82	18.09	−25.16	26.25	−1.13
1965	35.75	−11.58	26.30	45.38	29.79	13.48
Total		6.46		25.81		9.11

Source: Requena, M., T. Monreal (2)

Between 1962 and 1965 there has been an increase in the rate of induced abortion for all the country of 9.11 percent (6.46 percent in Santiago and 25.81 percent in the provinces). The annual increase was higher the year that followed the intensification of the activities, i.e., 1963 in Santiago, and 1965 in the provinces. Our interpretation, as seen in the following section, is that this is not a failure of the program but a displacement of those groups who resort to induced abortion.

Further evidence that the community was already motivated when the program was initiated, comes from the surveys carried out in Chile. In 1959, the Latin American Demographic Centre (7) carried out a survey on fertility and attitudes toward family formation in

---

* Information for the analysis of the repercussion that the program may have had on the incidence of induced abortion is based on the annual discharges from N.H.S. hospitals. Previous researches show that hospital patients account for only a fraction of the total abortions and that this fraction is dependent on the seriousness of the complications. In one of the surveys carried out, it was estimated that only a third, 31.6 percent, of the induced abortions have gone to hospitals because of complications. If this percentage continues without significant variations during the years of this analysis (and very probably it will), information on hospital discharges will be useful for discovering secular evolution and for estimating, as a consequence, the possible impact the plan would have on them.

Santiago with a sample of 1970 women in their fertile age. Data were not obtained about the use of contraceptives, but responses to the question, "Do you approve or disapprove of doctors giving information in their consulting rooms or at maternity clinics on methods of birth control?," showed that 71.4 percent approved, 24.6 percent disapproved, and 4.0 percent did not give any opinion. These answers were very similar to those given by French women interviewed in 1956: 62 percent approved, 29 percent disapproved, and 9 percent did not give any opinion (8). This is another indicator which proves our thesis that the community was already prepared.

It is also interesting to examine the general impression that Tabah and Samuel (7) developed about fertility dynamics in Chile. They assert that Chile at that time was in the initial moments of its third stage of demographic transition. An estimation based on the theory of a stable population and corrected for omissions in declaration of births to the civil registrar, shows that the birth rate would have begun to decline in 1940. That year, it would have reached 42 per thousand and in 1959, 36 per thousand. In Santiago, the decline would have commenced before 1940 and in 1959 the birth rate would have been 26 to 28 per thousand.

Although Santiago represents one third of Chile's population, we must know if the same situation occurs in provinces. In a survey (9) carried out in 1965 (previous to the initiation of the contraceptive program) in La Calera, a town located 100 km. north of Santiago, with a population of 25,000 inhabitants in the urban area and 25,000 in the rural area, 954 women were interviewed: 83.2 percent pronounced themselves in favor of a small family and 82.5 percent in favor of the use of contraceptives. Additional information revealing how aware people in Chile were, concerning these matters, comes from a small survey of 71 families in Colina, a town located 25 km. north of Santiago, with a population of 15,000 inhabitants, of which 7500 live in the rural area (10). Fertility in this area, measured by different indices, was 1.57 to 1.97 times higher than that of the city of Santiago, yet the women wished to wait some time after their marriage before having children and to space births (2.7 to 3.3 years between each one). Forty percent did not wish any children after they were 30 years old and 75 percent did not wish any after age 40. Eighty-five percent approved family planning and only 4 percent disapproved it. Fifty percent said they would accept abortion, if they did not have another possibility of fertility control and 44 percent said they would resort to it if it was legalized in Chile.

These two surveys carried out in rural areas (even though because of their proximity to Santiago these places cannot be considered as representatives of the rural patterns in Chile) document the striking contrast between the attitude of these women towards family planning and induced abortion and their high fertility. They indicate that the Chilean population, even in rural areas, was prepared and motivated to receive and adopt contraception.

The estimation we have made about the fertility changes that have taken place in Chile (2) shows that the general fertility rate declined from 144.7 per 1000 women in 1963, to 134.6 in 1965, and that during the same period, the birth rate declined from 34 to 32 per 1000 inhabitants. This impact is the product of a program that was progressively growing and that was developed in a community prepared to receive it. A brief analysis of some other conditions that could have also influenced fertility decline in Chile is given in the same paper (2).

Interpretative Hypothesis

We have demonstrated that Chile, previous to the intensification of family planning programmatic actions, had already initiated a decline in its fertility. Because of the lack of information and availability of contraceptives, induced abortion was generally used. Only those groups of a higher cultural level, who, consequently, had more means of gaining information and of reaching contraceptives, used them. But these groups were so limited in number that they did not have an important impact on fertility.

Of all intermediate variables, induced abortion and contraceptive usage are the ones that have most intensely influenced the fertility level in Chile. On the basis of results obtained from epidemiologic studies on induced abortion (11), Chilean women may be classified in three groups, according to these two variables and to their socioeconomic cultural level. The following diagram (11) gives a non-quantitative idea of this relationship:

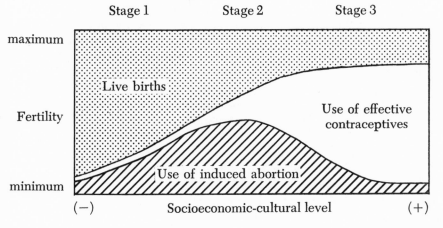

The group of high socioeconomic-cultural level resorted mainly to contraceptives. If they used induced abortion, they did it generally because of a failure of contraceptives. The women in the medium level group are the big users of induced abortion. This group was motivated to control family size but did not have the initiative or the necessary information to resort to contraceptive means. The lower level group had higher fertility and did not significantly use contraception or induced abortion. The relationship between the socioeconomic-cultural level and the use of induced abortion and contraceptives may be explained by the differences between these two methods. The contraceptive is a "preventive" means which implies a mature and conscious attitude toward the problem. Those of us who have cared about preventive medicine know how difficult is its practice. The lower the cultural level is, the more man needs the recognition of an immediate problem, in order to act. The one who deals with prevention plays with probabilities and it is inherent in human nature to assume that probabilities will be favorable to oneself. Abortion, on the contrary, is a "curative" means that solves a problem already existing and that always gives a definite result. That it involves risks, and that women are aware of them, is true, but again, the risk is only a probability that nobody expects to be unfavorable for himself.

During the period that has elapsed since the initiation of the program, fertility seems to have declined and the incidence of induced abortion seems to have increased. This phenomenon can be explained as a displacement of induced abortion usage towards those groups of a lower level. The group of medium level who used to resort to abortion at the initiation of the program is beginning to use contraceptives and those who did nothing are beginning to use abortion. What appears to have happened as a result of the program is that those women who previously used induced abortion have learned the possibility of changing to a more rational method and have adopted it; but those who had taken no action previously have been motivated by the program, and have resorted first to the "curative" means—abortion. This results in a fertility decline, since more women practice birth control, and in an increase of induced abortion because the group that adopts it is the most numerous. The significance of this phenomenon for the success of the program is favorable.

Forecast For the Next Decade
Making our forecast of what will happen in Chile during the next decade becomes easier now. If the reasoning we have put forward is accepted we may present the perspectives of the P.A.C.F.P. as follows:

(a) The program, administered and directed by the N.H.S. will be expanded. Its publicly proclaimed goals, the leadership of physicians, and the increasing pressure of the community are factors that assure the extension and promotion of educational activities and contraceptive services, in the near future, all over the country.

(b) Although at present physicians and other health personnel do not have favorable attitudes towards the aims stated by the N.H.S., the efforts in medical education to introduce these concepts and to teach contraceptive techniques, lead us to assume that rapid progress in the change of attitudes will be achieved.

(c) The community will go on adopting birth control in increasing numbers. The lowest level groups will temporarily adopt induced abortion, causing a temporary increase in its incidence or, at least, maintainance of its present level. The medium social-economic-cultural groups will begin to replace induced abortion by contraceptives.

(d) Controlled births—either by means of induced abortion or of contraceptives—will cause a fertility decrease. It is difficult to forecast the level that fertility will reach, but if the observed tendencies are maintained, it will decline to, at least, 25 births per 1000 inhabitants.

(e) It is possible that change in the age at marriage, in the percentage of celibates, in cultural development, in expansion of means of communications, in participation of the woman in working activities, and in other social factors, will help to decrease the fertility level.

Our conclusion is that Chile has entered into its third stage of demographic transition and that the next decade will begin a rapid decrease of fertility, which is characteristic of this stage.

REFERENCES

1. Alvarez, Leonel. *Proyección de la Poblacion de Chile por Sexo y Grupos de Edad, 1960-2000.* Centro Latinoamericano de Demografia, Serie C, No. 84, Santiago, Chile.

2. Requena B., Mariano and Tegualda Monreal, "Evaluation of the Induced Abortion Control and Family Planning Programs in Chile," *Milbank Memorial Fund Quarterly* (to be published).

3. (a) Matus, Victor. "El Problema del Aborto," *Boletin de la Sociedad Chilena de Obstetricia y Ginecologia,* April 3, 1938, pp. 184-205.

   (b) Manubens, Ricardo. "Estudio sobre Aborto Involuntario," thesis, University of Chile, 1952.

   (c) Mena, Victor. "Estudio sobre Aborto Provocada," thesis, University of Chile, 1952.

   (d) Walsen, Raúl. "Problema Médico, Social y Médico—legal del Aborto Provocada," *Boletin de la Sociedad Chilena de Obstetricia y Ginecologia,* Oct. 19, 1954, pp. 185-96.

   (e) Armijo, Rolando and Tegualda Monreal. "Epidemiology of Provoked Abortion in Santiago, Chile," *Population Dynamics,* eds. Minoru Muramatsu and Paul Harper, The Johns Hopkins Press, 1965, pp. 137-60.

   (f) Requena B., Mariano. "Social and Economic Correlates of Induced Abortion in Santiago, Chile," *Demography,* 2:33, 1965.

4. Requena B., Mariano. *First Report. Abortion Control Program,* Department "B" of Preventive Medicine, School of Medicine, University of Chile, Sept., 1964.

5. Viel, Benjamín. "Resultados del Programa de Planificación Familiar del Area Occidente de Santiago, April 1964 a Junio 1967." To be published in *The American Journal of Public Health.*

6. Valdivieso D., Ramón. "Normas de las Acciones de Regulación de la Natalidad," discurso del Minstro de Salud Pública en la Sesión Inaugural de la Octava Conferencia Mundial de la Federación Internacional de Planificación de la Familia, Ministerio de Salud Publica, Chile, Apr. 9, 1967.

7. Tabah, Leon and Raúl Samuel. "Preliminary Findings of a Survey on Fertility and Attitudes Toward Family Formation in Santiago, Chile," *Research in Family Planning,* ed. Clyde V. Kiser. Princeton University Press, 1962, pp. 263-304.

8. Girard, Alain and Raúl Samuel. "Une enquéte sur l'opinion a l'égard de la limitation des naissances," *Population,* Paris, July.-Sept. 1956, pp. 481-506.

9. Requena B., Mariano, and Ferdinand Rath. Unpublished data from the Latin American Demographic Center in conjunction with Department "B" of Preventive Medicine, School of Medicine, University of Chile.

10. Miró, Carmen, Juan Puga, and Donald Bogue. "La Fecundidad Rural en Latinoamerica: une Encuesta Experimental para Medir Actitudes, Conocimiento y Comportamiento," *Demography*, vol. 2, pp. 97-114, 1965.

11. Requena B., Mariano. "Condiciones Determinantes del Aborto Inducida," *Revista Medica de Chile*, 94, Nov., 1966, pp. 714-22.

VI. NEEDED PRIORITIES IN POPULATION CONTROL

THE CITIZEN'S VIEW OF PUBLIC
PROGRAMS FOR FAMILY LIMITATION

John D. Rockefeller, III
The Population Council

IF THIS GREAT UNIVERSITY HAD BEEN FOUNDED TEN YEARS EARLIER, if this sesquicentennial meeting on population were occurring in 1957 instead of 1967, our mood tonight would be altogether different. What an impressive decade it has been! One can scarcely overestimate what you and your colleagues around the world have accomplished in these few years.

If I had been asked to sound a keynote for this conference, it would have concerned a combination of satisfaction and profound awareness. We are like an army exultant at having won a battle, but fully aware that the war has yet to be won.

My own concern about the population problem took tangible form with the creation of the Population Council in 1952. In the opportunity to work with the Council, and in my frequent travels to study activities and progress in countries around the world, I have formed some impressions of where we stand. I would like to discuss them with you briefly in the belief that it is as useful at times to survey the field broadly through a telescope as it is to examine in detail its crucial aspects through a microscope.

In making appraisals, I shall divide the population field into broad constituent elements. These reflect the major concerns represented in the agenda for this conference and in the excellent program on population sponsored by this university. In making evaluations, I am concerned with where we stand at this cross-section in time— with assessing the current level of activity against the optimum level of what we ought to be doing today.

The first element of the population field I would mention is biomedical and contraceptive research. It is to this area that one looks for the innovations that can accelerate progress dramatically. Perhaps nothing is more important to successful family planning programs than modern contraceptives that are acceptable and highly effective. One has only to imagine where we would be today without the pill and the IUD.

Despite the excellent work under way, it is clear that biomedical and contraceptive research has not received high priority. It is not yet regarded as a prestige field. We need many more scientists in this field and we need to attract the best young scientists to it, both in the developed and lesser-developed countries.

In regard to overall effort, Doctors Oscar Harkavy and Anna Southam estimate that the worldwide annual expenditures in biomedical research are currently in the range of 35 to 40 million dollars. Since they postulate a reasonable optimum level of 150 million, they see current activity at only about 25 percent of need.

The second area is demographic research and evaluation, where there is an enormous amount of work to be done. The present state of census-taking does not provide a good basis for current estimates of population growth. In the developing world, tabulations are slow and analyses are inadequate. Even more serious is the fact that few developing countries have adequate vital statistics. Improvements are not given high priority and occur slowly.

Research and evaluation on family planning programs are poor except in two or three countries. It seems that only where there are good action programs do we get even moderately good research and evaluation.

We depend on demographic work to provide us with baseline data and with realistic possibilities of measuring progress in the population field. The ability to evaluate is crucial to success. At present, we have little data to work with and we are very short of skilled personnel. If I understand Dr. Dudley Kirk's analysis correctly, less than one-fifth of the people in the world live in areas adequately covered by demographic data.

Turning now from the underpinnings of research to the action areas, my third subdivision is a key motivational area—that of elite awareness and support. I refer to political, religious, and social leaders at the national level and to local leaders scattered throughout a national society.

Most of you are familiar, I am sure, with the World Leaders' Statement on Population, first announced by Secretary-General U Thant on December 10, 1966, Human Rights Day, at the United Nations. It had been signed by twelve heads of state. The second list of additional signatories will be announced this coming Human Rights Day by the Secretary-General. It, too, is an impressive list.

Despite such important progress, the fact remains that too many leaders still regard the population problem as too sensitive for bold and large-scale public action. Not more than a fourth of the heads of state in the developing world have come out publicly in support of population and family planning, and of these less than ten have put their full weight behind action programs.

In this regard, ironically, the leaders lag behind their people. From your work, it seems clear that women, in very large numbers, *want* to plan their families—to limit and space their childbearing. The surveys accord with what I have seen and heard in my travels. Nothing else augurs so well for long-term hope and success because it means that there is a basic congruence between our concern for the worldwide population problem and motivation within the individual family. But this widespread latent desire to limit family size will only have positive effect if supported and encouraged by national leadership.

It may well be that we will get forthright and effective leadership only when the population problem becomes visible in a dramatic and convincing way—when fear becomes a motivating rather than an inhibiting force. Thus far we have not had the population equivalent of an atomic explosion, a Sputnik, a Watts—the single critical incident that compels action. It may well come if, for example, tens of millions of persons die of starvation in a single year. Some observers believe that such a catastrophe is already foredoomed.

Even if world leaders were all as strongly motivated as we would wish, they would in turn have to depend on local leaders to translate awareness of the problem into effective action. It is a two-way relationship. Local leaders must have national support and guidance to be effective. And national leaders must motivate the decision-making and action structure of a national society—the thousands of state and local government officials, the school teachers and administrators, university scholars, community leaders.

My fourth subdivision is national programs. Approximately 20 countries in the developing world now have officially-proclaimed national programs of population and family planning. Many of these are in Asia. There are few programs in Africa, which is far behind in medical facilities and demography and where few leaders yet see the relevance of the population problem to their countries. In Latin America, of course, leaders are still inhibited by the position of the Church.

If it were only a matter of proclaiming the official existence of a national program, we could feel moderately satisfied since over half the people in the developing world live in countries with favoring policies. But there is often a great disparity between professed intent and actual performance. Of the national programs that have been proclaimed in 20 or so countries, my judgment is that not more than 5 of them are strong, meaningful programs with the full and energetic backing of top leadership.

Closely associated with the idea of national programs is the fifth area, that of organization and administration. This is a major problem. One may have elite support and a proclaimed national program, but there then remains the awesome responsibility of actually getting the job done.

One problem is that in many countries the top professional leadership of population programs is extremely thin. In many cases, the burden of developing a program rests too much and for too long on one or two people. They face the almost insurmountable tasks of mobilizing the national bureaucracy, of gaining priority for the effort in manpower and money, and of motivating local leaders.

There are fiscal problems, too. Typically, ministries of finance are so beset with short-term budgetary problems that they cannot see the longer-term urgency of population programs. Or there may be fiscal hindrances inherent in relationships between national and local levels of government.

The organization and administration of family planning programs form the crucial crossroads where all the other major elements of the problem come together at the point of action. They need our best attention. We are thin in manpower all the way down the line. Training is inadequate. We have not one-tenth the trained and qualified field workers that we need.

The sixth major element of the population problem is the field of information and education. It is another area of some progress but also of serious deficiencies. Information programs on population are not nearly good enough. We have not used the mass media effectively. The presence in school curricula of good, solid material is infinitesimal. Fortunately the motivation to limit family size has not been dependent on programs of information and education. But effective action to limit family size *is* dependent to a great degree on our ability to communicate and to educate. We must be more imaginative than ever before in finding effective channels of communication to large masses of people.

Even if we were to make rapid strides toward the goal of bringing to all women the knowledge and resources they need to plan their families, we would still face a problem of mass motivation. In the long run, it will not be enough to make it possible for women to avoid having unwanted children. Even in a world of wanted children, population may grow too fast. The most effective way to encourage a trend toward smaller families is in mass information and education—to speak out on the subject, to build understanding of the problem, to educate our children.

The seventh and last of the major elements of the population problem is funding. Currently, the field is woefully undernourished. One is tempted to think of other massive efforts to mobilize human and dollar resources, even though the analogies are to a considerable extent inexact. There is, for example, the race to land a man on the moon in which the United States has spent $16 billion, with the prospect that at least another $10 billion will be needed before a manned lunar landing is achieved.

In such efforts, the money begins to flow when the need is identified and the policy decisions are made. I believe this is beginning to happen in the population field, but there certainly is no room for complacency on this score. We have a long way to go. For example, in a recent Senate subcommittee hearing Dr. Harkavy reported on his study of the Department of Health, Education, and Welfare. He suggested that $100 million would be the level of expenditure that HEW should be reaching in family planning programs and support, but that only $19 million was currently available. I have seen the few private programs and university centers in the population field desperately in search of funds. I know of very few programs anywhere in the world that now are adequately funded.

Considering the situation in these seven major elements of the population field and examining our overall effort, where do we stand?

If we measure current effort against the optimum level—a high but realistically achievable goal—I believe that today we are doing less than one-fifth of what we should be doing.

I base this statement on judgment and observation as much as upon any documentation I can present to you. But where figures and reasonable estimates are available, they either fall in the range of 20 to 25 percent of the optimum level, or they are considerably less.

We are doing only one-fourth of the biomedical research that we should be doing. We have not one-tenth of the trained manpower we need. Less than a fourth of heads of state have given strong verbal support to population and family planning programs. Only about 20 developing countries have proclaimed programs, and of these as yet not more than five are strong, effective programs. Our funding of population programs is surely not one-fifth of what it should be. If one looks at the problem in terms of the number of women being served who need help, one-fifth is much too high an estimate. Even in the United States, the latest estimate of Planned Parenthood-World Federation is that only 700,000 of the 5.3 million women who need subsidized family planning services are in fact receiving them.

Some may feel that I am being generous when I say that we are doing less than one-fifth of what we could be doing—what we should be doing. Others might feel that one-fourth or one-third would be a more appropriate estimate. But I suspect that most of us would be reasonably close in order of magnitude. The main point is that the current worldwide level of action lags far behind the optimum level, far behind the urgency and magnitude of the problem.

Why does such an evaluation of how we are doing matter so much? Because the stakes are indeed so high. It seems to me clearer than ever that we are dealing here with the underlying social problem of our time. There will be no significant progress in any of the world's major areas of social problems unless we attain important successes in the population field. Population growth severely inhibits or negates man's efforts to cope with problems in such areas as education, urban decay, conservation, health, poverty, war, and peace.

Recognizing this fundamental importance of the population problem offers the best way of understanding that our purpose is positive and humanistic. Our concern is with the enrichment of human life. Only by curbing population growth rates can we have realistic hopes of attaining conditions that will enhance human dignity and provide men with a better chance to reach their full potential.

If these are the considerations at stake, then a performance level of one-fifth—or even a fourth or a third—is not nearly good enough. Great human problems demand commensurate effort—not necessarily at the fullest conceivable level, but much closer to it than we are now. There is a call to greatness in the population field and we dare not fall short. In stressing the lag between present need and present action, I mean to be realistic, not pessimistic. I recognize that we have made more progress in the past five years than we dared hope. But we must double and then redouble both the hope and the progress in the next five years.

CONTRIBUTORS

Ansley J. Coale, Ph. D.
Director, Office of Population Research, Princeton University; United State Representative—Population Commission of the United Nations; Member, Population Committee of the National Academy of Science; President Elect, Population Association of America, 1966-67; Member, Technical Advisory for Population, U.S. Bureau of the Census, 1965-   ; Member, American Philosophical Society; William Church Osborn Professor of Public Affairs, 1964-

David V. Glass, Ph.D.
Professor, London School of Economics and Political Science, University of London; Research Secretary, Population Investigation Committee (1936-1940; 1945-1946); Martin White Professor of Sociology, 1949-   ; Fellow, British Academy; Member, International Statistical Institute; Honorary President (formerly President), International Union for the Scientific Study of Population; Chairman, I.S.A. Committee on Research into Social Stratification and Social Mobility; Past-President, Sociology Section, British Association for the Advancement of Science.

Dudley Kirk, Ph.D.
Professor of Demography, Food Research Institute, Stanford University; Chief, Planning Staff, Research & Intelligence, Department of State, 1953-54; Member, U.S. Delegation to U.N. Population Commission, 1948-53; Chief, Division of Research for Near East, South Asia, and Africa, 1952; Department of State, President's Commission on Immigration and Naturalization, 1952; Demographic Director, The Population Council, 1954-   ; Board of Directors, American Eugenics Society, 1955-   ; American Sociological Association (Fellow) Committee on Social Statistics, 1955- (Chairman, 1957-59); Eastern Sociological Society, Committee on Social Statistics, 1959-   ; International Union for the Scientific Study of Population; Population Association of America, Board of Directors, 1947-53; President, 1960; Social Science Research Council, Chairman, Committee on Population Census Monographs, 1959-   ; American Association for the Advancement of Science (Fellow).

Norman B. Ryder, Ph.D.
Director, Center for Demography and Ecology, Department of Sociology, University of Wisconsin; Co-director, National Fertility

Study; Editor, *American Sociological Review;* Demographer, Canadian Bureau of Statistics, 1950-51; Demographer, Scripps Foundation for Research in Population Problems, 1954-56.

Richard A. Easterlin, Ph.D.

Professor of Economics, Department of Economics, University of Pennsylvania; Board of Directors, Population Association of America, 1964-65; Economic History Association; International Union for the Scientific Study of Population; Regional Science Association; Conference on Research in Income and Wealth (Executive Committee, 1963-   ); Editorial Board, *American Economic Review,* 1965-   ; National Bureau of Economic Research; S.S.R.C. Fellow, 1951-52; N.S.F. Economics Advisory Panel, 1963-65; Editorial Board, *Demography,* 1965-   ; Editorial Board, *Journal of Economic History,* 1965-

Simon Kuznets, Ph.D.

George F. Baker Professor of Economics, Department of Economics, Harvard University; Fellow, Royal Statistical Society; Member, American Statistical Association (President, 1949); Member, American Economics Association (President, 1954); Member, Royal Academy of Sciences, Sweden; Staff, National Bureau of Economic Research, 1927-   .

Harrison Brown, Ph.D.

Professor of Geochemistry, Division of Geological Sciences, California Institute of Technology: Assistant Director of Chemistry, Plutonium Project, University of Chicago, 1942-43; Associate Profess. Institute for Nuclear Studies, University of Chicago; American Association for the Advancement of Science, Annual Award in Pure Science, 1946: American Chemical Society Annual Award in Pure Chemistry, 1952; Lasker Award, 1958; L.LD., University of Alberta, 1961; D.Sc., Rutgers University, 1964; National Academy of Sciences, Member; Foreign Secretary, National Academy of Sciences; Editor-at-large, *Saturday Review.*

Amos H. Hawley, Ph.D.

Professor of Sociology, Department of Sociology, University of North Carolina; Chairman, Department of Sociology, University of Michigan, 1952-61; Member Population Association of America (First Vice-President, 1955-56); Member, American Sociological Society; Member, American Association of University Professors; Human Relations Research Institute, Department of Air Force, 1951-

Jean Sutter, M.D., Ph.D.

Ministere de la Sante Publique et de la Population Institut National D'Etudes Demographiques; Member, Council on "French Foundation for the Study of Human Problems," 1943; Chief of Qualitative Demography Section, National Institut of Demographic Studies, 1945: President, French Genetic Society, 1960-63; Member, Council of Biometrics Society, 1964-65.

Celso-Ramon Garcia, M.D.

Professor of Obstetrics and Gynecology, Department of Obstetrics and Gynecology, Hospital of the University of Pennsylvania; Chief, Fertility and Endocrine Clinic, Hospital of the University of Pennsylvania; Consultant in Obstetrics and Gynecology, Philadelphia General Hospital; Consultant, The Worcester Foundation or Experimental Biology, Shrewsbury, Mass.; Carl G. Hartman Award, American Society for the Study of Sterility—1961.

Sheldon J. Segal, Ph.D.
Director, Bio-Medical Division, The Population Council, Rockefeller University; Honorable Mention Award for Exhibit on Anti-spermatozoal Immunologie Factors in Infertility; Scientific Exhibit, American Medical Association, 1960; Guest Investigator, Brookhaven National Laboratory and Marine Biological Laboratories, Woods Hole, Massachusetts; Consultant on Reproduction Biology, Ford Foundation, New Delhi, India, 1962-63, Visiting Professor of Reproduction Biology, All-India Institute of Medical Sciences, New Delhi, India, 1962-3; Officership positions in the following: American Society of Zoologists, American Eugenics Society, American Fertility Society, American Association for the Advancement of Science, Indian Society for Scientific Study of Reproduction.

Christopher Tietze, M.D.
Associate Director, Biomedical Division, The Population Council; Chief, Population and Labor Staff, Division of Functional Intelligence, Department of State 1949-57; Director of Research, National Committee on Maternal Health, Inc., New York, New York, 1958- ; Lecturer in Obstetrics and Gynecology, College of Physicians and Surgeons, Columbia University; Advisor, U.S. Delegation to 8th and 9th Sessions, United Nations Population Commission, 1955 and 1957; Statistician for Family Planning, United Nations Technical Assistance Administration, Barbados, West Indies, 1956 and 1958; U.S. Delegate to the Conference on Demographic Problems of the Area Served by the Caribbean Commission, Port-of-Spain, Trinidad, 1957; Rapporteur, World Health Organization Scientific Groups on Clinical Aspects of Oral Gestogens and on Basic and Clinical Aspects of Intrauterine Devices, Geneva, 1965 and 1966; Member, Advisory Committee on Obstetrics and Gynecology, Food and Drug Administration, Washington, D. C.

Bernard Berelson, Ph.D.
Vice-President, The Population Council; American Sociological Association; President, American Association for Public Opinion Research (1951-52); American Academy of Arts and Sciences; National Academy of Sciences Committees; Phi Beta Kappa Nominations Committee; Director, Behavioral Sciences Program, the Ford Foundation, 1951-57; Director, Bureau of Applied Social Research, Columbia University, 1960-61.

Charles F. Westoff, Ph.D.
Associate Director, Office of Population Research and Professor of Sociology, Chairman, Department of Sociology, Princeton University; Statistical Consultant, U.S. Public Health Service, Cardiovascular Mortality Project Puerto Rico, 1962-63; Statistical Consultant, Study of the Economics of the Performing Arts for the Twentieth Century

Fund; Consultant in Demography and Survey Research, TriState Transportation Committee; Milbank Memorial Fund Fellowship; Participant, Hungarian Academy of Science, Second International Demographic Symposium, Budapest, 1965; Fellow, American Sociological Association; Member Board of Directors, Population Association of America (1960-62); International Union for the Scientific Study of Population; Amercian Statistical Association; American Association of University Professors.

Robert G. Potter, Jr., Ph.D.

Research Professor, Department of Soiology and Anthropology, Brown University; Schick Population Fellow, Princeton University, 1952-53; Population Council Fellow, Princeton University, 1953-54; American Eugenics Society; American Public Health Association; American Sociological Society; American Statistical Association; International Planned Parenthood Federation; International Union for the Scientific Study of Population; Population Association of America.

Leona Baumgartner, M.D.

Visiting Professor of Social Medicine, Harvard Medical School; Clinical Professor of Public Health, Cornell Medical College; Special Advisor to Agency for International Development, Department of State; John Lovett Morse Prize in Pediatrics, New England Pediatric Society, 1934; American Design Award for creative work in designs for living for children, 1946; Distinguished Service Award, Kansas University, 1947; Elizabeth Blackwell Citation, New York Infirmary; Albert Lasker Award for Distinguished Achievement in Public Health Administration, 1954; Award to Outstanding Leaders of New York City, Lord & Taylor, 1955; Citation for Distinguished Work in the Promotion of Health, Royal Society of Health (England) 1956; Citation "Outstanding Professional Woman of the Year," New York State Medical Women's Society, 1957; William J. Schieffelen Public Service Award, Citizen's Union of New York City, 1960; Citation "Medical Woman of the Year in New York State," New York State Medical Women's Society, 1960; Elizabeth Blackwell Award, Hobart and William Smith Colleges, 1961; Samuel J. Crumbine Award, Kansas Public Health Association, 1962; Albert Einstein Award for Distinguished Service to Humanity, 1964; New York State Academy of Preventive Medicine Award, 1964; Sedwick Award in Public Health, American Public Health Association, 1964; Chapin Medal (Charles V.), 1966. Honorary Degrees: Sc. D. Women's Medical College of Pennsylvania, 1950; Sc. D. New York University, 1954; Sc. D. Russell Sage College, 1955; Sc. D. Smith College, 1956; Ll. D. Skidmore College, 1959; Sc. D. Western College for Women, 1960; Sc. D. University of Massachusetts, 1963; L.H.D. Keuka College, 1963; Ll. D. Oberlin College, 1965.

L. P. Chow, M.D., Dr. P. H.

Director, Taiwan Population Studies Center, Taiwan, China; and Deputy Health Commissioner, Province of Taiwan, China; Non-resident Lecturer in Population Planning, School of Public Health, University of Michigan; Visiting Professor, Johns Hopkins University.

S. C. Hsu, M.D., M.P.H.

Chief, Rural Health Division, Joint Commission on Rural Reconstruction, Taipei, Taiwan; Non-resident Lecturer in Population Planning, School of Public Health, University of Michigan.

Nusret H. Fisek, M.D., Ph.D.

Director, Hacettepe Institute of Population Studies, Hacettepe Science Center, Ankara, Turkey; Member, Turkish Academy of Medicine; Honorary Member, American Medical Association; Honorary Fellow, American Public Health Association; Member, Excutive Board, World Health Organization, 1964-67; Coopter, Medical Committee, International Planned Parenthood Federation.

Mariano Requena B. (Bichet), M.D., M.P.H.

Professor, Latin American Demographic Center; Director, Program of Comparative Studies on Induced Abortion and Use of Contraceptives in Latin America; Professor, University of Chile School of Public Health and Co-Director, Latin American Course on Health and Population Dynamics; Milbank Memorial Fund, 1967; Vice-President, Chilean Society of Public Health; American Public Health Association, Member; Member, Association of Teachers of Preventive Medicine; Member, Population Association of America; Member, American Eugenics Society; Fellow, Royal Society of Health.

Edward E. Wallach, M.D.

Assistant Professor, Department of Obstetrics and Gynecology, Hospital of the University of Pennsylvania; Member, American Fertility Society; Diplomate, American Board of Obstetrics and Gynecology; Fellow, American College of Obstetricians and Gynecologists; Member, Endocrine Society; Member, Philadelphia Endocrine Society; Member, Obstetrical Society of Philadelphia; Member, American Association for Advancement of Science; Surgeon, United States Public Health Service, Division of Indian Health; Chief of Obstetrics and Gynecology, USPHS, Indian Hospital, Tuba City, Arizona, 1963-1965.